GABBE'S

OBSTETRICS ESSENTIALS
Normal and Problem Pregnancies

OBSTETRICS ESSENTIALS
Normal and Problem Pregnancies

MARK B. LANDON, MD
Richard L. Meiling Professor and Chair
Department of Obstetrics and Gynecology
Ohio State University College of Medicine
Columbus, Ohio

HENRY L. GALAN, MD
Professor
Department of Obstetrics and Gynecology
University of Colorado School of Medicine;
Co-Director
Colorado Fetal Health Center
Aurora, Colorado

ERIC R.M. JAUNIAUX, MD,PhD, FRCOG
Professor of Obstetrics and Fetal Medicine
EGA Institute for Women's Health
Faculty of Population Health Sciences
University College London
London, United Kingdom

DEBORAH A. DRISCOLL, MD
Luigi Mastroianni Professor and Chair
Department of Obstetrics and Gynecology
Perelman School of Medicine
  at the University of Pennsylvania
Philadelphia, Pennsylvania

VINCENZO BERGHELLA, MD, FACOG
Professor
Department of Obstetrics and Gynecology
Director, Division of Maternal-Fetal Medicine
Thomas Jefferson University
Philadelphia, Pennsylvania

WILLIAM A. GROBMAN, MD, MBA
Arthur Hale Curtis Professor of Obstetrics
  and Gynecology
Department of Obstetrics and Gynecology
Feinberg School of Medicine
Northwestern University
Chicago, Illinois

STEVEN G. GABBE, MD
Emeritus Chief Executive Officer
Ohio State University Wexner
  Medical Center
Professor of Obstetrics and Gynecology
Ohio State University College of Medicine
Columbus, Ohio

JENNIFER R. NIEBYL, MD
Professor
Department of Obstetrics and Gynecology
University of Iowa Hospitals and Clinics
Iowa City, Iowa

JOE LEIGH SIMPSON, MD
Senior Vice President for Research
  and Global Programs
March of Dimes Foundation
White Plains, New York;
Professor of Obstetrics and Gynecology
Professor of Human and Molecular Genetics
Herbert Wertheim College of Medicine
Florida International University
Miami, Florida

ELSEVIER

ELSEVIER

1600 John F. Kennedy Blvd.
Ste 1800
Philadelphia, PA 19103-2899

GABBE'S OBSTETRICS ESSENTIALS: NORMAL AND PROBLEM PREGNANCIES

ISBN: 978-0-323-60974-6

Library of Congress Cataloging-in-Publication Data

Names: Landon, Mark B., editor.
Title: Gabbe's obstetrics essentials : normal and problem pregnancies /
    [edited by] Mark B. Landon [and 5 others].
Other titles: Obstetrics essentials | Abridgement of (work): Obstetrics
    (Gabbe) 7th edition
Description: Philadelphia, PA : Elsevier, [2019] | Abridgement of Obstetrics
    / [edited by] Steven G. Gabbe [and 8 others]. Seventh edition. 2017. |
    Includes bibliographical references and index.
Identifiers: LCCN 2018007618 | ISBN 9780323609746 (pbk. : alk. paper)
Subjects: | MESH: Pregnancy Complications | Pregnancy | Prenatal Care
Classification: LCC RG524 | NLM WQ 240 | DDC 618.2--dc23 LC record available at
https://lccn.loc.gov/2018007618

Senior Content Strategist: Sarah Barth
Content Development Specialist: Meghan Andress
Publishing Services Manager: Patricia Tannian
Senior Project Manager: Carrie Stetz
Design Direction: Patrick Ferguson

Printed in China

Last digit is the print number: 9   8   7   6   5   4   3   2   1

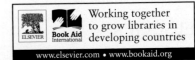

Working together
to grow libraries in
developing countries

www.elsevier.com • www.bookaid.org

Kjersti Aagaard, MD, PhD, MSCI
Associate Professor
Department of Obstetrics and Gynecology
Baylor College of Medicine
Houston, Texas

Kristina M. Adams Waldorf, MD
Associate Professor
Department of Obstetrics and Gynecology
University of Washington
Seattle, Washington

Margaret Altemus, MD
Associate Professor
Department of Psychiatry
Yale University School of Medicine
New Haven, Connecticut

George J. Annas, JD, MPH
Professor and Chair
Department of Health Law, Bioethics &
 Human Rights
Boston University School of Public Health
Boston, Massachusetts

Kathleen M. Antony, MD, MSCI
Department of Obstetrics and Gynecology
University of Wisconsin School of Medicine
 and Public Health
Madison, Wisconsin

Jennifer L. Bailit, MD, MPH
Clinical Director
Family Care Service Line
Metrohealth Medical Center
Cleveland, Ohio

Ahmet Alexander Baschat, MD
Director
Johns Hopkins Center for Fetal Therapy
Department of Gynecology and Obstetrics
Johns Hopkins Hospital
Baltimore, Maryland

Vincenzo Berghella, MD
Professor
Department of Obstetrics and Gynecology
Director
Maternal-Fetal Medicine
Jefferson Medical College of Thomas
 Jefferson University
Philadelphia, Pennsylvania

Helene B. Bernstein, MD, PhD
Director, Division of Maternal-Fetal
 Medicine
Departments of Obstetrics and Gynecology,
 Microbiology, and Immunology
SUNY Upstate Medical University
Syracuse, New York

Amar Bhide, MD
Consultant in Fetal Medicine
Fetal Medicine Unit
St. George's Hospital
London, United Kingdom

Meredith Birsner, MD
Assistant Professor
Department of Maternal-Fetal Medicine
Thomas Jefferson University
Philadelphia, Pennsylvania

Debra L. Bogen, MD
Associate Professor of Pediatrics
Department of Psychiatry and Clinical and
 Translational Sciences
University of Pittsburgh School of Medicine
Division of General Academic Pediatrics
Children's Hospital of Pittsburgh of UPMC
Pittsburgh, Pennsylvania

D. Ware Branch, MD
Professor
Department of Obstetrics and Gynecology
University of Utah School of Medicine
Salt Lake City, Utah

Gerald G. Briggs, AB, BPharm
Clinical Professor of Pharmacy
University of California–San Francisco
San Francisco, California;
Adjunct Professor of Pharmacy Practice
University of Southern California–Los
 Angeles
Los Angeles, California;
Adjunct Professor
Department of Pharmacotherapy
Washington State University
Spokane, Washington

Haywood L. Brown, MD
Professor and Chair
Department of Obstetrics and Gynecology
Duke University
Durham, North Carolina

Brenda A. Bucklin, MD
Professor of Anesthesiology and Assistant
 Dean
Clinical Core Curriculum
Department of Anesthesiology
University of Colorado School of Medicine
Denver, Colorado

Graham J. Burton, MD, DSc
Centre for Trophoblast Research
Physiology, Development and Neuroscience
University of Cambridge
Cambridge, United Kingdom

Mitchell S. Cappell, MD, PhD
Chief
Division of Gastroenterology and Hepatology
William Beaumont Hospital;
Professor of Medicine
Oakland University William Beaumont
 School of Medicine
Royal Oak, Michigan

Jeanette R. Carpenter, MD
Department of Maternal-Fetal Medicine
Obstetric Medical Group of the Mountain
 States
Salt Lake City, Utah

Patrick M. Catalano, MD
Dierker-Biscotti Women's Health and
 Wellness Professor
Director, Center for Reproductive Health at
 MetroHealth
Director, Clinical Research Unit of the Case
 Western Reserve University CTSC at
 MetroHealth
Professor of Reproductive Biology
MetroHealth Medical Center/Case Western
 Reserve University
Cleveland, Ohio

Suchitra Chandrasekaran, MD, MSCE
Assistant Professor
Department of Obstetrics and Gynecology
University of Washington
Seattle, Washington

David F. Colombo, MD
Department of Obstetrics, Gynecology, and
 Reproductive Biology
Spectrum Health
College of Human Medicine
Michigan State University
Grand Rapids, Michigan

Larry J. Copeland, MD
Professor
Department of Obstetrics and Gynecology
The Ohio State University
Columbus, Ohio

Jason Deen, MD
Assistant Professor of Pediatrics
Adjunct Assistant Professor of Medicine
Division of Cardiology
Seattle Children's Hospital
University of Washington Medical Center
Seattle, Washington

COL Shad H. Deering, MD
Chair, Department of Obstetrics and
 Gynecology
Assistant Dean for Simulation Education
F. Edward Hebert School of Medicine
Uniformed Services University of the Health
 Sciences
Chair, Army Central Simulation Committee
Bethesda, Maryland

Mina Desai, MSc, PhD
Associate Professor
Department of Obstetrics and Gynecology
David Geffen School of Medicine at Harbor-
   UCLA Medical Center
Los Angeles, California

Gary A. Dildy III, MD
Professor and Vice Chair of Quality and
   Patient Safety
Director, Division of Maternal-Fetal
   Medicine
Department of Obstetrics and Gynecology
Baylor College of Medicine;
Chief Quality Officer, Obstetrics and
   Gynecology
Service Chief, Maternal-Fetal Medicine
Texas Children's Hospital
Houston, Texas

Mitchell P. Dombrowski, MD
Professor and Chief
Department of Obstetrics and Gynecology
St. John Hospital
Detroit, Michigan

Deborah A. Driscoll, MD
Luigi Mastroianni Professor and Chair
Department of Obstetrics and Gynecology
Perelman School of Medicine at the
   University of Pennsylvania
Philadelphia, Pennsylvania

Maurice L. Druzin, MD
Professor and Vice Chair
Department of Obstetrics and Gynecology
Stanford University School of Medicine
Stanford, California

Patrick Duff, MD
Professor
Associate Dean for Student Affairs
Department of Obstetrics and Gynecology
University of Florida
Gainesville, Florida

Thomas Easterling, MD
Professor
Department of Obstetrics and Gynecology
University of Washington
Seattle, Washington

Sherman Elias, MD[†]
John J. Sciarra Professor and Chair
Department of Obstetrics and Gynecology
Feinberg School of Medicine
Northwestern University
Chicago, Illinois

M. Gore Ervin, PhD
Professor of Biology
Middle Tennessee State University
Murfreesboro, Tennessee

Michael R. Foley, MD
Chairman
Department of Obstetrics and Gynecology
Banner University Medical Center
Professor
University of Arizona College of Medicine
Phoenix, Arizona

Karrie E. Francois, MD
Perinatal Medical Director
Obstetrics and Gynecology
HonorHealth
Scottsdale, Arizona

Steven G. Gabbe, MD
Emeritus Chief Executive Officer
The Ohio State University Wexner Medical
   Center
Professor of Obstetrics and Gynecology
The Ohio State University College of
   Medicine
Columbus, Ohio

Henry L. Galan, MD
Professor
Department of Obstetrics and Gynecology
University of Colorado School of Medicine;
Co-Director
Colorado Fetal Care Center
Colorado Institute for Maternal and Fetal
   Health
Aurora, Colorado

Etoi Garrison, MD, PhD
Associate Professor, Division of Maternal-
   Fetal Medicine
Department of Obstetrics and Gynecology
Vanderbilt Medical Center
Nashville, Tennessee

[†] Deceased.

Elizabeth E. Gerard, MD
Associate Professor
Department of Neurology
Northwestern University
Chicago, Illinois

Robert Gherman, MD
Associate Director
Prenatal Diagnostic Center and Antepartum
    Testing Unit
Division of Maternal-Fetal Medicine
Franklin Square Medical Center
Baltimore, Maryland

William M. Gilbert, MD
Regional Medical Director
Women's Services
Department of Obstetrics and Gynecology
Sutter Medical Center Sacramento;
Clinical Professor
Department of Obstetrics and Gynecology
University of California–Davis
Sacramento, California

Laura Goetzl, MD, MPH
Professor and Vice Chair
Department of Obstetrics and Gynecology
Temple University
Philadelphia, Pennsylvania

Bernard Gonik, MD
Professor and Fann Srere Endowed Chair of
    Perinatal Medicine
Department of Obstetrics and Gynecology
Division of Maternal-Fetal Medicine
Wayne State University School of Medicine
Detroit, Michigan

Mara B. Greenberg, MD
Director of Inpatient Perinatology
Obstetrics and Gynecology
Kaiser Permanente Northern California
Oakland Medical Center
Oakland, California

Kimberly D. Gregory, MD, MPH
Vice Chair
Women's Healthcare Quality & Performance
    Improvement
Department of Obstetrics and Gynecology
Cedars Sinai Medical Center
Los Angeles, California

William A. Grobman, MD, MBA
Arthur Hale Curtis Professor
Department of Obstetrics and Gynecology
The Center for Healthcare Studies
Feinberg School of Medicine
Northwestern University
Chicago, Illinois

Lisa Hark, PhD, RD
Director
Department of Research
Wills Eye Hospital
Philadelphia, Pennsylvania

Joy L. Hawkins, MD
Professor
Department of Anesthesiology
University of Colorado School of Medicine
Aurora, Colorado

Wolfgang Holzgreve, MD, MBA
Professor of Obstetrics and Gynaecology
Medical Director and CEO
University Hospital Bonn
Bonn, Germany

Jay D. Iams, MD
OB Lead
Ohio Perinatal Quality Collaborative
Emeritus Professor of Obstetrics and
    Gynecology
The Ohio State University
Columbus, Ohio

Michelle M. Isley, MD, MPH
Assistant Professor
Department of Obstetrics and Gynecology
The Ohio State University
Columbus, Ohio

Eric R.M. Jauniaux, MD, PhD
Professor of Obstetrics and Fetal Medicine
Institute for Women's Health
University College London
London, United Kingdom

Vern L. Katz, MD
Clinical Professor
Department of Obstetrics and Gynecology
Oregon Health Science University
Eugene, Oregon

Sarah Kilpatrick, MD, PhD
Head and Vice Dean
Department of Obstetrics and Gynecology
Director
Division of Maternal-Fetal Medicine
University of Minnesota
Minneapolis, Minnesota

George Kroumpouzos, MD, PhD
Clinical Associate Professor
Department of Dermatology
Alpert Medical School of Brown University
Providence, Rhode Island

Daniel V. Landers, MD
Professor and Vice Chair
Department of Obstetrics, Gynecology, and
  Women's Health
University of Minnesota
Minneapolis, Minnesota

Mark B. Landon, MD
Richard L. Meiling Professor and Chair
Department of Obstetrics and Gynecology
The Ohio State University College of
  Medicine
Columbus, Ohio

Susan M. Lanni, MD
Associate Professor of OBGYN and
  Maternal-Fetal Medicine
Director, Labor and Delivery
Virginia Commonwealth University
Richmond, Virginia

Gwyneth Lewis, OBE, MBBS, DSc, MPH
Leader
International Women's Health Research
Institute for Women's Health
University College London
London, United Kingdom

Charles J. Lockwood, MD, MHCM
Dean, Morsani College of Medicine
Senior Vice President
USF Health
Professor of Obstetrics & Gynecology and
  Public Health
University of South Florida
Tampa, Florida

Jack Ludmir, MD
Professor
Department of Obstetrics and Gynecology
Perelman School of Medicine at the
  University of Pennsylvania
Philadelphia, Pennsylvania

A. Dhanya Mackeen, MD, MPH
Clinical Assistant Professor
Temple University School of Medicine
Department of Obstetrics, Gynecology, and
  Reproductive Services
Director of Research
Division of Maternal-Fetal Medicine
Geisinger Health System
Danville, Pennsylvania

George A. Macones, MD, MSCE
Professor and Chair
Department of Obstetrics and Gynecology
Washington University in St. Louis School of
  Medicine
St. Louis, Missouri

Brian M. Mercer, MD
Professor and Chairman
Department of Reproductive Biology
Case Western Reserve University–
  MetroHealth Campus
Chairman, Department of Obstetrics and
  Gynecology
Director, Women's Center
MetroHealth Medical Center
Cleveland, Ohio

Jorge H. Mestman, MD
Professor
Departments of Medicine and Obstetrics &
  Gynecology
Keck School of Medicine of the University of
  Southern California
Los Angeles, California

David Arthur Miller, MD
Professor of Obstetrics, Gynecology, and
  Pediatrics
Keck School of Medicine of the University of
  Southern California
Children's Hospital of Los Angeles
Los Angeles, California

Emily S. Miller, MD, MPH
Assistant Professor
Department of Obstetrics and Gynecology
Division of Maternal-Fetal Medicine
Feinberg School of Medicine
Northwestern University
Chicago, Illinois

Dawn Misra, MHS, PhD
Professor and Associate Chair for Research
Department of Family Medicine & Public
    Health Sciences
Wayne State University School of Medicine
Detroit, Michigan

Kenneth J. Moise Jr, MD
Professor of Obstetrics, Gynecology, and
    Reproductive Sciences and Pediatric
    Surgery
Director
Fetal Intervention Fellowship
UTHealth School of Medicine at Houston;
Co-Director
The Fetal Center
Children's Memorial Hermann Hospital
Houston, Texas

Mark E. Molitch, MD
Martha Leland Sherwin Professor of
    Endocrinology
Division of Endocrinology, Metabolism, and
    Molecular Medicine
Northwestern University Feinberg School of
    Medicine
Chicago, Illinois

Chelsea Morroni, MBChB, DTM&H, DFSRH, Mphil, MPH, PhD
Clinical Lecturer
EGA Institute for Women's Health and
    Institute for Global Health
University College London
London, United Kingdom;
Senior Researcher
Wits Reproductive Health and HIV Institute
    (Wits RHI)
University of the Witwatersrand
Johannesburg, South Africa

Roger B. Newman, MD
Professor and Maas Chair for Reproductive
    Sciences
Department of Obstetrics and Gynecology
Medical University of South Carolina
Charleston, South Carolina

Edward R. Newton, MD
Professor
Department of Obstetrics and Gynecology
Brody School of Medicine
Greenville, North Carolina

Jennifer R. Niebyl, MD
Professor
Department of Obstetrics and Gynecology
University of Iowa Hospitals and Clinics
Iowa City, Iowa

COL Peter E. Nielsen, MD
Commander
General Leonard Wood Army Community
    Hospital
MFM Division Director
Obstetrics and Gynecology
Fort Leonard Wood, Missouri

Jessica L. Nyholm, MD
Assistant Professor
Department of Obstetrics, Gynecology and
    Women's Health
University of Minnesota
Minneapolis, Minnesota

Lucas Otaño, MD, PhD
Head, Division of Obstetrics and Fetal
    Medicine Unit
Department of Obstetrics and Gynecology
Hospital Italiano de Buenos Aires
Buenos Aires, Argentina

John Owen, MD, MSPH
Professor
Department of Obstetrics and Gynecology
Division of Maternal-Fetal Medicine
University of Alabama at Birmingham
Birmingham, Alabama

Teri B. Pearlstein, MD
Associate Professor of Psychiatry and Human
  Behavior and Medicine
Alpert Medical School of Brown University;
Director
Women's Behavioral Medicine
Women's Medicine Collaborative, a Lifespan
  Partner
Providence, Rhode Island

Christian M. Pettker, MD
Associate Professor
Department of Obstetrics, Gynecology, and
  Reproductive Sciences
Yale University School of Medicine
New Haven, Connecticut

Diana A. Racusin, MD
Maternal Fetal Medicine Fellow
Department of Obstetrics and Gynecology
Baylor College of Medicine
Houston, Texas

Kirk D. Ramin, MD
Professor
Department of Obstetrics, Gynecology, and
  Women's Health
University of Minnesota
Minneapolis, Minnesota

Diana E. Ramos, MD, MPH
Director
Reproductive Health
Los Angeles County Public Health;
Adjunct Assistant Clinical Professor
Keck University of Southern California
  School of Medicine
Los Angeles, California

Roxane Rampersad, MD
Associate Professor
Department of Obstetrics and Gynecology
Washington University in St. Louis School of
  Medicine
St. Louis, Missouri

Leslie Regan, MD, DSc
Chair and Head
Department of Obstetrics and Gynaecology at
  St. Mary's Campus
Imperial College;
Vice President, Royal College of Obstetricians
  & Gynaecologists
Chair, FIGO Women's Sexual &
  Reproductive Rights Committee
Chair, National Confidential Enquiry into
  Patient Outcome and Death
London, United Kingdom

Douglas S. Richards, MD
Clinical Professor
Division of Maternal-Fetal Medicine
Intermountain Medical Center
Murray, Utah;
Clinical Professor
Division of Maternal-Fetal Medicine
University of Utah School of Medicine
Salt Lake City, Utah

Roberto Romero, MD, DMedSci
Chief, Program for Perinatal Research and
  Obstetrics
Division of Intramural Research
Eunice Kennedy Shriver National Institute of
  Child Health and Human Development
Perinatology Research Branch
National Institutes of Health
Bethesda, Maryland;
Professor, Department of Obstetrics and
  Gynecology
University of Michigan
Ann Arbor, Michigan;
Professor, Department of Epidemiology and
  Biostatistics
Michigan State University
East Lansing, Michigan

Adam A. Rosenberg, MD
Professor
Department of Pediatrics
Children's Hospital of Colorado
University of Colorado School of Medicine
Aurora, Colorado

Michael G. Ross, MD, MPH
Distinguished Professor
Department of Obstetrics and Gynecology
David Geffen School of Medicine at Harbor-
  UCLA Medical Center;
Distinguished Professor
Community Health Sciences
Fielding School of Public Health at UCLA
Los Angeles, California

Paul J. Rozance, MD
Associate Professor
Department of Pediatrics
University of Colorado School of Medicine
Aurora, Colorado

Ritu Salani, MD, MBA
Associate Professor
Department of Obstetrics and Gynecology
The Ohio State University
Columbus, Ohio

Philip Samuels, MD
Professor
Residency Program Director
Department of Obstetrics and Gynecology,
  Maternal-Fetal Medicine
The Ohio State University Wexner Medical
  Center
Columbus, Ohio

Nadav Schwartz, MD
Assistant Professor
Department of Obstetrics and Gynecology
Perelman School of Medicine at the
  University of Pennsylvania
Philadelphia, Pennsylvania

Lili Sheibani, MD
Peter E. Nielsen, MD, Clinical Instructor
Obstetrics and Gynecology
University of California–Irvine
Orange, California

Baha M. Sibai, MD
Director
Maternal-Fetal Medicine Fellowship Program
Department of Obstetrics, Gynecology and
  Reproductive Sciences
University of Texas Medical School at
  Houston
Houston, Texas

Colin P. Sibley, PhD, DSc
Professor of Child Health and Physiology
Maternal and Fetal Health Research Centre
University of Manchester
Manchester, United Kingdom

Hyagriv N. Simhan, MD
Professor and Chief
Division of Maternal-Fetal Medicine
Executive Vice Chair
Obstetrical Services Department
University of Pittsburgh School of Medicine;
Medical Director of Obstetric Services
Magee-Women's Hospital of UPMC
Pittsburgh, Pennsylvania

Joe Leigh Simpson, MD
Senior Vice President for Research and
  Global Programs
March of Dimes Foundation
White Plains, New York;
Professor of Obstetrics and Gynecology
Professor of Human and Molecular Genetics
Herbert Wertheim College of Medicine
Florida International University
Miami, Florida

Dorothy K.Y. Sit, MD
Department of Psychiatry
University of Pittsburgh Medical Center
Pittsburgh, Pennsylvania

Karen Stout, MD
Director
Adult Congenital Heart Disease Program
Department of Internal Medicine
Division of Cardiology
University of Washington;
Professor of Internal Medicine/Pediatrics
Department of Pediatrics
Division of Cardiology
Seattle Children's Hospital
Seattle, Washington

Dace S. Svikis, PhD
Professor
Department of Psychology
Institute for Women's Health
Virginia Commonwealth University
Richmond, Virginia

Elizabeth Ramsey Unal, MD, MSCR
Assistant Professor
Department of Obstetrics and Gynecology
Division of Maternal-Fetal Medicine
Southern Illinois University School of
  Medicine
Springfield, Illinois

Annie R. Wang, MD
Department of Dermatology
Alpert Medical School of Brown University
Providence, Rhode Island

Robert J. Weber, MS, PharmD
Administrator
Pharmacy Services
Assistant Dean
College of Pharmacy
The Ohio State University Wexner Medical
  Center
Columbus, Ohio

Elizabeth Horvitz West, MD
Resident Physician
Department of Obstetrics and Gynecology
University of California–Irvine
Irvine, California

Janice E. Whitty, MD
Professor and Director of Maternal-Fetal
  Medicine
Department of Obstetrics and Gynecology
Meharry Medical College
Nashville, Tennessee

Deborah A. Wing, MD, MBA
Professor
Department of Obstetrics and Gynecology
University of California–Irvine
Orange, California

Katherine L. Wisner, MD
Asher Professor of Psychiatry and Obstetrics
  and Gynecology
Director
Asher Center for Research and Treatment of
  Depressive Disorders
Department of Psychiatry
Feinberg School of Medicine
Northwestern University
Chicago, Illinois

Jason D. Wright, MD
Sol Goldman Associate Professor
Chief, Division of Gynecologic Oncology
Department of Obstetrics and Gynecology
Columbia University College of Physicians
  and Surgeons
New York, New Yor

CONTENTS

PART I Physiology

1   Placental Anatomy and Physiology*   2
Graham J. Burton ■ Colin P. Sibley ■ Eric R.M. Jauniaux

2   Fetal Development and Physiology*   3
Michael G. Ross ■ M. Gore Ervin

3   Maternal Physiology*   4
Kathleen M. Antony ■ Diana A. Racusin ■ Kjersti Aagaard ■ Gary A. Dildy III

4   Maternal-Fetal Immunology   5
Kristina M. Adams Waldorf

5   Developmental Origins of Adult Health and Disease   13
Michael G. Ross ■ Mina Desai

PART II Prenatal Care

6   Preconception and Prenatal Care   22
Kimberly D. Gregory ■ Diana E. Ramos ■ Eric R.M. Jauniaux

7   Nutrition During Pregnancy   30
Elizabeth Horvitz West ■ Lisa Hark ■ Patrick M. Catalano

8   Drugs and Environmental Agents in Pregnancy and Lactation: Teratology and Epidemiology   38
Jennifer R. Niebyl ■ Robert J. Weber ■ Gerald G. Briggs

9   Obstetric Ultrasound: Imaging, Dating, Growth, and Anomaly   48
Douglas S. Richards

10   Genetic Screening and Prenatal Genetic Diagnosis   59
Deborah A. Driscoll ■ Joe Leigh Simpson ■ Wolfgang Holzgreve ■ Lucas Otaño

11   Antepartum Fetal Evaluation   69
Mara B. Greenberg ■ Maurice L. Druzin

PART III Intrapartum Care

12   Normal Labor and Delivery   80
Sarah Kilpatrick ■ Etoi Garrison

13   Abnormal Labor and Induction of Labor   90
Lili Sheibani ■ Deborah A. Wing

14   Operative Vaginal Delivery   93
Peter E. Nielsen ■ Shad H. Deering ■ Henry L. Galan

15   Intrapartum Fetal Evaluation   97
David Arthur Miller

16   Obstetric Anesthesia   106
      Joy L. Hawkins ■ Brenda A. Bucklin

17   Malpresentations   112
      Susan M. Lanni ■ Robert Gherman ■ Bernard Gonik

18   Antepartum and Postpartum Hemorrhage   123
      Karrie E. Francois ■ Michael R. Foley

19   Cesarean Delivery   137
      Vincenzo Berghella ■ A. Dhanya Mackeen ■ Eric R.M. Jauniaux

20   Vaginal Birth After Cesarean Delivery   145
      Mark B. Landon ■ William A. Grobman

21   Placenta Accreta   151
      Eric R.M. Jauniaux ■ Amar Bhide ■ Jason D. Wright

PART IV   **Postpartum Care**

22   The Neonate   158
      Paul J. Rozance ■ Adam A. Rosenberg

23   Postpartum Care and Long-Term Health Considerations   165
      Michelle M. Isley ■ Vern L. Katz

24   Lactation and Breastfeeding   171
      Edward R. Newton

PART V   **Complicated Pregnancy**

25   Surgery During Pregnancy   178
      Nadav Schwartz ■ Jack Ludmir

26   Trauma and Related Surgery in Pregnancy   182
      Haywood L. Brown

27   Early Pregnancy Loss and Stillbirth   189
      Joe Leigh Simpson ■ Eric R.M. Jauniaux

28   Cervical Insufficiency   198
      Jack Ludmir ■ John Owen ■ Vincenzo Berghella

29   Preterm Labor and Birth   203
      Hyagriv N. Simhan ■ Jay D. Iams ■ Roberto Romero

30   Premature Rupture of the Membranes   212
      Brian M. Mercer

31   Preeclampsia and Hypertensive Disorders   217
      Baha M. Sibai

32   Multiple Gestations   233
      Roger B. Newman ■ Elizabeth Ramsey Unal

33   Intrauterine Growth Restriction   245
      Ahmet Alexander Baschat ■ Henry L. Galan

34 Red Cell Alloimmunization 257
Kenneth J. Moise Jr

35 Amniotic Fluid Disorders 263
William M. Gilbert

PART VI Pregnancy and Coexisting Disease

36 Prolonged and Postterm Pregnancy 270
Roxane Rampersad ▪ George A. Macones

37 Heart Disease in Pregnancy 274
Jason Deen ▪ Suchitra Chandrasekaran ▪ Karen Stout ▪ Thomas Easterling

38 Respiratory Disease in Pregnancy 282
Janice E. Whitty ▪ Mitchell P. Dombrowski

39 Renal Disease in Pregnancy 294
David F. Colombo

40 Diabetes Mellitus Complicating Pregnancy 300
Mark B. Landon ▪ Patrick M. Catalano ▪ Steven G. Gabbe

41 Obesity in Pregnancy 310
Patrick M. Catalano

42 Thyroid and Parathyroid Diseases in Pregnancy 313
Jorge H. Mestman

43 Pituitary and Adrenal Disorders in Pregnancy 318
Mark E. Molitch

44 Hematologic Complications of Pregnancy 322
Philip Samuels

45 Thromboembolic Disorders in Pregnancy 329
Christian M. Pettker ▪ Charles J. Lockwood

46 Collagen Vascular Diseases in Pregnancy 333
Jeanette R. Carpenter ▪ D. Ware Branch

47 Hepatic Disorders During Pregnancy 342
Mitchell S. Cappell

48 Gastrointestinal Disorders During Pregnancy 347
Mitchell S. Cappell

49 Neurologic Disorders in Pregnancy 355
Elizabeth E. Gerard ▪ Philip Samuels

50 Malignant Diseases and Pregnancy 363
Ritu Salani ▪ Larry J. Copeland

51 Skin Disease and Pregnancy 374
Annie R. Wang ▪ George Kroumpouzos

52 Maternal and Perinatal Infection: *Chlamydia,* Gonorrhea, and Syphilis in Pregnancy 382
Jessica L. Nyholm ▪ Kirk D. Ramin ▪ Daniel V. Landers

53   Maternal and Perinatal Infection in Pregnancy: Viral   388
      Helene B. Bernstein

54   Maternal and Perinatal Infection in Pregnancy: Bacterial   402
      Patrick Duff ▪ Meredith Birsner

55   Mental Health and Behavioral Disorders in Pregnancy*   409
      Katherine L. Wisner ▪ Dorothy K.Y. Sit ▪ Debra L. Bogen ▪ Margaret Altemus ▪
      Teri B. Pearlstein ▪ Dace S. Svikis ▪ Dawn Misra ▪ Emily S. Miller

PART VII   Legal and Ethical Issues in Perinatology

56   Patient Safety and Quality Measurement in Obstetric Care*   412
      William A. Grobman ▪ Jennifer L. Bailit

57   Ethical and Legal Issues in Perinatology*   413
      George J. Annas ▪ Sherman Elias†

58   Improving Global Maternal Health: Challenges and Opportunities*   414
      Gwyneth Lewis ▪ Lesley Regan ▪ Chelsea Morroni ▪ Eric R.M. Jauniaux

APPENDIX

A   Normal Values in Pregnancy and Ultrasound Measurements   415
      Henry L. Galan ▪ Laura Goetzl

B   Anatomy of the Pelvis*   432
      Steven G. Gabbe

C   Glossary of Key Abbreviations*   433

      Index   434

---

*Full text available at ExpertConsult.com.
†Deceased

PART I

Physiology

CHAPTER 1

Placental Anatomy and Physiology*

Graham J. Burton ■ Colin P. Sibley ■ Eric R.M. Jauniaux

KEY POINTS

- The mature human placenta is a discoid organ that consists of an elaborately branched fetal villous tree bathed directly by maternal blood of the villous hemochorial type. Normal term placental weight averages 450 g and represents approximately one seventh (one sixth with cord and membranes) of the fetal weight.
- Continual development throughout pregnancy leads to progressive enlargement of the surface area for exchange (12 to 14 m² at term) and reduction in the mean diffusion distance between the maternal and fetal circulations (approximately 5 to 6 μm at term).
- The maternal circulation to the placenta is not fully established until the end of the first trimester; hence organogenesis takes place in a low-oxygen environment of approximately 20 mm Hg, which may protect against free radical–mediated teratogenesis. Uterine blood flow at term averages 750 mL/min, or 10% to 15% of maternal cardiac output.
- During the first trimester, the uterine glands discharge their secretions into the placental intervillous space and represent an important supply of nutrients, cytokines, and growth factors prior to the onset of the maternal-fetal circulation.
- The exocoelomic cavity acts as an important reservoir of nutrients during early pregnancy, and the secondary yolk sac is important in the uptake of nutrients and their transfer to the fetus.
- Oxygen is a powerful mediator of trophoblast proliferation and invasion, villous remodeling, and placental angiogenesis.
- Ensuring an adequate maternal blood supply to the placenta during the second and third trimesters is an essential aspect of placentation and is dependent upon physiologic conversion of the spiral arteries induced by invasion of the endometrium by extravillous trophoblast during early pregnancy. Many complications of pregnancy, such as preeclampsia, appear to be secondary to deficient invasion.
- All transport across the placenta must take place across the syncytial covering of the villous tree, the syncytiotrophoblast, the villous matrix, and the fetal endothelium, each of which may impose its own restriction and selectivity. Exchange will occur via one of four basic processes: (1) bulk flow/solvent drag, (2) diffusion, (3) transporter-mediated mechanisms, and (4) endocytosis/exocytosis.
- The rate of transplacental exchange will depend on many factors, such as the surface area available, the concentration gradient, the rates of maternal and fetal blood flows, and the density of transporter proteins. Changes in villous surface area, diffusion distance, and transporter expression have been linked with IUGR.
- The placenta is an important endocrine gland that produces both steroid and peptide hormones, principally from the syncytiotrophoblast. Concentrations of some hormones are altered in pathologic conditions—for example, human chorionic gonadotropin in trisomy 21—but in general, little is known regarding control of endocrine activity.

---

*Text for this chapter is available at ExpertConsult.com.

CHAPTER 2

Fetal Development and Physiology*

Michael G. Ross ■ M. Gore Ervin

KEY POINTS

- Mean amniotic fluid volume increases from 250 to 800 mL between 16 and 32 weeks and decreases to 500 mL at term.
- Fetal urine production ranges from 400 to 1200 mL/day and is the primary source of amniotic fluid.
- The fetal umbilical circulation receives approximately 40% of fetal combined ventricular output (300 mL/mg/min).
- Umbilical blood flow is 70 to 130 mL/min after 30 weeks' gestation.
- Fetal cardiac output is constant over a heart rate range of 120 to 180 beats/min.
- The fetus exists in a state of aerobic metabolism, with arterial P_{O_2} values in the 20 to 25 mm Hg range.
- Glucose, amino acids, and lactate are the major substrates for fetal oxidative metabolism.
- Approximately 20% of the fetal oxygen consumption of 8 mL/kg/min is required in the acquisition of new tissue.
- By week 12 of gestation, thyrotropin-releasing hormone is present in the fetal hypothalamus.
- Fetal activity periods in late gestation are often termed *active* or *reactive* and *quiet* or *nonreactive*.

---

*Text for this chapter is available at ExpertConsult.com.

CHAPTER 3

Maternal Physiology*

Kathleen M. Antony ■ Diana A. Racusin ■ Kjersti Aagaard ■ Gary A. Dildy III

KEY POINTS

- The "healthy" amount of weight to gain during pregnancy is BMI specific.
- Maternal cardiac output increases 30% to 50% during pregnancy. Supine positioning and standing are both associated with a fall in cardiac output, which is highest during labor and in the immediate postpartum period.
- As a result of the marked fall in systemic vascular resistance and pulmonary vascular resistance, pulmonary capillary wedge pressure does not rise despite an increase in blood volume.
- Maternal BP decreases early in pregnancy. The diastolic BP and the mean arterial pressure reach a nadir at midpregnancy (16 to 20 weeks) and return to prepregnancy levels by term.
- Maternal plasma volume increases 50% during pregnancy. Red blood cell volume increases about 18% to 30%, and the hematocrit normally decreases during gestation but not below 30%.
- Pregnancy is a hypercoagulable state that is accompanied by increases in the levels of most of the procoagulant factors and decreases in the fibrinolytic system and in some of the natural inhibitors of coagulation.
- Pao_2 and $Paco_2$ fall during pregnancy because of increased minute ventilation. This facilitates transfer of CO_2 from the fetus to the mother and results in a mild respiratory alkalosis.
- Blood urea nitrogen and creatinine normally decrease during pregnancy as a result of the increased glomerular filtration rate.
- Plasma osmolality decreases during pregnancy as a result of a reduction in the serum concentration of sodium and associated anions. The osmolality set points for AVP release and thirst are also decreased.
- Despite alterations in thyroid morphology, histology, and laboratory indices, the normal pregnant woman is euthyroid, with levels of free T_4 within nonpregnant norms.
- Pregnancy is associated with a peripheral resistance to insulin, primarily mediated by tumor necrosis factor alpha and human placental lactogen. Insulin resistance increases as pregnancy advances; this results in hyperglycemia, hyperinsulinemia, and hyperlipidemia in response to feeding, especially in the third trimester.
- Physiologic changes in the vagina interact with the vaginal microbiome to protect against infection and promote pregnancy maintenance.

---

*Text for this chapter is available at ExpertConsult.com.

CHAPTER 4

Maternal-Fetal Immunology

Kristina M. Adams Waldorf

KEY POINTS

- The innate immune system uses fast, nonspecific methods of pathogen detection to prevent and control an initial infection and includes macrophages, NK cells, the complement system, and cytokines. Macrophages have critical scavenger functions that likely help to prevent bacteria from establishing an intrauterine infection during pregnancy. Decidual NK (dNK) cells are thought to play a major role in remodeling of the spiral arteries to establish normal placentation.

- Proinflammatory cytokines such as IL-1β, TNF-α, and IL-6 have been identified in the amniotic fluid, maternal and fetal blood, and vaginal fluid of women with intraamniotic infection at much higher levels than those observed during normal pregnancy. These cytokines not only serve as a marker of intraamniotic infection, they trigger preterm labor and can lead to neonatal complications.

- Adaptive immunity results in the clonal expansion of lymphocytes (T cells and B cells) and an increase in antibodies against a specific antigen. Although slower to respond, adaptive immunity targets specific components of a pathogen and is capable of eradicating an infection that has overwhelmed the innate immune system.

- The function of B cells is to protect the extracellular spaces in the body (e.g., plasma, vagina) through which infectious pathogens usually spread by secreting antibodies (immunoglobulins). Antibodies control infection by several mechanisms, including neutralization, opsonization, and complement activation. Autoantibodies produced by B cells against angiotensin receptor 1 are thought to play a role in inducing hypertension and proteinuria in women with preeclampsia and intrauterine fetal growth restriction.

- When pathogens replicate inside cells (all viruses, some bacteria, and parasites), they are inaccessible to antibodies and must be destroyed by T cells. A variety of T cells are recognized based on their expression of different cell surface markers that include those of CD8+ (effector or cytotoxic T cells), CD4+ (helper T cells), and CD4+CD25+ (T_{REG} cells). CD8+ T cells kill cells directly, whereas helper T cells activate B cells to produce antibodies. T_{REG} cells are now recognized as master regulators of the immune system that work by downregulating antigen-specific T-cell responses to diminish tissue damage during inflammation and to prevent autoimmunity.

- The fetal immune system, even very early in gestation, has innate immune capacity. Acquired immunity, particularly the capacity to produce antibodies, develops more slowly and is not completely functional until well after birth. CD71+ cells appear to protect the neonate from excessive inflammation that would occur from commensal microbes during bacterial colonization of the gut at the expense of impairing neonatal immunity to systemic infections.

- Fetal blood contains a high number of hematopoietic stem cells, making it an ideal source of cells for hematopoietic stem cell transplantation. The estimated need for the use of privately banked cord blood is between 1 in 1000 and 1 in 200,000, which is cost effective only for children with a very high likelihood of needing a transplant.

- Maintaining tolerance to the fetus requires several immunologic mechanisms, both at the maternal-fetal interface and in the maternal periphery. A critical interface is within the secondary lymphoid organs (lymph nodes and spleen), where fetal antigens are presented to maternal immune cells. Some of these mechanisms include generation of paternal-specific T_{REG} and B_{REG} cells in the maternal periphery, T-cell deletion, tryptophan depletion, presence of FasL or TNF-related apoptosis-inducing ligand/Apo-2L on trophoblast cells, HLA-G expression by the placenta, and inhibition of complement activation by the placenta.
- Among the many mechanisms identified to maintain tolerance of the fetus, T_{REG} cells are unique because fetal antigen–specific T_{REG} cells are maintained after delivery, which may benefit the next pregnancy. T_{REG} cells suppress antigen-specific immune responses and are elevated in the maternal circulation of women and mice during pregnancy. Pregnancy selectively drives expansion of maternal T_{REG} cells (>100-fold), which are maintained after delivery and are rapidly expanded in subsequent pregnancies. In addition, hCG acts as a chemoattractant for T_{REG} to the maternal-fetal interface and, in the mouse, stimulates T_{REG} cell numbers and their suppressive activity.
- Unexplained preterm fetal death has been linked to a loss of fetal tolerance and chronic chorioamnionitis, which refers to an influx of T cells into the fetal membranes. A related observation in mice connects maternal T-cell infiltration of the placenta with a loss of maternal T_{REG} cells and perinatal death during infection with *L. monocytogenes*.
- A pregnant woman with a solid organ transplant has at least three and possibly more sources of small foreign cell populations (Mc) to which she must maintain tolerance: fetal Mc, maternal Mc (her own mother's cells that entered when she was a fetus), and cells from the donor allograft. In a few cases, transplant rejection has been linked to antifetal antibodies that developed during pregnancy.
- Remarkably, uterine transplantation has now been performed in at least 11 women with one live birth reported following transplantation.
- Pregnancy has a remarkable effect on the disease course of some autoimmune or inflammatory diseases, such as RA and multiple sclerosis, that results in a temporary amelioration or remission of symptoms. Amelioration of RA during pregnancy may occur as a secondary benefit from the maternal T- and B-cell tolerance that develops to fetal antigens during pregnancy.

Introduction

- Pregnancy poses unique immunologic challenges to the mother, who must become tolerant to a genetically foreign fetus yet remain immunocompetent to fight infection.
- *Microchimerism Mc:* Small populations of fetal cells in the mother and maternal cells in the fetus can persist for decades after pregnancy.[1]

Immune System Overview: Innate and Adaptive Immunity

- The immune system is classically divided into two arms, the innate and adaptive immune systems.
- Innate immunity consists of immune cells such as macrophages, dendritic cells (DCs), natural killer (NK) cells, eosinophils, and basophils.

Innate Immunity: First Line of Host Defense

- After a pathogen enters the tissues, it is often recognized and killed by phagocytes, a process mediated by macrophages and neutrophils. Toll-like receptors, a family of pattern-recognition receptors on the surface of macrophages and other innate immune and epithelial cells, represent a primary mechanism of pathogen detection.

ANTIMICROBIAL PEPTIDES

- Defensins are a major family of antimicrobial peptides that protect against bacterial, fungal, and viral pathogens.
- Elevated concentrations of vaginal and amniotic fluid defensins have been associated with intraamniotic infection and preterm birth.

MACROPHAGES

- Uterine macrophages represent up to one third of the total leukocytes in pregnancy-associated tissue during the later parts of pregnancy and perform many critical functions to support the pregnancy.

NATURAL KILLER CELLS

- NK cells differ from T and B cells in that they do not express clonally distributed receptors for foreign antigens and can lyse target cells without prior sensitization.
- During pregnancy, dNK cells are the predominant decidual immune cell with peak levels (~85%) in early pregnancy.[2]

TOLL-LIKE RECEPTORS

- Toll-like receptors are now recognized as the principal early sensors of pathogens that can activate both the innate and adaptive immune system (Fig. 4.1).

COMPLEMENT SYSTEM

- An important component of the innate immune system is the complement system, which consists of a large number of plasma proteins that cooperate to destroy and facilitate the removal of pathogens.

CYTOKINES

- The release of cytokines and chemokines by macrophages and other immune cells represents an important induced innate immune response.
- These cytokines are often referred to as *proinflammatory* because they mediate fever, lymphocyte activation, tissue destruction, and shock.
- The *fetal inflammatory response syndrome* describes the connection between elevated proinflammatory cytokines in fetal blood, preterm labor, and increased adverse fetal outcomes.[3]
- Interleukin (IL)-1β and TNF-α serve a primary role in the induction of infection-associated preterm birth.
- IL-6 plays a role in triggering normal parturition, perhaps in activation of labor pathways.

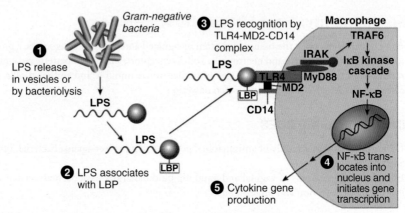

Fig. 4.1 Toll-like receptor 4 (TLR4) recognition of lipopolysaccharide (LPS). Recognition of LPS by TLR4 occurs through several steps. *(1)* LPS is released from intact or lysed bacteria. *(2)* LPS binds to LPS-binding protein (LBP). *(3)* The LPS-LBP complex is recognized by a cell surface receptor complex TLR4, CD14, and MD-2. Binding of LPS-LBP to the TLR4-CD14-MD-2 receptor recruits the intracellular adapter molecule, myeloid differentiation factor 88 (MyD88). Binding of MyD88 promotes the association of IL-1 receptor–associated protein kinase 4 (IRAK). Next, tumor necrosis factor receptor–associated kinase 6 (TRAF6) initiates a signaling cascade that results in degradation of Iκ-B, which releases nuclear factor κB (NF-κB), a transcription factor, into the cytoplasm. *(4)* NF-κB translocates into the nucleus and activates cytokine gene expression. Although the figure depicts TLR4 activation in a macrophage, many other immunologic and epithelial cells express TLR4 and induce cytokine production *(5)* through this mechanism.

CHEMOKINES

- Chemokines are a class of cytokines that act primarily as chemoattractants that direct leukocytes to sites of infection.
- Increases in IL-8 levels have been described in the amniotic fluid, maternal blood, and vaginal fluid with infection-associated preterm birth.[4] IL-8 and CCL2 have also been implicated in uterine stretch-induced preterm labor thought to occur in multiple gestation.

Adaptive Immunity

- The function of the adaptive immune system is to eliminate infection as the second line of immune defense and to provide increased protection against reinfection through immunologic "memory." Adaptive immunity comprises primarily B cells and T cells (lymphocytes).

MAJOR HISTOCOMPATIBILITY COMPLEX

- The ability of a lymphocyte to distinguish self from nonself is based on the expression of unique major histocompatibility complex molecules on a cell's surface, which present small peptides from within the cell.

HUMORAL IMMUNE RESPONSES: B CELLS AND ANTIBODIES

- Antibodies control infection by several mechanisms that include neutralization, opsonization, and complement activation.
- Overall, pregnancy is associated with profound changes in the numbers of B cells in several compartments.

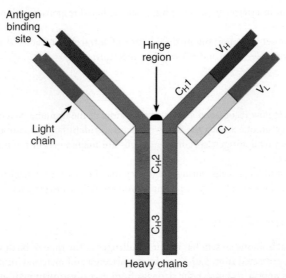

Fig. 4.2 Structure of immunoglobulin. Immunoglobulins are produced by B cells to neutralize foreign substances, such as bacteria and viruses. They are large, Y-shaped proteins found in the serum and plasma. C_H, constant domain of the heavy chain; C_L, constant domain of the light chain; V_H, variable domain of the heavy chain; V_L, variable domain of the light chain.

ANTIBODY ISOTYPES

- Antibodies share the same general structure produced by the interaction and binding of four separate polypeptides (Fig. 4.2). These include two identical light chains (23 kDa) and two identical heavy chains (55 kDa).
- The first antibody to be produced during an immune response is immunoglobulin M (IgM).
- IgM is highly efficient at activating the complement system, which is critical during the earliest stages of controlling an infection.
- IgG represents about 75% of serum immunoglobulin in adults and is further divided into four subclasses: IgG1, IgG2, IgG3, and IgG4. IgG1 and IgG3 are transported across the placenta and are important for the fetus after birth.
- IgA is the principal antibody in breast milk, which provides the neonate with humoral immunity from the mother.

T CELLS

- T cells are lymphocytes responsible for the cell-mediated immune responses of adaptive immunity, which require direct interactions between T lymphocytes and cells bearing the antigen that the T cells recognize.
- Cytotoxic T cells kill infected cells directly and express a variety of cell surface antigen and specific receptors.
- HIV uses multiple strategies to disable T-cell responses, mainly by targeting CD4⁺ T cells.

HELPER T-CELL SUBSETS

- CD4⁺ T cells were originally classified into T-helper 1 (Th1) and T-helper 2 (Th2) subsets depending on whether their main function involved cell-mediated responses and selective production of interferon-γ (Th1) or humoral-mediated responses with production of IL-4 (Th2).

- The Th1 subset is important in the control of intracellular bacterial infections such as *Mycobacterium tuberculosis* and *Chlamydia trachomatis*.

Regulatory T Cells

- T_{REG} cells are now recognized as master regulators of the immune system.
- T_{REG} cells are unique among the many mechanisms identified to maintain tolerance of the fetus, because fetal antigen-specific T_{REG} cells are maintained in the maternal circulation after delivery.[5]
- The function of T_{REG} cells during pregnancy may be critical for fetal tolerance but could also underlie the susceptibility of pregnant women to *L. monocytogenes*.

Fetal Immune System

- The neonatal immune system has unique challenges at the time of birth when the newborn is no longer protected from pathogens by the placenta and maternal immune system.
- CD71+ cells appear to protect the neonate from excessive inflammation that would occur from commensal microbes during bacterial colonization of the gut at the expense of impairing neonatal immunity to systemic infections.

CORD BLOOD TRANSPLANTATION

- The American Congress of Obstetricians and Gynecologists recommends that if a patient requests information regarding collection and banking of umbilical cord blood, balanced and accurate information regarding the advantages and disadvantages of public versus private banking should be provided.
- The obstetrician-gynecologist can play an important role in improving the availability of cord blood units internationally by encouraging pregnant women to donate to a public cord blood bank.

Maternal Tolerance of the Fetus

- Pregnancy is a unique immunologic phenomenon in which the normal immune rejection of foreign tissues does not occur.
- Achieving fetal tolerance requires changes to maternal immunity in multiple locations and by many different cell types because maternal and fetal cells are in direct contact with each other (Fig. 4.3).
- The complex nature of the cells and many locations of the maternal-fetal interface necessitate a number of different immune mechanisms to prevent fetal rejection.

TOLERANCE THROUGH REGULATION OF MATERNAL T CELLS

- Maternal T cells acquire a state of tolerance for fetal alloantigens during pregnancy.
- Several mechanisms exist to suppress maternal T-cell responses.
- Pregnancy selectively drives expansion of maternal T_{REG} cells (>100-fold), which are maintained after delivery and are rapidly expanded in a subsequent pregnancy.[5] This preexisting pool of fetal-specific maternal T_{REG} cells is poised to impart tolerance and benefit the next pregnancy.

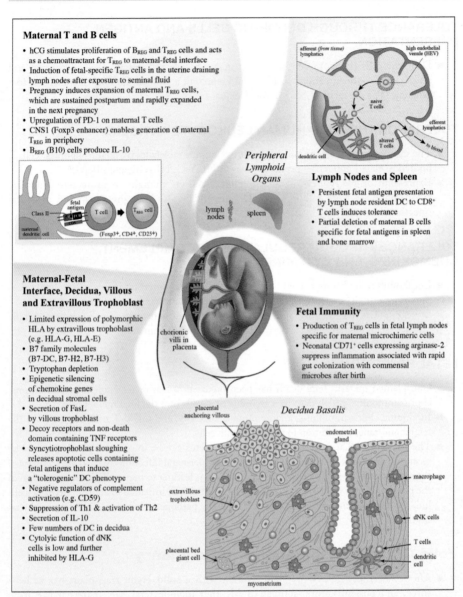

Maternal T and B cells

- hCG stimulates proliferation of B_{REG} and T_{REG} cells and acts as a chemoattractant for T_{REG} to maternal-fetal interface
- Induction of fetal-specific T_{REG} cells in the uterine draining lymph nodes after exposure to seminal fluid
- Pregnancy induces expansion of maternal T_{REG} cells, which are sustained postpartum and rapidly expanded in the next pregnancy
- Upregulation of PD-1 on maternal T cells
- CNS1 (Foxp3 enhancer) enables generation of maternal T_{REG} in periphery
- B_{REG} (B10) cells produce IL-10

Peripheral Lymphoid Organs

Lymph Nodes and Spleen

- Persistent fetal antigen presentation by lymph node resident DC to $CD8^+$ T cells induces tolerance
- Partial deletion of maternal B cells specific for fetal antigens in spleen and bone marrow

Maternal-Fetal Interface, Decidua, Villous and Extravillous Trophoblast

- Limited expression of polymorphic HLA by extravillous trophoblast (e.g. HLA-G, HLA-E)
- B7 family molecules (B7-DC, B7-H2, B7-H3)
- Tryptophan depletion
- Epigenetic silencing of chemokine genes in decidual stromal cells
- Secretion of FasL by villous trophoblast
- Decoy receptors and non-death domain containing TNF receptors
- Syncytiotrophoblast sloughing releases apoptotic cells containing fetal antigens that induce a "tolerogenic" DC phenotype
- Negative regulators of complement activation (e.g. CD59)
- Suppression of Th1 & activation of Th2
- Secretion of IL-10
- Few numbers of DC in decidua
- Cytolyic function of dNK cells is low and further inhibited by HLA-G

Fetal Immunity

- Production of T_{REG} cells in fetal lymph nodes specific for maternal microchimeric cells
- Neonatal $CD71^+$ cells expressing arginase-2 suppress inflammation associated with rapid gut colonization with commensal microbes after birth

Decidua Basalis

Fig. 4.3 Mechanisms that promote maternal-fetal tolerance. Many different mechanisms and cell types have been identified that prevent rejection or dangerous immune responses during pregnancy. We have illustrated some of these mechanisms that operate within the maternal-fetal interface, maternal B- and T-cell populations, secondary lymphoid organs, and the fetus. The term *maternal-fetal interface* may refer to several locations where maternal and fetal cells come into direct contact, including the decidua and the intervillous space.

TOLERANCE THROUGH REGULATION OF MATERNAL B CELLS

■ An important cofactor for B_{REG} cells is hCG, and the rise of hCG in early pregnancy is likely to stimulate proliferation of B_{REG} cells to support early tolerance of the fetus.

TOLERANCE THROUGH DENDRITIC CELLS AND ANTIGEN PRESENTATION

- Dendritic cells (DCs) present antigen to naïve T cells and initiate T-cell expansion and polarization to foreign antigens. This could represent a problem for fetal tolerance but fortunately, DCs are relatively rare in the decidua.

TOLERANCE THROUGH HUMAN LEUKOCYTE ANTIGENS

- The expression of major histocompatibility complex molecules by fetal trophoblast cells is limited to class I antigens—primarily class Ib HLA-G, HLA-E, and HLA-F.
- Expression of HLA-G by fetal trophoblast cells is thought to protect the invasive cytotrophoblast from killing by dNK cells and is also thought to contain placental infection.

TOLERANCE THROUGH REGULATION OF COMPLEMENT, CHEMOKINES, AND CYTOKINES

- Local inhibition of complement in the placenta may be important in preventing fetal rejection or preterm labor, particularly in the setting of inflammation or infection.
- Several studies suggest that inhibition of complement activation may contribute significantly to fetal tolerance, particularly in the setting of inflammation.

FETAL REJECTION

- Unexplained preterm fetal death has been linked to a loss of fetal tolerance and chronic chorioamnionitis, which describes an influx of T cells into the fetal membranes.
- In chronic chorioamnionitis, a large number of $CD3^+$ and $CD8^+$ T cells are found in the fetal membranes in addition to some $CD4^+$ T cells.
- The conclusion that maternal tolerance of the fetus can be impaired is also supported by recent observations and hypotheses surrounding perinatal infections (e.g., *L. monocytogenes*) through an infection-associated reduction in T_{REG} leading to maternal T-cell infiltration of the placenta. Once maternal-fetal tolerance is sufficiently impaired to allow maternal T cells into the placenta, inflammation can then facilitate pathogenic invasion of the fetus and fetal death.

Solid Organ Transplantation in Pregnancy

- *Microchimerism (Mc).* A pregnant woman with a solid organ transplant has at least three, and possibly more, sources of Mc that include fetal Mc, maternal Mc from her own mother's cells that entered when she was a fetus, and cells from the donor allograft.

Amelioration of Rheumatoid Arthritis in Pregnancy

- Nearly three quarters of pregnant women with RA experience improvement in symptoms during the second and third trimesters with a return of symptoms postpartum.

References for this chapter are available at ExpertConsult.com.

CHAPTER 5

Developmental Origins of Adult Health and Disease

Michael G. Ross ■ Mina Desai

KEY POINTS

- Maternal influences on the in utero environment (nutrition, hormonal, metabolic, stress, environmental toxins, and drugs) are critical determinants of fetal growth and influence a wide variety of metabolic, developmental, and pathologic processes in adulthood.
- Both ends of the growth spectrum (i.e., both low and high birthweight) are associated with increased risk of adult obesity, metabolic syndrome, cardiovascular disease, insulin resistance, and neuroendocrine disorders.
- The mechanisms that link early developmental events to the later manifestation of disease states involve "programmed" changes in organ structure, cellular responses, gene expression, the epigenome, and/or stem cells.
- Gestational programming events may have immediate effects or are deferred and expressed at a later age, with potential transmission to multiple generations.
- Transmission of gestational programming effects to multiple generations may occur via epigenomic modulation that causes heritable and persistent changes in gene expression without altering the DNA sequence.
- Prenatal care is evolving to provide essential goals to optimizing maternal, fetal, and neonatal health and prevent or reduce the long-term consequences on adult health and adult-onset diseases.
- Guiding policies regarding optimal pregnancy nutrition and weight gain, management of low- and high-fetal-weight pregnancies, use of maternal glucocorticoids, and newborn feeding strategies, among others, have yet to be comprehensively integrated in prenatal management protocols.

Introduction

- An understanding of the developmental origins of adult health and disease provides an appreciation of the critical role of perinatal care and may ultimately guide our treatment paradigms.
- A variety of mechanisms may "program" the phenotype of the offspring via aberrations in cellular signaling or epigenetic function.

Epigenetics and Programming

- "Gestational programming" signifies that the nutritional, hormonal, and metabolic environment provided by the mother may permanently alters organ structure, cellular responses, and gene expression that ultimately impact the metabolism and physiology of her offspring (Fig. 5.1).

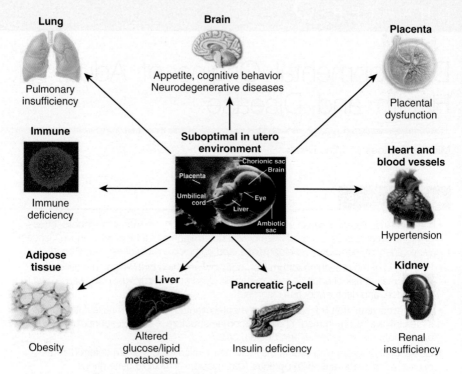

Fig. 5.1 Impact of gestational programming on organ systems.

- Epigenetic phenomena are fundamental features of mammalian development that cause heritable and persistent changes in gene expression without altering DNA sequence.
- DNA methylation is a primary epigenetic mechanism.
- Changes in epigenetic markers are associated with inflammation and multiple human diseases, including many cancers and neurologic disorders.
- Another essential mechanism of gene expression and silencing is the packaging of chromatin into open (euchromatic) or closed (heterochromatic) states, respectively. Chromatin consists of DNA packaged around histones into a nucleoprotein complex.
- Noncoding RNAs are emerging as a potential third epigenetic mediator.
- Both human and animal studies provide evidence of epigenomic modulation by the maternal milieu, which is implicated in the transmission of gestational programming effects to multiple generations.[1]

Fetal Nutrition and Growth

- Nutrition is unquestionably one of the cornerstones of health.
- Good evidence suggests that appropriate nutritional supplementation before conception and during pregnancy may reduce the risk of some birth defects. For example, iodine deficiency–induced cretinism and folate deficiency are linked to the development of spina bifida and anencephaly (see Chapters 6 and 7).
- Obesity now represents a major public health problem and is considered a health epidemic (see Chapter 41).

- The risks of obesity in metabolic syndrome can be markedly influenced by early life events, particularly prenatal and neonatal growth and early childhood environmental exposures.
- Nutritional insufficiency during embryonic and fetal development results in latent disease, including obesity, in adulthood.
- The relationship between birthweight and adult obesity, cardiovascular disease, and insulin resistance is in fact a U-shaped curve, with increasing risks at both the low and high ends of the birthweight spectrum.
- The field of developmental origins of adult disease has grown from studying short-term toxic or teratogenic effects to evaluating the long-term adult sequelae of low or high birthweight and, more recently, at the impact of environmental toxins (e.g., bisphenol A [BPA]).

Energy-Balance Programming

- Obesity results from an imbalance in energy intake and expenditure as regulated by appetite, metabolism, adipogenic propensity, and energy utilization.
- In response to an impaired nutrient supply in utero, the growing fetus adapts to maximize metabolic efficiency because it will increase its survival likelihood in the postnatal environment.
- Low birthweight (LBW) appears to predispose to excess central adiposity and thus increases the risk of obesity, a phenotype specifically associated with a high risk for cardiovascular disease.
- Contrary to current practice, it may be advisable to limit rapid weight gain or "catch-up growth" in the neonatal and early childhood period among the LBW infants.
- Breastfeeding results in a lower obesity risk compared with formula feeding.[2]
- Obesity, glucose intolerance, and a high-fat diet—and their outcomes (large for gestational age [LGA]) may individually contribute to the programming of adult obesity.

PROGRAMMING BY ENVIRONMENTAL AGENTS

- BPA levels are associated strongly with levels of the adipokines adiponectin and leptin. Higher BPA urinary concentrations are associated with increased adiposity at 9 years of age.[3]
- Low-dose maternal BPA exposure has been shown to accelerate neurogenesis and neuronal migration in mice and results in aberrant neuronal network formation.
- Gender-specific effects of BPA are well documented; in utero BPA exposure has been found to alter offspring rat brain structure and behavior, including sexually dimorphic behaviors, with effects more apparent in females than in males.

Mechanisms of Programmed Obesity: Appetite and Adiposity

- Early-life leptin exposure is likely to be a putative programming mechanism in small-for-gestational-age and LGA human newborns.
- Leptin binding to its receptor activates proopiomelanocortin neurons and downstream anorexigenic pathways. Obesity is often associated with leptin resistance, which results in an inability to balance food intake with actual energy needs.
- Mechanisms that regulate adipose tissue development and function (lipogenesis) may be a key factor in the development of programmed obesity. LBW preadipocytes exhibit early differentiation and premature induction of adipogenic genes, because the signaling pathways of adipogenesis and lipogenesis are upregulated prior to the development of obesity.[4,5]
- The potential transdifferentiation of white adipose tissue toward a brown-fat phenotype, which can expend energy via thermogenesis, offers an alternative preventive strategy for programmed obesity.

HEPATIC PROGRAMMING

- Children and adolescents now have an increased risk of developing nonalcoholic fatty liver disease (NAFLD), or nonalcoholic steatohepatitis, and type 2 diabetes.
- Cases of cirrhosis associated with NAFLD in obese children have been described recently.
- Poor weight gain in infancy is associated with altered adult liver function.
- An undiagnosed increase in liver adiposity may exist among normal-weight offspring of mothers exposed to Western, high-fat diets.

PANCREATIC PROGRAMMING

- In utero nutrition and environmental exposures directly impact the pancreas. LGA human neonates have pancreatic β-cell hyperplasia and increased vascularization, whereas SGA infants have reduced plasma insulin concentrations and pancreatic β-cell numbers.[6]
- Reduced β-cell growth and insulin secretion have been observed in LBW offspring,[7] whereas accelerated β-cell mass and excess insulin secretion was observed in offspring of obese pregnant women.[8]
- In humans, growth in utero is directly associated with fetal insulin levels. Beyond the regulation of glucose uptake, insulin has important developmental functions in systems that include skeletal and connective tissues and neural development.
- Extremes in weight are critical because the risk of insulin resistance in adult life is twofold greater among men who weighed less than 8.2 kg at 1 year of age and in those who weighed 12.3 kg or more.[9]
- Approximately 25% of individuals with normal glucose tolerance have insulin resistance similar to that seen in type 2 diabetes, but they compensate for this with enhanced insulin secretion.
- Antenatal exposure to betamethasone may result in insulin resistance in adult offspring. No differences in body size, blood lipids, blood pressure, or cardiovascular disease have been observed among those exposed to betamethasone or placebo. However, offspring exposed to betamethasone demonstrated higher plasma insulin concentrations at 30 minutes in a 75 g oral glucose tolerance test, and lower glucose concentrations were observed at 120 minutes.[10]
- Maternal gestational diabetes and the resultant intrauterine hyperglycemia can transmit the diabetogenic phenotype to a subsequent generation ("transgeneration diabetogenic effect").[11] Consequently, the incidence of mothers who exhibit gestational diabetes has increased.[12]
- There is an association between birthweight and adult coronary heart disease. Small body size at birth and low weight gain during infancy followed by a rapid gain in body mass index during childhood is associated with an increase in coronary heart disease as adults.
- The association between LBW and coronary heart disease has been replicated among men and women throughout North America, the Indian subcontinent, and Europe.
- Left ventricular hypertrophy has also been reported in growth-restricted infants.
- Poor body growth in utero and throughout infancy, followed by a persistent small body size at adolescence, result in an increased risk of stroke and an atherogenic lipid profile. Prevention of fetal growth restriction, rather than modulation of infant growth rates, is key in preventing these adult diseases.
- Preterm birth also significantly affects the elastin content and viscoelastic properties of the vascular extracellular matrix in human arteries.

- Evidence suggests that maternal betamethasone treatment of preterm infants is associated with long-term adverse cardiac outcomes, including hypertrophic cardiomyopathy.[13]
- Prenatal cocaine exposure has been demonstrated to have significant effects on cardiac function in newborns and potentially a longer-term impact on cardiac function in adults.

OSTEOPOROSIS PROGRAMMING

- Bone mass in the elderly is largely determined by peak bone mass that occurs much earlier in life; thus fetal and neonatal life may be a critical factor in the development of osteoporosis.
- The mechanisms by which the fetal and neonatal period can influence peak bone mineral content include the interaction between vitamin D and calcium and additional factors, such as fetal and neonatal growth hormone, cortisol, and insulin-like growth factor 1.
- Low maternal fat stores, maternal smoking or increased physical exercise in late pregnancy, and low maternal birthweight all predict lower whole-body bone marrow content in the neonate.[14]

BRAIN PROGRAMMING

- In utero exposure to cocaine, and perhaps methamphetamine, demonstrates a number of cerebral effects.[15]
- Prenatal cocaine use may affect the development of brain systems involved in the regulation of attention and response inhibition.[15] Heavy cocaine use is related to worse outcome in regard to behavior, language, and IQ in offspring.[15]
- Animal studies have indicated that prenatal nicotine or cocaine exposure targets specific neurotransmitter receptors in the fetal brain and elicits abnormalities in cell proliferation and differentiation and thus leads to reduced neurogenesis and altered synaptic activity.[16] The underlying mechanism may involve increased apoptosis of neuronal cells.

Maternal Stress and Anxiety

- Maternal nurturing impacts the offspring's epigenome and behavior.
- Neonates of mothers with high anxiety demonstrate altered auditory evoked responses, which suggests differences in attention allocation. Prenatal anxiety has also been associated with childhood asthma, whereas stress-related maternal factors have been linked to increased eczema during early childhood.
- Children of mothers with posttraumatic stress disorder during pregnancy display altered cortisol levels accompanied by signs of behavioral distress during the first 9 months of life.[17]
- The role of the maternal hypothalamic-pituitary-adrenal (HPA) axis is recognized as contributing to maternal stress-mediated effects on fetal development.
- A reduction in placental 11β-HSD2 may increase fetal exposure to maternal cortisol levels and thus may have secondary effects on brain maturation and development.
- A generational effect of fetal programming on the HPA axis is suggested by findings that LBW babies have elevated cortisol concentrations in umbilical cord blood and have elevated urinary cortisol secretion in childhood.[18]

Glucocorticoids and Prematurity

- Children exposed to multiple doses of dexamethasone before term because of a high prenatal risk of congenital adrenal hyperplasia who are born at term have increased emotionality, general behavioral problems, and impairments in verbal working memory.[19]
- Offspring of women given multiple doses of antenatal glucocorticoids have reduced head circumference and significantly increased aggressive violent behavior and attention deficits.[20]
- Infants delivered preterm are exposed to increased endogenous cortisol prior to the time at which they would normally experience this increase—that is, at term.
- In view of the consequences of exogenous and endogenous glucocorticoids, maternal glucocorticoid use should be directed only at fetuses most likely to benefit and those most likely to deliver preterm.
- High exposure to glycyrrhiza from maternal licorice ingestion increases the risks of deficits in verbal and visual spatial abilities and in narrative memory. They also increase the incidence of externalizing symptoms and in aggression-related problems.
- Women who were born before 37 weeks of gestational age have a 2.5-fold increased risk of developing gestational hypertension in their own pregnancies.[21]
- LBW predicts depression in adolescent girls (38.1% vs. 8.4% among girls with normal birthweight) but not boys. LBW is associated with an increased risk of social phobia, post-traumatic stress symptoms, and generalized anxiety disorder—all of which are far more common in girls than in boys.[22]

Immune Function

- Prenatal stress may influence the developing immune system, particularly as related to asthma and atopic diseases.
- Responses to typhoid vaccination are positively associated with birthweight. These findings suggest that atopy-related immune function may be enhanced in either LBW offspring or offspring associated with maternal prenatal stress, although LBW may well result in significant impairment in offspring infectious disease–related immune function.
- Both the maternal allergic phenotype and the maternal environmental exposures during pregnancy affect the risk of subsequent allergic disease in childhood.
- Maternal exposure to microbials may influence fetal immune competence.
- Factors that determine fetal growth may also be associated with wheezing in childhood.

Other Programming

ENDOCRINE PROGRAMMING

- Reduced fetal growth results in exaggerated adrenarche, early puberty, and small ovarian size with the subsequent development of ovarian hyperandrogenism.[23]
- Children who present with precocious puberty, particularly those with a history of LBW, have an increased risk of developing ovarian hyperandrogenism and other features of polycystic ovary syndrome during or soon after menarche.[23]
- LBW does not appear to advance the age of menopause in women.[24]

SEXUALITY PROGRAMMING

- Significant research demonstrates a major role for gonadal steroidal androgens in regulating sexual dimorphism in the brain and subsequent behavior.

- The *fraternal birth order effect* indicates that homosexual men have a greater number of older brothers than heterosexual men do, with the estimated odds of being homosexual increasing by 33% with each older brother.[25]
- Little conclusive evidence exists of specific neurodevelopmental mechanisms that produce homosexuality or heterosexuality.

RENAL PROGRAMMING

- Select genes that regulate renal signaling and transcription permutation have been associated with renal hypoplasia. Thus most congenital renal anomalies have an inheritable component.
- Environmental exposures and stresses are well demonstrated to alter nephron number. The developmental impact on nephron number may play an important role in programmed hypertension.
- Low glomerular number and high glomerular size have been associated with the development of hypertension, cardiovascular diseases, and an increased susceptibility to renal disease in later life.
- Very LBW infants exhibit a high rate of hypertension during adolescence.[26]
- Nephrotoxic drugs, including nonsteroidal antiinflammatory drugs (NSAIDs), ampicillin/penicillin, and aminoglycosides, may lead to renal hypoperfusion during critical nephrogenic periods, resulting in cystic changes in developing nephrons.[27]
- Whether a reduced nephron number is etiologic of hypertension, a consequence of hypertension, or a coincident finding may depend upon the individual.

References for this chapter are available at ExpertConsult.com.

PART II

Prenatal Care

CHAPTER 6

Preconception and Prenatal Care

Kimberly D. Gregory ■ Diana E. Ramos ■ Eric R.M. Jauniaux

KEY POINTS

- The breadth of prenatal care includes both preconception and postpartum care, which extends up to 1 year after the infant's birth.
- *Interconception care* is defined as care provided between the end of a woman's pregnancy to the beginning of her next pregnancy and is an opportunity to assess risk, promote healthy lifestyle behaviors, and identify and treat medical and psychosocial issues that could impact pregnancy and the lifetime health of the mother and child.
- During the interconception period, intensive interventions are provided to women who have had a previous pregnancy that ended in an adverse outcome (i.e., fetal loss, PTB, LBW, infant death, or birth defect).
- When specific conditions are detected such that pregnancy is not recommended or intended, reliable contraception should be prescribed, and the importance of compliance should be reinforced. Many women with complex medical problems who are advised against pregnancy conceive unintentionally and/or do not use contraception because of a low perceived risk of conceiving.
- Age, weight (BMI), and changes in weight during pregnancy and over time impact pregnancy outcome and long-term maternal health.
- All reproductive-age women should be current with immunizations as recommended by ACIP and the CDC.
- The time to screen appropriate populations for genetic disease-carrier status, congenital malformations, or familial diseases with major genetic components is *before* pregnancy. If patients screen positive, referral for genetic counseling is indicated because consideration of additional preconception options may be warranted.
- Smoking and alcohol and drug use by pregnant women are all harmful to the developing fetus, but because these substances are often used in combination, teasing apart the specific contributions of each substance to adverse child outcomes can prove difficult. Overall, the risks to the neonate include IUGR, birth defects, altered neuropsychological behavior, and for some drugs, withdrawal symptoms. Subsequent behavior, development, and neurologic function may also be impaired from health problems that started during the preconception period.
- A study based on the National Health and Nutrition Examination Survey demonstrated that all pregnant women are exposed to and have detectable levels of chemicals that can be harmful to reproduction or human development. Because exposure to environmental agents can be mitigated or prevented, it is important for women to be made aware of known toxic substances and to inform them as to how to access resources to gain additional information.
- Clear evidence shows that for some conditions—such as diabetes mellitus, phenylketonuria, and inflammatory bowel disease—medical disease management before conception can positively influence pregnancy outcome. Medical management should be discussed with the patient, and appropriate management plans should be outlined before conception. Advice should also be given about specific medications to avoid during the first trimester (e.g., isotretinoin).

Definition and Goals of Prenatal Care

- The aim of preconception care is to promote the health of women before conception in order to reduce preventable adverse pregnancy outcomes by facilitating risk screening, health promotion, and effective interventions as part of routine health care.
- During the interconception period, intensive interventions are provided to women who have had a previous pregnancy that ended in an adverse outcome (i.e., fetal loss, preterm birth [PTB], low birthweight [LBW], birth defects, or infant death).
- Specifically, for those planning pregnancy, preconception/interconception visits provide an opportunity for teachable moments, and data suggest couples planning pregnancy are more likely to change behaviors.

Components of Preconception Care and Well-Woman Visits

- Preconception care is included as a preventive health service in well-woman visits covered by the Patient Protection and Affordable Care Act.
- Table 6.1 lists representative examples of potential topic areas pertinent for a preconception care visit, and it gives examples of medical conditions that could be optimized prior to conception, assuming pregnancy is planned.

Preconception Health Counseling

ADVANCED MATERNAL AGE

- The average maternal age at first birth has been steadily increasing over the past three decades in developed countries and is a contributing factor to maternal mortality.
- With advancing maternal age comes an increased likelihood of preexisting chronic medical diseases such as arthritis, hypertension, and diabetes.
- Women aged 50 years or more are at increased risk for preeclampsia and gestational diabetes mellitus (GDM), and the vast majority of them can expect to deliver via cesarean delivery.

TABLE 6.1 ■ **Pertinent Topics for Preconception/Interconception Counseling and of Medical Conditions That Can Be Optimized When Pregnancy Is Planned**

Clinical Condition	Comment
General Health	
Age	**<18 years:** Teenage pregnancy is associated with adverse maternal and familial consequences and increased risk of preterm birth.
	>18 to 34 years: This is the ideal age group, especially if part of the reproductive life plan.
	>35 years: Increased genetic risks; increase in complications, risk of cesarean delivery, obstetric morbidity, and mortality; general health, not age, should guide recommendations for pregnancy.
Weight	**Underweight:** Advise weight gain before conceiving and/or greater weight gain with pregnancy.
	Overweight: Advise weight loss before conceiving; increased BMI is associated with multiple adverse outcomes that include pregnancy loss, stillbirth, diabetes, preeclampsia, and cesarean delivery.
Psychiatric/ Neurologic	
Depression, anxiety	Adjust medications to those most favorable to pregnancy at the lowest possible dose; counsel about fetal echocardiography and neonatal withdrawal syndrome for some medications; reassure that risk/benefit profile favors treatment.
Seizure disorders	Start folic acid 4 mg when considering pregnancy to decrease risk of NTD; if no seizure in 2 years, consider trial off medication; adjust medications to those most favorable to pregnancy to avoid risk of dysmorphic structural malformation syndromes; close serum monitoring is required during pregnancy; reassure that risk/benefit profile favors treatment.
Migraines	Migraine pattern can change with pregnancy. Most migraine-specific medications are not contraindicated.
Cardiac	
Congenital cardiac disease or valve disease	Coordinate with cardiologist; pregnancy may be contraindicated with some conditions depending on severity (NYHA classification) or medications needed.
Coronary artery disease	Coordinate with cardiologist.
Hypertension	Adjust medications to optimize blood pressure. Discontinue ACE inhibitors and ARBs; these drugs are associated with congenital abnormalities.
Respiratory	
Asthma	Optimize treatment regimen per stepped protocol; if steroid dependent, use early ultrasound to evaluate for fetal cleft; advise patients at increased risk for gestational diabetes that medications, including steroids, are not contraindicated; emphasize that benefits of treatment exceed risks.
Gastrointestinal	
Inflammatory bowel disease	Optimize treatment regimen, advise that it is ideal to conceive while in remission; some medications have absolute versus relative contraindications.
Genitourinary	
Uterine malformations	Coordinate with reproductive endocrinologist if indicated.
Metabolic/Endocrine	
Diabetes	Achieve euglycemia before conception (hemoglobin A <7%); dose-dependent relationship regarding risk of congenital anomalies with medications; with type 1 and long-standing type 2 diabetes, insulin therapy is best; sulfonylureas are usually reserved for gestational diabetes mellitus.

TABLE 6.1 ■ Pertinent Topics for Preconception/Interconception Counseling and of Medical Conditions That Can Be Optimized When Pregnancy Is Planned—cont'd

Clinical Condition	Comment
Hematologic	
Sickle cell/thalassemia	Genetic counseling; advise sickle cell patient that crises can be exacerbated by pregnancy, and a risk of preterm birth/low birthweight is present.
History of DVT/PE, known hereditary thrombophilias	Risk of recurrent DVT/PE requires prophylaxis during pregnancy
Infectious	
STIs, TORCH, parvovirus	Establish risk factors, counsel to avoid infection, and treat as appropriate.
Rheumatologic	
SLE	It is ideal to conceive while SLE is in remission; some medications may be contraindicated.
Genetic	
Known genetic disorder in patient or partner	Genetic counseling, medical records to confirm diagnosis, and evaluation are warranted for prenatal diagnosis or assisted reproduction to avoid inheritance risk based on parents' preferences and values.

ACE, angiotensin-converting enzyme; *ARB,* angiotensin II receptor blockers; *BMI,* body mass index; *DVT,* deep vein thrombosis; *NTD,* neural tube defect; *NYHA,* New York Hospital Association; *PE,* pulmonary embolism; *STI,* sexually transmitted infection; *SLE,* systemic lupus erythematosus; *TORCH,* toxoplasmosis, other infections, rubella, cytomegalovirus, herpes.

TEEN PREGNANCIES

- A higher risk of prematurity has been consistently reported by other authors and seems to be the only significant obstetric risk of late teen pregnancy.
- Adolescent parenthood is associated with a range of adverse outcomes for young mothers, including mental health problems such as depression, substance abuse, and posttraumatic stress disorder (PTSD).

WEIGHT GAIN

- In the United States, the total weight gain recommended in pregnancy is 11 to 16 kg (25 to 35 lb) for women at a healthy weight.
- Underweight women can gain up to 18 kg (40 lb), but overweight women should limit weight gain to 7 kg (15 lb), although they do not need to gain any weight if they are morbidly obese.
- Inadequate weight gain is associated with an increased risk of an LBW infant.
- When excess weight gain is noted, patients should be counseled to avoid foods that are high in fats and carbohydrates, to limit sugar intake, and to increase their physical activity.

IMMUNIZATIONS

- All reproductive-age women should be current with immunizations recommended by the Advisory Committee on Immunization Practices (ACIP) and the CDC.
- This is the time to draw and document protective titers for rubella, varicella, and hepatitis B and to immunize the susceptible patient against influenza and tetanus, diphtheria and pertussis.

GENETIC AND FAMILY HISTORY

- The time to screen appropriate populations for genetic disease-carrier status and multifactorial congenital malformations or familial diseases with major genetic components is *before* pregnancy.
- If patients screen positive, referral for genetic counseling is indicated, and consideration of additional preconception options may be warranted (see Chapter 10).

SUBSTANCE ABUSE AND OTHER HAZARDS

- Smoking and use of alcohol and drugs by pregnant women are all harmful to the developing fetus, but because these substances are often used in combination, teasing apart the specific contributions of each substance to adverse child outcomes can prove difficult when analyzing epidemiologic data (see Chapter 8).
- Overall, the risks to the neonate include IUGR, birth defects, altered neuropsychological behavior, and, for some drugs, withdrawal symptoms.
- Subsequent behavior, development, and neurologic function may also be impaired by behaviors that occurred during the preconception period.

Active and Passive Smoking

- In many countries, smoking has replaced poverty as the most important risk factor for PTB, IUGR, and sudden infant death syndrome (SIDS).
- The use of or exposure to tobacco products by pregnant women is associated with placenta previa, placental abruption, placenta accreta, pregnancy bleeding of unknown origin, and preterm premature rupture of membranes.
- Because most of the placental and fetal damage is done in the first trimester of pregnancy, helping women to quit smoking before conceiving should be a primary objective in prepregnancy counseling.

Alcohol

- Alcohol is a well-established teratogen, and alcohol used during pregnancy can lead to fetal alcohol syndrome, which includes specific morphologic features, such as microcephaly, and long-term abnormal neuropsychological outcomes.
- The main issue with alcohol use during pregnancy is that no amount of alcohol consumption has been found to be safe during pregnancy.

Other Substance Abuse

- *Cannabis* use can lead to IUGR and withdrawal symptoms in the neonate.
- A recent case-control study has also found that cannabis use, cigarette smoking, illicit drug use, and apparent exposure to second-hand cigarette smoke separately or in combination during pregnancy were associated with an increased risk of stillbirth.
- Cocaine use in pregnancy can lead to spontaneous abortion, PTB, placental abruption, and preeclampsia. Neonatal issues include poor feeding, lethargy, and seizures.
- Poor obstetric outcomes can be up to six times higher in patients who abuse opiates such as heroin and methadone.

Mercury Exposure

- Data regarding the accumulation of mercury in fish has led to warnings advising pregnant women to avoid or decrease fish consumption since mercury has been associated with a dose-dependent impact on neurologic development.

Environmental Exposures

- A study based on the National Health and Nutrition Examination Survey demonstrated that all pregnant women are exposed to and have detectable levels of chemicals that can be harmful to reproduction or human development.
- Because exposure to environmental agents can be mitigated or prevented, it is important for women to be made aware of known toxic substances and to be informed as to how to access resources to gain additional information.

Screening for Chronic Disease, Optimizing Care, and Managing Medication Exposure

- Clear evidence shows that for some conditions—such as diabetes mellitus, phenylketonuria, and inflammatory bowel disease—medical disease management before conception can positively influence pregnancy outcome.
- Medical management to normalize the intrauterine biochemical environment should be discussed with the patient, and appropriate management plans should be outlined before conception; advice can also be given about avoiding specific medications in the first trimester (e.g., isotretinoin).

Prenatal Care

COMPONENTS OF PRENATAL CARE

- Prevention of morbidity and mortality is now the goal of prenatal care.
- Obstetricians must optimize their efforts by resourceful use of other professionals and support groups that include nutritionists, childbirth educators, public health nurses, nurse practitioners, family physicians, nurse midwives, and specialty medical consultants.
- Education about pregnancy, childbearing, and childrearing is an important part of prenatal care, as are detection and treatment of abnormalities.

RISK ASSESSMENT

- All the problems that arise in pregnancy, whether common complaints or more hazardous diseases, convey some risk to the pregnancy depending on how they are managed by the patient and her care provider.
- It has been shown that most women and infants who suffer morbidity and mortality will come from a small segment of those with high-risk factors; by reassessing risk factors before pregnancy, during pregnancy, and again in labor, the ability to identify those at highest risk increases.

INITIAL PRENATAL VISIT

- The initial visit should include a detailed history (medical, surgical, obstetric, reproductive), family history along with physical and laboratory examinations.
- If a patient has a history of a previous neonatal death, stillbirth, or PTB, records should be carefully reviewed so that the correct diagnosis is made and recurrence risk is appropriately assessed.
- A history of drug abuse or recent blood transfusion should be elicited.

REPEAT PRENATAL VISITS

- Traditionally, this has been every 4 weeks for the first 28 weeks of pregnancy, every 2 to 3 weeks until 36 weeks, and weekly thereafter if the pregnancy progresses normally.

- If any complications are present, the intervals can be increased appropriately. The goal of subsequent pregnancy visits is to assess fetal growth and maternal well-being (i.e., blood pressure, proteinuria, bacteriuria).

COMMON PATIENT-CENTERED ISSUES

- Most patients are able to maintain their normal activity levels in pregnancy; however, heavy lifting and excessive physical activity should be avoided.
- In the absence of medical or obstetric complications, current ACOG recommendations advocate for 30 minutes or more of moderate exercise daily.
- If the job presents hazards no greater than those encountered in daily life, healthy pregnant women may work until their delivery.
- A pregnant woman should be advised against prolonged sitting during car or airplane travel because of the risk of venous stasis and possible thromboembolism.
- Nausea and vomiting are common in pregnancy and affect approximately 75% of pregnancies.
- Hyperemesis gravidarum is an extreme form characterized by vomiting, dehydration, and weight loss that frequently results in hospitalization. These patients may benefit from enteral or parenteral nutrition.
- Back pain is a common complaint in pregnancy that affects over 50% of women. Backache can be prevented to a large degree by avoidance of excessive weight gain and a regular exercise program before pregnancy.

PREPARED PARENTHOOD AND SUPPORT GROUPS

- Routine classes on newborn child care and parenting should be part of the prenatal care program.

PRENATAL RECORD

- The prenatal care record should describe the comprehensive care provided and should allow for systematic documentation of coordinated services.

Components of the Postpartum Visit

- Most patients should be seen approximately 6 weeks postpartum, sooner for complicated deliveries and cesarean deliveries.
- The goal of this visit is to evaluate the physical, psychosocial, and mental well-being of the mother; to provide support and referral for breastfeeding; and to initiate or encourage compliance with the preferred family planning option and preconception care for the next pregnancy.

BIRTH SPACING

- An important goal of the postpartum visit and interconception care is to encourage birth spacing—specifically, to educate women about the importance of waiting at least 24 months to conceive again to decrease the risk of PTB/LBW and risk for uterine rupture among women attempting a vaginal birth after a cesarean delivery.
- Educating women on the most appropriate contraception based on medical conditions and discharging patients with an effective contraception method is essential to assist women in achieving the recommended 24-month interval.

COUNSELING REGARDING MEDICAL CONDITIONS AND OBSTETRIC COMPLICATIONS

- Follow-up is needed for medical complications such as heart disease, hypertension, diabetes, and depression—conditions that may have been exacerbated by pregnancy—as well as thyroid disease and epilepsy, conditions in which postpartum medication adjustments may be required.
- Women with a history of PTB, preeclampsia, and GDM should be informed that they are at increased risk of recurrence with subsequent pregnancies in addition to being at risk for subsequent development of hypertension, cardiovascular disease, and type 2 diabetes.

References for this chapter are available at ExpertConsult.com.

CHAPTER 7

Nutrition During Pregnancy

Elizabeth Horvitz West ■ Lisa Hark ■ Patrick M. Catalano

KEY POINTS

- Pregnant women may need as much as an additional 300 kcal/day for the entire pregnancy, but requirements may vary among individuals.
- The IOM recommendations for gestational weight gain for women are set by weight category: underweight (BMI <18.5; 28 to 40 lb), normal weight (BMI 18.5 to 24.9; 25 to 35 lb), overweight (BMI 25.0 to 29.9; 15 to 35 lb), and obese (BMI >30; 11 to 20 lb).
- Protein requirements during pregnancy increase from 0.8 g/kg/day for nonpregnant women to 1.1 g/kg/day during pregnancy.
- The daily recommended intake for folate in women of childbearing age is 400 µg/day; for pregnant women, it is 600 µg/day. Women whose fetuses are at high risk of an NTD should be prescribed a higher dose of folate (4 mg/day) both before conception and in early pregnancy.
- Iron supplementation is often prescribed during pregnancy because of the (20% to 30%) expanded maternal red cell mass as well as for fetal and placental tissue production. Iron supplements can cause gastrointestinal side effects such as constipation.
- Vitamin D supplementation is often required during pregnancy in particular for those with minimal exposure to sunlight, in vegan women, and those from minority populations with dark skin. To evaluate vitamin D concentrations before and during pregnancy, check serum 25(OH)D levels and aim for concentrations of 25(OH)D of greater than 20 nmol/L. The DRI for vitamin D is 600 IU/day in all pregnant and reproductive-age women.
- The DRI for calcium in nonpregnant and pregnant women 19 to 50 years of age is 1000 mg/day, and it is 1300 mg/day for females 9 to 19 years of age.
- Many common gastrointestinal problems during pregnancy—such as heartburn, nausea and vomiting, and constipation—are improved with proper nutritional counseling.

Overview

- The increase in obesity disproportionately affects minority populations, such as Hispanics and blacks, and especially women.[1]
- Excessive weight gain during pregnancy significantly increases the risk of postpartum weight retention and contributes to the accretion of excess adipose tissue in the fetus and diabetes in subsequent pregnancy and later in life.

Integrating Nutrition Into the Obstetric History

- The purpose of this assessment is to identify the quality of a patient's diet and to assess any nutritional risk factors that could jeopardize her health or the health of her developing baby.
- A patient's diet can be assessed by asking about intake over the previous 24 hours or by administering a diet history questionnaire in the waiting room.

- Women with a short interpregnancy interval (e.g., <1 year between pregnancies) may have depleted nutrient reserves, which is associated with increased preterm birth, intrauterine growth restriction, and maternal morbidity and mortality.[2,3]

Maternal Weight Gain Recommendations

- There are many general recommendations regarding diets for pregnant women to avoid problems such as excessive gestational weight gain and potential complications such as gestational diabetes and fetal overgrowth.
- Consuming healthy food is the goal to meet the Institute of Medicine (IOM) gestational weight guidelines and address the individual needs of the patient.

LOW OR UNDERWEIGHT PRECONCEPTION BODY MASS INDEX

- Based on the available data, there is strong support that women with low pregnancy body mass index (BMI) and low gestational weight gain have an increased risk (<10%) for having small-for-gestational-age infants, preterm birth, and perinatal mortality.[4]

OVERWEIGHT AND OBESE PREPREGNANCY BODY MASS INDEX

- Approximately 60% of reproductive-age women are overweight (BMI >25 kg/m^2), and of these, half are obese (BMI >30 kg/m^2). BMI varies widely within the United States (Fig. 7.1).

Prevalence* of Self-Reported Obesity Among U.S. Adults by State and Territory, BRFSS, 2013

*Prevalence estimates reflect BRFSS methodological changes started in 2011. These estimates should not be compared to prevalence estimates before 2011.

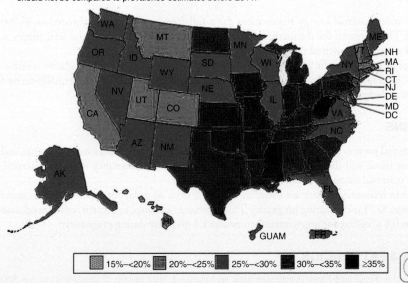

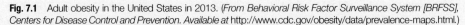

Fig. 7.1 Adult obesity in the United States in 2013. (*From Behavioral Risk Factor Surveillance System [BRFSS], Centers for Disease Control and Prevention. Available at* http://www.cdc.gov/obesity/data/prevalence-maps.html.)

- The 2009 IOM guidelines recommend that overweight women with a singleton pregnancy gain a total of 15 to 25 lb during pregnancy (compared with 25 with 35 lb for normal-weight women). Obese women are advised to gain only 11 to 20 lb during the course of their pregnancy.

Maternal Weight Gain Recommendations for Special Populations

MULTIPLE GESTATIONS

- For twin pregnancy, the IOM recommends a gestational weight gain of 37 to 54 lb for women of normal weight, 31 to 50 lb for overweight women, and 25 to 42 lb for obese women.
- For triplet and higher-order gestations, the data on ideal gestational weight gain are insufficient and thus there are no specific recommendations.

ADOLESCENTS

- Approximately 17% of teenage girls ages 12 through 19 are obese in America, and these obese teens face the same obstetric risks that adult obese women face.
- The 2009 IOM recommendations state that adolescents should follow the adult BMI categories to guide their weight gain.

OTHER GROUPS

- There are no specific recommendations for gestational weight gain in women of short stature, specific racial or ethnic groups, or those who smoke cigarettes.

Maternal Nutrient Needs: Current Recommendations

ENERGY

- The total maternal energy requirement for a full-term pregnancy is estimated at 80,000 kcal. This accounts for the increased metabolic activity of the maternal and fetal tissues as well as for the growth of the fetus and placenta
- Later in pregnancy, the basal or fasting contribution of carbohydrates to oxidative metabolism increases. Fetal growth and lactation are dependent on energy preferentially derived from carbohydrates.[5]

PROTEINS

- Maternal protein synthesis increases to support expansion of the blood volume, uterus, and breast tissue and thus additional protein is required during pregnancy for fetal, placental, and maternal tissue development.
- Protein recommendations are therefore increased from 46 g/day for an adult, nonpregnant woman to 71 g/day during pregnancy. This represents a change in protein recommendation from 0.8 g/kg/day for nonpregnant women to 1.1 g/kg/day during pregnancy.[6]

OMEGA-3 FATTY ACIDS

- The U.S. Food and Drug Administration recommends that pregnant women consume 200 to 300 mg/day of DHA, which can be achieved by consuming 1 to 2 servings (8 to 12 ounces) of fish per week. However, the average pregnant or lactating woman consumes only 52 mg/day of docasahexaenoic acid and 20 mg/day of eicosapentaenoic acid.[7]

- Avoid fish with the highest mercury concentration—specifically, tilefish, shark, swordfish, and king mackerel. They should also limit consumption of white albacore tuna to 6 oz/week.[8]
- The best evidence in support of polyunsaturated fatty acid (PUFA) supplementation comes from studies that show a positive relationship between PUFA supplementation and neurodevelopmental outcomes in children.[9,10]
- Maternal Fetal Medicine Network trial did not find evidence that fish oil supplementation decreased the risk of preterm delivery in high-risk patients.[11]

Vitamin and Mineral Supplementation Guidelines

DIETARY REFERENCE INTAKES

- The daily recommended intakes (DRIs) provide a range for safe and appropriate intake, as well as tolerable upper limit, based on the available research. The DRIs include four dietary reference values for every life stage and gender group.[12]

TOLERABLE UPPER INTAKE LEVEL

- Most health care providers prescribe a prenatal vitamin and mineral supplement because many women do not meet their nutritional requirements during the first trimester, especially with regard to folic acid and iron.

VITAMINS

Vitamin A

- Over-the-counter multivitamin supplements may contain excessive doses of vitamin A and therefore should be discontinued during pregnancy if above the recommended daily intake.
- Topical creams that contain retinol derivatives, commonly used to treat acne, should be avoided during pregnancy and in women trying to conceive (see Chapter 8).

Vitamin D

- During pregnancy, vitamin D is also critically important for fetal growth and development as well as for regulation of genes associated with normal implantation and angiogenesis.
- Vitamin D supplementation is advised for women who are strict vegetarians, those with limited exposure to sunlight, and those from minority populations with dark/black skin. To evaluate vitamin D levels during a preconception or prenatal visit, serum 25-hydroxy-D levels may be evaluated.

Vitamins C and E

- The hypothesis that oxidative stress contributes to development of preeclampsia has spurred interest in the use of antioxidants such as vitamins C and E for prevention of the disease.
- Several large, randomized placebo-controlled studies and a Cochrane review have shown no benefit.[13] Thus supplementation with antioxidant vitamins C and E for the prevention of preeclampsia is *not* recommended.[14]

Vitamin B$_6$

- Research shows that supplemental vitamin B$_6$ is effective at relieving nausea and vomiting during pregnancy.[15]
- Because excessive amounts of vitamin B$_6$ can cause numbness and nerve damage, the tolerable upper intake level for pregnant women was established at 100 mg/day.

Vitamin K

■ The DRI for vitamin K is 90 mg for pregnant and nonpregnant women and the tolerable upper intake has not been established.

Folate

■ Adequate levels of dietary folate are important for fetal and placental development and are needed to support rapid cell growth, replication, cell division, and nucleotide synthesis.

■ Because embryonic neural tube closure is complete by 18 to 28 days after conception, it is critical that pregnant women consume adequate folate before and during the first 4 weeks of embryologic development (6 weeks gestational age by last menstrual period).

■ The DRI for folate in women of childbearing age is 400 µg/day; for pregnant women it is 600 µg/day.

Folate and Neural Tube Defects

■ The etiology of NTDs is thought to be insufficient folate intake coupled with the increased folate demands of pregnancy.

■ The early formation and the detrimental effects of folate deficiency on neural tube formation are the basis behind the recommendation that folate supplementation begin prior to conception and be continued at least through the first trimester of pregnancy.[16]

Folate Supplementation

■ Several randomized, controlled, and observational trials have shown that periconceptional and early pregnancy consumption of folate supplements can reduce a woman's risk for having an infant with an NTD by as much as 50% to 70%.[17]

■ In women with a previous pregnancy affected by an NTD, research has shown that supplementation with 4000 µg/day (4 mg/day) of folate initiated at least 1 month prior to attempting to conceive and continued throughout the first trimester of pregnancy reduced the risk of a repeat NTD by 72%.[18]

■ No definitive evidence proves that other high-risk groups such as close family members of affected individuals, diabetics, or women on antiseizure medications will benefit from higher levels of supplementation; many experts recommend a higher dose of folate, at least 1000 µg/day before conception and in early pregnancy.

MINERALS
Iron

■ Additional iron is needed to expand maternal red cell volume by 20% to 30%, and iron is also required for fetal and placental tissue production.

■ As shown in Table 7.1, hemoglobin less than 11 g/dL or hematocrit below 33% in the first or third trimester indicates anemia. Hemoglobin less than 10.5 g/dL or hematocrit below 32% in the second trimester also indicates anemia.

■ Prenatal care providers generally recommend daily iron supplementation with 30 mg of elemental iron in the form of simple salts beginning around the twelfth week of pregnancy for women who have normal preconception hemoglobin measurements (Table 7.2).

■ Women with severe iron deficiency, those who cannot tolerate oral iron, or those with malabsorption syndromes, parenteral iron can be used. Parenteral iron is especially valuable for increasing hemoglobin levels faster than oral iron.

TABLE 7.1 ■ **Diagnosis of Anemia in Pregnancy**

Lab Test	First Trimester	Second Trimester	Third Trimester
Hemoglobin (g/dL)	<11	10.5	<11
Hematocrit (%)	<33	32	<33

Data from U.S. Centers for Disease Control and Prevention (www.cdc.gov).

TABLE 7.2 ■ **Oral Iron Supplements**

Oral Supplement	Elemental Iron
Ferrous fumarate	106 mg/tablet
Ferrous sulfate	65 mg/tablet
Ferrous gluconate	28-36 mg/tablet

Data from the American College of Obstetricians and Gynecologists. ACOG practice bulletin No. 95: Anemia in pregnancy. *Obstet Gynecol.* 2008;112(1):201-207.

Calcium

- Large quantities of calcium are essential for the development of the fetal skeleton, fetal tissues, and hormonal adaptations during pregnancy. Evidence has also shown that calcium supplementation reduces the risk of developing hypertension during pregnancy, but only in women who did not have adequate calcium intake prior to supplementation.
- The DRI for calcium in pregnant women 19 to 50 years old is 1000 mg/day; and 1300 mg/day for adolescent females age 9 to 19 years. Adolescents may need additional calcium during pregnancy since their own bones still require calcium deposition to ensure adequate bone density.
- The standard prenatal vitamin typically contains 150 to 300 mg per tablet.

Zinc

- More than 100 enzymes require zinc, and maternal zinc deficiency can lead to prolonged labor, intrauterine growth restriction, teratogenesis, and embryonic or fetal death.[19]
- The DRI for pregnant women is 11 mg/day and may be higher for vegetarians or vegans since phytates from whole grains and beans bind with zinc and can reduce absorption.

Choline

- Adequate choline is needed for normal fetal neural development, function, and memory.[20] Choline is derived not only from the diet, but also from de novo synthesis.
- The current recommendation for choline during pregnancy is 450 mg/day and 550 mg/day for breastfeeding patients.

Nutrition-Related Problems During Pregnancy

NAUSEA AND VOMITING

- Women with hyperemesis may vomit multiple times throughout the day, lose more than 5% of their prepregnancy body weight, and usually require hospitalization for dehydration and electrolyte replacement.

- Strategies for managing nausea and vomiting during pregnancy are shown in Box 7.1. After following these recommendations, vitamin B_6 (10 to 25 mg three times daily) can be considered as first-line treatment for nausea and vomiting during pregnancy.

HEARTBURN AND INDIGESTION

- Heartburn and indigestion affect two-thirds of pregnant women.
- Strategies for managing nausea and vomiting during pregnancy are shown in Box 7.1.

CONSTIPATION

- Fifty percent of pregnant women experience constipation at some point during their pregnancy.
- Strategies for managing constipation during pregnancy are shown in Box 7.2.

FOOD CONTAMINATION

- Pathogens of special concern during pregnancy include *Listeria monocytogenes, Toxoplasma gondii, Salmonella* species, and *Campylobacter jejuni.*
- To avoid listeriosis, pregnant women should be advised to wash vegetables and fruits well, cook all meats to minimum safe internal temperatures, avoid processed, precooked meats (cold cuts, smoked seafood, pâté) and soft cheeses (brie, blue cheese, Camembert, and Mexican queso blanco), and to consume only pasteurized dairy products.

BOX 7.1 ■ Strategies for Managing Nausea, Vomiting, Heartburn, and Indigestion in Pregnancy

- Eat small, low-fat meals and snacks (fruits, pretzels, crackers, nonfat yogurt).
- Eat slowly and frequently.
- Avoid strong food odors by eating room temperature or cold foods and using good ventilation while cooking.
- Drink fluids between meals rather than with meals.
- Avoid foods that may cause stomach irritation such as spearmint, peppermint, caffeine, citrus fruits, spicy foods, high-fat foods, or tomato products.
- Wait 1-2 hours after eating a meal before lying down.
- Take a walk after meals.
- Wear loose-fitting clothes.
- Brush teeth after eating to prevent symptoms.

Courtesy Lisa Hark, PhD, RD.

BOX 7.2 ■ Strategies for Managing Constipation in Pregnancy

- Increase fluid intake by drinking water, herbal teas, and noncaffeinated beverages.
- Increase daily fiber intake by eating high-fiber cereals, whole grains, legumes, and bran.
- Use a psyllium fiber supplement (e.g., Metamucil).
- Increase consumption of fresh, frozen, or dried fruits and vegetables.
- Participate in moderate physical activity such as walking, swimming, or yoga.
- Take stool softeners in conjunction with iron supplementation.

Courtesy Lisa Hark, PhD, RD.

- Toxoplasmosis can be passed to humans by water, dust, soil and eating contaminated foods. Cats are the main host of *T. gondii*. Toxoplasmosis most often results from eating raw or uncooked meat or unwashed fruits and vegetables, cleaning a cat litter box, or handling contaminated soil.

Special Nutritional Considerations During Pregnancy

CAFFEINE

- Moderate caffeine consumption (less than 200 mg per day) is not a major contributing factor to miscarriage or preterm birth.

VEGETARIAN AND VEGAN DIETS

- Vegan diets—those that exclude all animal products, including eggs and dairy—may provide insufficient iron, essential amino acids, trace minerals (zinc), vitamin B_{12}, vitamin D, calcium, and PUFAs to support normal embryonic and fetal development.
- It is recommended that patients who follow a vegan diet meet with a dietitian early during the pregnancy to analyze their nutritional intake and assess any necessary supplementation that should be added.

HERBAL SUPPLEMENTS

- Whereas countless other herbs and supplements certainly hold potential benefits, more research is needed before any of these supplements can be safely recommended in pregnancy.

References for this chapter are available at ExpertConsult.com.

CHAPTER 8

Drugs and Environmental Agents in Pregnancy and Lactation: Teratology and Epidemiology

Jennifer R. Niebyl ■ Robert J. Weber ■ Gerald G. Briggs

KEY POINTS

- The critical period of organ development extends from day 31 to day 71 after the first day of the LMP.
- Infants of epileptic women taking certain anticonvulsants, such as valproic acid, have double the rate of malformations of unexposed infants. The risk of fetal hydantoin syndrome is less than 10%.
- The risk of malformations after in utero exposure to isotretinoin is 25%, and an additional 25% of infants will develop mental retardation.
- Heparin is the drug of choice for anticoagulation during pregnancy except for women with artificial heart valves, who should receive coumadin despite the 5% risk of warfarin embryopathy.
- Angiotensin-converting enzyme inhibitors and angiotensin receptor blockers can cause fetal renal failure in the second and third trimesters, leading to oligohydramnios and hypoplastic lungs.
- Vitamin B_6 25 mg three times a day is a safe and effective therapy for first-trimester nausea and vomiting. Doxylamine 12.5 mg three times a day is also effective in combination with B_6.
- Most antibiotics are generally safe in pregnancy, although aminoglycosides are known to be ototoxic to the fetus. Trimethoprim may carry an increased risk in the first trimester, and tetracyclines taken in the second and third trimesters may cause tooth discoloration.
- Aspirin in analgesic doses inhibits platelet function and prolongs bleeding time, increasing the risk of peripartum hemorrhage but is not associated with congenital defects.
- Fetal alcohol syndrome occurs in infants of mothers who drink heavily during pregnancy. A safe level of alcohol intake during pregnancy has not been determined.
- Cocaine has been associated with increased risk of miscarriage, abruptio placentae, and congenital malformations, in particular, microcephaly and limb defects.
- Most drugs are safe during lactation because subtherapeutic amounts, approximately 1% to 2% of the maternal dose, appear in breast milk. Short-term (<2 days) use of codeine is safe during breastfeeding.
- Only a small amount of prednisone crosses the placenta, so it is the preferred corticosteroid for most chronic maternal illnesses such as lupus. In contrast, betamethasone and dexamethasone readily cross the placenta and are preferred for acceleration of fetal lung maturity.
- Exposure to high-dose ionizing radiation at any stage during gestation causes microcephaly and mental retardation Diagnostic exposures below 5 rads after 12 weeks of gestation do not pose increased teratogenic risks.

KEY POINTS—cont'd

- Lead levels in blood have decreased in recent years in all except some immigrant populations. Blood levels below 25 µg/dL in women of reproductive age minimizes the risk of fetal growth restriction during pregnancy.
- Mercury in high levels deleteriously affects the fetal nervous system. For this reason pregnant and nursing women should avoid shark, swordfish, king mackerel, and tilefish. Exposures to mercury can further be limited by restricting ingestion of certain other seafood (shrimp, canned tuna, salmon, pollock, catfish) to 12 oz/week.

Overview

- Virtually all drugs cross the placenta to some degree, with the exception of large molecules such as heparin and insulin but also vaccines.
- The incidence of major malformations in the general population is 2% to 3%.[1]
- The classic teratogenic period is from day 31 after the last menstrual period (LMP) in a 28-day cycle to 71 days from the LMP. During this critical period, organs are forming, and teratogens may cause malformations that are usually overt at birth.
- Before day 31, exposure to a teratogen produces an all-or-none effect.
- FDA categories lists five categories of labeling for drug use during pregnancy. The risk increases from A (controlled studies show no risk) to X (contraindicated during pregnancy). These categories were designed for prescribing physicians and not to address inadvertent exposure. For example, isotretinoin and oral contraceptives are both category X based on lack of benefit for oral contraceptives during pregnancy, yet oral contraceptives do not have any teratogenic risk with inadvertent exposure.

Basic Principles of Teratology

- Wilson's six general principles of teratogenesis[2] provide a framework for understanding how structural or functional teratogens may act.

GENOTYPE AND INTERACTION WITH ENVIRONMENTAL FACTORS

- The first principle is based on the concept that susceptibility to a teratogen depends on the *genotype of the conceptus* and on the manner in which the genotype interacts with environmental factors. Not all fetuses exposed to a specific drug at a similar dose and gestational age will develop congenital malformations.

TIMING OF EXPOSURE

- The second principle is that susceptibility of the conceptus to teratogenic agents varies with the developmental stage at the time of exposure. Most structural defects occur during the second to the eighth weeks of development after conception, during the embryonic period.

MECHANISMS OF TERATOGENESIS

- The third principle is that teratogenic agents act in specific ways—that is, via specific *mechanisms*—on developing cells and tissues in initiating abnormal embryogenesis (pathogenesis).

MANIFESTATIONS

■ The fourth principle is that irrespective of the specific deleterious agent, the final manifestations of abnormal development are malformation, growth restriction, functional disorder, and death.

AGENT

■ The fifth principle is that access of adverse environmental influences to developing tissues depends on the nature of the influence (*agent*).

DOSE EFFECT

■ The final principle is that manifestations of abnormal development increase in degree from the no-effect level to the lethal level as *dosage* increases.

Medical Drug Use

EFFECTS OF SPECIFIC DRUGS

Estrogens and Progestins

■ Studies have not confirmed any teratogenic risk for oral contraceptives or progestins.

Androgenic Steroids

■ Androgens may masculinize a developing female fetus.

Spermicides

■ A meta-analysis of reports of spermicide exposure has concluded that the risk of birth defects is not increased.[4]

Antiepileptic Drugs

■ Women with epilepsy who take antiepileptic drugs (AEDs) during pregnancy have approximately double the general population risk of malformations in offspring.
■ Valproic acid and carbamazepine each carry approximately a 1% risk of neural tube defects (NTDs) and other anomalies.
■ Fewer than 10% of offspring show the fetal hydantoin syndrome, which consists of microcephaly, growth deficiency, developmental delays, mental retardation, and dysmorphic craniofacial features.
■ Valproate should not be used as a first-choice drug in women of reproductive age.
■ Of 1532 infant exposures to newer-generation antiepileptic drugs, 1019 were to lamotrigine, and 3.7% presented with major birth defects. Of 393 infants exposed to oxcarbazepine, the rate was 2.8%, and for 108 exposed to topiramate, the rate was 4.6%. None of these differences were statistically different from controls.
■ Most authorities agree that the benefits of AEDs during pregnancy outweigh the risks of discontinuation of the drug if the patient is first seen during pregnancy.

Isotretinoin

■ Isotretinoin is a significant human teratogen.
■ The risk of structural anomalies in patients studied prospectively is now estimated to be about 25%, and an additional 25% have mental retardation alone.

- In 88 pregnancies prospectively ascertained after discontinuation of isotretinoin, no increased risk of anomalies was noted.

Vitamin A

- Cases of birth defects have been reported after exposure to levels of 25,000 IU or more of vitamin A during pregnancy.

Psychoactive Drugs

- No clear risk has been documented for most psychoactive drugs with respect to overt birth defects.

Lithium

- A prospective study of 148 women exposed to lithium in the first trimester showed no difference in the incidence of major anomalies compared with controls.[5] Polyhydramnios may be a sign of fetal lithium toxicity.
- Discontinuation of lithium may pose an unacceptable risk of increased morbidity in women who have had multiple episodes of affective instability. These women should be offered appropriate prenatal diagnosis with ultrasound, including fetal echocardiography.
- We recommend that women exposed to lithium be offered a detailed fetal ultrasound examination including fetal echocardiography.

Antidepressants

- No increased risk of major malformations has been found after first-trimester exposure to fluoxetine in several studies.[6] However, one study showed a twofold increased risk of ventricular septal defects and two other studies found an increased risk of cardiac defects after exposure to paroxetine.[7]
- When considering the use of antidepressant drugs during pregnancy, it should be noted that among women who maintained their medication throughout pregnancy, 26% relapsed compared with 68% who discontinued medication.[8]
- Fetal alcohol spectrum disorders are 10 times more common in offspring exposed to selective serotonin reuptake inhibitors than in unexposed offspring.

Anticoagulants

- Warfarin embryopathy occurs in about 5% of exposed pregnancies and includes nasal hypoplasia, bone stippling seen on radiologic examination, ophthalmologic abnormalities including bilateral optic atrophy, and mental retardation.
- The risk for pregnancy complications is higher when the mean daily dose of warfarin is more than 5 mg.
- Because heparin does not have an adverse effect on the fetus, it should be the drug of choice for patients who require anticoagulation during pregnancy, except in women with artificial heart valves.
- Women with mechanical heart valves, especially the first-generation valves, require warfarin anticoagulation because heparin is neither safe nor effective.
- Low-molecular-weight heparins may have substantial benefits over standard unfractionated heparin. Enoxaparin is cleared more rapidly during pregnancy, so twice-daily dosing is advised.

Thyroid and Antithyroid Drugs

- Methimazole has been associated with scalp defects in infants and choanal or esophageal atresia.[9]

- In 2009 the FDA released a black box warning highlighting serious liver injury with propylthiouracil (PTU) treatment, to a greater extent than with methimazole. The Endocrine Society is now advocating treatment with PTU only during the first trimester and switching to methimazole for the remainder of the pregnancy.[10, 11]
- It is recommended that women with hypothyroidism increase their levothyroxine dose by approximately 30% as soon as pregnancy is confirmed (two extra doses each week) and then have dosing adjustments based on thyroid-stimulating hormone levels.[12]

Digoxin

- Digoxin has not been associated with significant teratogenic effects.

Antihypertensive Drugs

- Antihypertensive drugs are used for treatment of chronic hypertension in pregnancy. In particular α-methyldopa has been widely used and no unusual fetal effect has been observed.

Sympathetic Blocking Agents

Angiotensin-Converting Enzyme Inhibitors and Angiotensin Receptor Blockers

- Angiotensin-converting enzyme inhibitors inhibitors such as enalapril and captopril and angiotensin II receptor antagonists such as valsartan can cause fetal renal tubular dysplasia in the second and third trimesters, leading to oligohydramnios, fetal limb contractures, craniofacial deformities, and hypoplastic lung development.
- Women taking these medications who plan a pregnancy should be switched to other agents before conception.

Antineoplastic Drugs and Immunosuppressants

- **Mycophenolate mofetil** carries a moderate teratogenic risk.[13]
- **Methotrexate**, a folic acid antagonist, appears to be a human teratogen, although experience is limited.

Antiasthmatics

- **Terbutaline, cromolyn sodium, isoproterenol,** and **metaproterenol** have not been associated with significant teratogenic effects.
- A meta-analysis of chronic exposure to **corticosteroids** in the first trimester showed an odds ratio of 3.0 for cleft lip and/or cleft palate.
- **Iodide** is found in some cough medicines and may produce a fetal goiter.

Antiemetics

- None of the current medications used to treat nausea and vomiting have been found to be teratogenic except possibly methylprednisolone when used before 10 weeks of gestation.
- **Vitamin B$_6$** has not been associated with significant teratogenic effects in randomized controlled trials.
- **Doxylamine** is an effective antihistamine for nausea and vomiting of pregnancy and can be combined with vitamin B$_6$ to produce a therapeutic effect similar to Diclegis.

Meclizine, Dimenhydrinate, Diphenhydramine, and Phenothiazines

- These drugs have not been associated with significant teratogenic effects.

Metoclopramide

- Of 3458 infants exposed to metoclopramide during the first trimester, no increased risk of malformations, low birthweight, or preterm delivery was reported.[14]

Ondansetron

- This drug has not been evaluated in large studies for teratogenicity.

Methylprednisolone

- This drug should not be use before 10 weeks because of the potential risks of cleft lip and palate.

Ginger

- Ginger has been used with success for treating nausea, vomiting, and hyperemesis in the outpatient setting with no evidence of fetal effects.

Acid-Suppressing Drugs

- These drugs have not been associated with significant teratogenic effects.

Antihistamines and Decongestants

- Most of these drugs have not been associated with significant teratogenic effects. Terfenadine may be associated with fetal polydactyly.

Antibiotics and Antiinfective Agents

- Penicillins are safe during pregnancy.
- When clavulanate is added to amoxicillin, it increases the risks of necrotizing enterocolitis in premature newborns; thus these preparations should be avoided in women at risk for preterm delivery.
- Cephalosporins are considered safe during pregnancy.
- Sulfonamides have not been associated with significant teratogenic effects.
- In one retrospective study of trimethoprim with sulfamethoxazole, the odds ratio for birth defects was 2.3, whereas in another study it was 2.5 to 3.4.
- Nitrofurantoin has not been associated with significant teratogenic effects.
- Tetracyclines readily cross the placenta and are firmly bound by chelation to calcium in developing bone and tooth structures. This produces brown discoloration of the deciduous teeth, hypoplasia of the enamel, and inhibition of bone growth. The staining of the teeth takes place in the second or third trimesters of pregnancy, whereas bone incorporation can occur earlier.
- First-trimester exposure to doxycycline is not known to carry any risk. First-trimester exposure to tetracyclines was not found to have any teratogenic risk in 341 women in the Collaborative Perinatal Project or in 174 women in another study. Alternative antibiotics are currently recommended during pregnancy.
- Aminoglycosides have not been associated with significant teratogenic effects.
- Antituberculosis drugs have not been associated with significant teratogenic effects.
- Erythromycin has not been associated with significant teratogenic effects.
- Clarithromycin has not been associated with significant teratogenic effects.
- Fluoroquinolones have not been associated with significant teratogenic effects.
- Metronidazole has not been associated with significant teratogenic effects during early or late gestation

Antiviral Agents

- Antiviral agents such as acyclovir have not been associated with significant teratogenic effects.

- Lindane is not associated with obvious fetal damage but it is a potent neurotoxin and should be avoided during pregnancy.

Antiretroviral Agents

- Agents such as zidovudine have not been associated with significant teratogenic effects.
- Efavirenz is associated with malformations in monkeys and should be avoided during pregnancy.
- Zidovudine should be included as a component in the antiretroviral regimen whenever possible because of its record of safety and efficacy.

Antifungal Agents

- These agents have not been associated with significant teratogenic effects.

Induction of Ovulation

- These drugs have not been associated with significant teratogenic effects.

Mild Analgesics

Aspirin

- Aspirin does have significant perinatal effects, however, because it inhibits prostaglandin synthesis. Uterine contractility is decreased, and patients taking aspirin in analgesic doses have delayed onset of labor, longer duration of labor, and an increased risk of a prolonged pregnancy.
- Aspirin also decreases platelet aggregation, which can increase the risk of bleeding before as well as at delivery but has not been associated with significant teratogenic effects.

Acetaminophen

- In contrast to aspirin, bleeding time is not prolonged with acetaminophen but is not toxic to the fetus.

Other Nonsteroidal Antiinflammatory Agents

- Codeine has not been associated with significant teratogenic effects but can cause addiction and newborn withdrawal symptoms if used to excess perinatally.
- Sumatriptan has not been associated with significant teratogenic effects and may be used during pregnancy for women whose severe headaches do not respond to other therapy.[15]

Drugs of Abuse

- Tobacco and nicotine products are associated with increased risks of miscarriage, abruptio placentae, placenta previa, premature labor and IUGR, leading to high perinatal mortality rates.

NICOTINE

- Maternal smoking is the most preventable cause of premature delivery in the United States, and nicotine medications are indicated for patients with nicotine dependence.
- Although the propriety of prescribing nicotine during pregnancy might be questioned, cessation of smoking eliminates many other toxins, including carbon monoxide; nicotine blood levels are not increased over that of smokers.

ALCOHOL

- In heavy drinkers (average daily intake of 3 oz of 100-proof liquor or more), 32% of the infants have anomalies.
- Heavy drinking remains a major risk to the fetus, and reduction even from midpregnancy can benefit the infant.[16]
- Fetal alcohol syndrome occurs in 6% of infants of heavy drinkers, and less severe birth defects and neurocognitive deficits occur in a larger proportion of children whose mothers drank heavily during pregnancy.

CANNABIS/MARIJUANA

- This drug has not been associated with significant teratogenic effects.

COCAINE

- Cocaine-using women have a higher rate of miscarriage than controls. Other studies have suggested an increased risk of congenital anomalies after first-trimester cocaine use, most frequently those of the cardiac and central nervous systems, limb defects and IUGR.
- Abruptio placentae has been reported to occur immediately after nasal or IV administration.[17]
- The most common brain abnormality in infants exposed to cocaine in utero is impairment of intrauterine brain growth as manifested by microcephaly.[18]

NARCOTICS AND METHADONE

- Narcotics addicts are at increased risk for miscarriage, premature birth, and IUGR. Withdrawal should be watched for carefully in the neonatal period.[19]

OTHER SUBSTANCES
Caffeine

- No evidence of teratogenic effects of caffeine in humans has been found.
- In one report that controlled for smoking and other habits, demographic characteristics, and medical history, no relationship was found between malformations, low birth weight, or short gestation and heavy coffee consumption.
- The American College of Obstetricians and Gynecologists concluded that moderate caffeine consumption (less than 200 mg/day) does not appear to be a major contributing factor in miscarriage or preterm birth, but the relationship to intrauterine growth restriction remains undetermined.[20]

Aspartame

- This chemical has not been associated with significant teratogenic effects.

Drugs in Breast Milk

- Most drugs are detected in breast milk at low levels and short-term effects, if any, of most maternal medications on breastfed infants are mild and pose little risk to the infants.[21]

DRUGS COMMONLY LISTED AS CONTRAINDICATED DURING BREASTFEEDING

- Drugs of abuse for which adverse effects on the infant during breastfeeding have been reported include amphetamines, cocaine, heroin, marijuana, and phencyclidine and are thus contraindicated.
- Radiopharmaceuticals require variable intervals of interruption of breastfeeding.

DRUGS WITH UNKNOWN EFFECTS ON NURSING INFANTS BUT POSSIBLY OF CONCERN

- Sertraline causes a decline in 5-hydroxytryptamine levels in mothers but not in their breastfed infants.[22] This implies that the small amount of drug the infant ingests in breast milk is not enough to have a pharmacologic effect. Infants of mothers taking psychotropic drugs should be monitored for sedation during use and for withdrawal after cessation of the drug.
- The benefits of nursing should be weighed against the negative effect on bonding that would result from untreated postpartum depression.

DRUGS ASSOCIATED WITH SIGNIFICANT EFFECTS (ADMINISTER WITH CAUTION)

- Administer bromocriptine, ergotamine, and lithium to nursing mothers with caution.

DRUGS USUALLY COMPATIBLE WITH BREASTFEEDING

- Narcotics, sedatives, and anticonvulsants
- Cold preparations
- Antihypertensives:
  - Thiazides
  - β-Blockers
  - Angiotensin-converting enzyme inhibitors
  - Calcium channel blockers
- Corticosteroids
- Digoxin
- Antibiotics
- Acyclovir
- Antifungal agents
- Oral contraceptives
- H2–Receptor blockers
- Anticoagulants are generally safe but require careful monitoring of maternal prothrombin time, so that the dosage is minimized, and of neonatal prothrombin times to ensure lack of drug accumulation. Warfarin may be safely administered to nursing mothers.
- Alcohol, when used occasionally, has not been associated with significant harmful effects on the infant.
- Propylthiouracil (PTU) is preferred to methimazole because of low breast milk concentrations; mothers taking PTU can thus continue nursing with close supervision of the infant.
- Caffeine has been reported to have no adverse effects on the nursing infant, even if the mother consumes five cups of coffee per day.
- Nicotine and its metabolite cotinine enter breast milk.

Occupational and Environmental Hazards

IONIZING RADIATION

- Ionizing radiation has mutagenic effects that are sometimes manifested years after birth such as infant leukemia.
- The greatest number of children with microcephaly, mental retardation, and growth restriction were found in the group of pregnant women exposed at 15 weeks' gestation or earlier.
- Effects of chronic low-dose radiation on reproduction have not been identified in animals or humans.
- Virtually no single diagnostic test produces a substantive risk.
- Video display terminals use does not increase the risk of adverse reproductive outcomes.

LEAD

- In high concentrations, lead has been associated with IUGR and NTDs.
- Ideally, the maternal blood lead level should be less than 10 μg/dL to ensure that a child begins life with minimal lead exposure. A dose-response relationship is strongly supported by numerous epidemiologic studies of children showing a reduction in IQ with increasing blood lead concentrations above 10 μg/dL.
- Other neurologic impairments associated with increased blood lead concentrations include attention-deficit/hyperactivity disorder, hearing deficits, and learning disabilities. Shorter stature has also been noted.

MERCURY

- Pregnant women, those who may become pregnant, and nursing mothers should avoid shark, swordfish, king mackerel, and tilefish because they contain high levels of mercury.[23]

References for this chapter are available at ExpertConsult.com.

CHAPTER 9

Obstetric Ultrasound: Imaging, Dating, Growth, and Anomaly

Douglas S. Richards

KEY POINTS

- Sonographers should become familiar with the basic physics of ultrasound, equipment controls, and scanning techniques to optimize ultrasound images.
- All of the elements of the standard obstetric ultrasound exam are important for clinical management and should not be neglected.
- Because most birth defects occur in fetuses of low-risk women, all standard exams should include a full anatomic survey.
- Physicians who perform and interpret obstetric ultrasound examinations should have appropriate training and experience.
- Appropriate documentation of ultrasound studies is important for good medical care.
- Pregnancy dating by ultrasound measurements is most accurate early in pregnancy. Guidelines have been established for when ultrasound dates should be used in preference to menstrual dates.
- Ultrasound for fetal weight estimation is of limited usefulness for the prevention of shoulder dystocia and other complications associated with fetal macrosomia.
- The AIUM and ACOG strongly discourage nonmedical use of ultrasound for entertainment purposes.
- It is not expected that all birth defects will be diagnosed by prenatal ultrasound.
- The sensitivity of ultrasound for the detection of birth defects depends on the level of training of examiners and the maintenance of a structured approach to the fetal examination.
- Performance of the first-trimester ultrasound component of the aneuploidy screen requires formal training and certification.
- Individuals who perform prenatal sonography should be aware of conditions that can be detected with a standard examination.

Biophysics of Ultrasound

- The underlying basis of ultrasound image production relies on the piezoelectric effect: when electrical impulses are applied to certain ceramic crystals, mechanical oscillations are induced.
- Ultrasound machines used in obstetrics operate at frequencies between about 2 and 9 MHz.
- Highly reflective tissues, such as bone, generate relatively more intense echoes.

Optimizing the Ultrasound Image

FREQUENCY

- The highest frequency probe that allows adequate penetration should be used.
- For obese patients, a lower-frequency probe must be chosen. The frequency for most transabdominal obstetric probes is about 3 to 5 MHz. and transvaginal probes usually operate at a frequency of 5 to 10 MHz.

POWER

- Increasing power output increases the amplitude of energy waves in the ultrasound beam and results in stronger returning echoes.

GAIN

- Signals from the weak echoes returning to the transducer elements must be amplified before being used for display. The amplification is referred to as gain.

ATTENUATION

- Attenuation of ultrasound waves is affected by the medium through which the sound waves pass. Virtually no pulses pass through gas. This is why there must be a coupling agent (e.g., ultrasound gel).
- In patients with a thick, dense abdominal wall, image quality is greatly reduced.

FOCUS

- Image resolution is optimal when the structure of interest lies within the zone of optimal focus, which can be adjusted by the sonographer.

DEPTH AND ZOOM

- Limiting the size of the scanned area allows a higher frame rate and resolution. Honing-in on the area of interest draws attention to important detail within that scanned area.

Special Ultrasound Modalities

M-MODE

- M-mode is sometimes used for specialized echocardiography applications.

COLOR AND PULSE-WAVE DOPPLER

- Doppler ultrasound is primarily used to demonstrate the presence, direction, and velocity of blood flow. Flow velocity waveforms are used to calculate the systolic/diastolic ratio, the pulsatility index, and the resistance index. These indexes are primarily used to assess downstream resistance in the vessel being interrogated. When screening for fetal anemia, the peak flow velocity in the fetal middle cerebral artery is measured, as this correlates with the degree of fetal anemia.

THREE-DIMENSIONAL ULTRASOUND

- Despite the demonstrated capabilities of 3D ultrasound, no proof exists of an advantage of this technology over standard 2D imaging for prenatal diagnosis.

Scanning Technique

ORIENTATION

- The probe is held in such a way that the image on the screen is properly oriented. For sagittal views, the right of the screen corresponds to the inferior aspect of the patient. For transverse views, the patient's right is shown on the left of the screen.
- To establish the position of the fetus, the orientation of the probe must obviously be correct.

USING NATURAL WINDOWS

- Thickness is also decreased lateral to the central pannus.
- Scanning through amniotic fluid improves the image quality below or deep to the amniotic fluid.

First-Trimester Ultrasound

- Transvaginal ultrasound is almost always superior to transabdominal ultrasound for evaluation very early in pregnancy.
- At 10 to 12 weeks' gestation, the uterus has grown enough and the fetus is far enough away from the transducer that advantages of transvaginal scanning are lost.

FIRST-TRIMESTER NORMAL FINDINGS

- M-mode ultrasound is used to document cardiac activity during this time.
- The cerebral falx is visible at 9 weeks, and the appearance and disappearance of physiologic gut herniation are noted between 8 and 11 weeks. The diagnosis of an abdominal wall defect should be made with caution at this age.
- Until 12 weeks, the crown-rump length (CRL) should be measured for gestational age determination.

FIRST-TRIMESTER ABNORMAL FINDINGS

- When cardiac activity has been demonstrated, the miscarriage rate is reduced to 2% to 3% in asymptomatic low-risk women.[1]
- In younger women who present with bleeding, only 5% miscarry if the ultrasound is normal and shows a live embryo.
- If there are borderline findings and uterine evacuation is being considered, it is prudent to repeat the ultrasound in 7 to 10 days to be absolutely sure that a viable pregnancy is not interrupted.
- First-trimester ultrasound findings predictive of a chromosome abnormality include a thick nuchal translucency, absent nasal bone, abnormally fast or slow fetal heart rate, and some structural malformations.[2]

Second- and Third-Trimester Ultrasound

TYPES OF EXAMINATIONS

- Components of a standard obstetric examination are shown in Box 9.1.
- Limited ultrasound examinations are used to obtain a specific piece of information about the pregnancy.

BOX 9.1 ■ Suggested Components of the Standard Obstetric Ultrasound Performed in the Second and Third Trimesters

- Standard biometry
- Fetal cardiac activity (present or absent, normal or abnormal)
- Number of fetuses (if multiples, document chorionicity, amnionicity, comparison of fetal sizes, estimation of amniotic fluid normality in each sac, and fetal genitalia)
- Presentation
- Qualitative or semiquantitative estimate of amniotic fluid volume
- Placental location, especially its relationship to the internal os, and placental cord insertion site
- Evaluation of the uterus that includes fibroids, adnexal structures, and the cervix
- Cervix when clinically appropriate and technically feasible
- Anatomic survey to include:

Head and neck
- Cerebellum
- Choroid plexus
- Cisterna magna
- Lateral cerebral ventricles
- Midline falx
- Cavum septum pellucidum
- Fetal lip
- Nuchal skin fold may be helpful for aneuploidy risk

Chest
- Four-chamber view of the heart
- Outflow tracts (if possible)

Abdomen
- Stomach (presence, size, and situs)
- Kidneys
- Bladder
- Umbilical cord insertion into the abdomen
- Number of umbilical cord vessels

Spine
- Extremities (presence or absence of legs and arms)

Gender

Data from American College of Obstetricians and Gynecologists. ACOG Practice Bulletin No. 101: ultrasonography in pregnancy. Obstet Gynecol. 2009; 113:451-461; American Institute of Ultrasound in Medicine (AIUM). AIUM practice guidelines for the performance of an antepartum obstetric ultrasound examination. J Ultrasound Med. 2003;22:1116-1125; and Reddy UM, Abuhamad AZ, Levine D. Saade GR. Fetal imaging: executive summary of a joint Eunice Kennedy Shriver National Institute of Child Health and Human Development, Society for Maternal-Fetal Medicine, American Institute of Ultrasound in Medicine, American College of Obstetricians and Gynecologists, American College of Radiology, Society for Pediatric Radiology, and Society of Radiologists in Ultrasound Fetal Imaging Workshop. Obstet Gynecol. 2014;123:1070-1082.

■ All the aspects of the standard obstetric examination listed in Box 9.1 are important for clinical management and should not be neglected.

QUALIFICATIONS FOR PERFORMING AND INTERPRETING DIAGNOSTIC ULTRASOUND EXAMINATIONS

■ The AIUM has published guidelines on the training and experience needed for physicians to perform or interpret ultrasound examinations.

Components of the Examination

■ Confirming the absence of a heartbeat with color or pulse-wave Doppler is recommended.
■ When a multiple pregnancy is diagnosed, the number of amnions and chorions should always be determined. Determination of chorionicity is most easily accomplished in early pregnancy. The presence of unlike sex twins, separate placentae, or a thick membrane dividing the sacs with a twin peak or "lambda sign" all indicate the presence of two chorions.
■ In all twin pregnancies, periodic ultrasound examinations should be performed to assess fetal growth.

AMNIOTIC FLUID VOLUME

■ The amniotic fluid index (AFI) is the sum of the measurements of the deepest vertical pocket of fluid in each of the uterine quadrants. The line between the calipers should not cross through loops of cord or fetal parts.
■ Polyhydramnios and oligohydramnios can be defined either by an AFI greater than 24 cm or less than 5 cm, respectively. A simpler semiquantitative method is to diagnose *polyhydramnios* when the single deepest pool measures greater than 8 cm and *oligohydramnios* when the shallowest pool measures less than 2 cm in two dimensions.
■ Deficit of amniotic fluid that occurs before the mid second trimester can result in the oligohydramnios sequence, which includes pulmonary hypoplasia, fetal deformations, and flexion contractures of the extremities.
■ With less than a 1-cm pocket of fluid, perinatal mortality increased 40-fold. The incidence of intrauterine growth restriction is also much higher.
■ In 2014, ACOG recommended using a deepest vertical pocket of 2 cm or less as the definition of oligohydramnios. This method has been shown to reduce the rate of obstetric interventions for oligohydramnios with no difference in perinatal outcomes compared with using an AFI of less than 5.[3]
■ The chance of a malformation or genetic syndrome being present with mild, moderate, or severe polyhydramnios is approximately 8%, 12%, and 30%, respectively. The chance of a fetus with polyhydramnios having aneuploidy is 10% when other anomalies are present.
■ With polyhydramnios, an increase in preterm birth is observed when the patient has diabetes (22%) or the fetus has anomalies (39%) but not when it is idiopathic.
■ At the time of the routine screening ultrasound (beyond 18 weeks), it should be determined whether the placenta covers the internal cervical os. If the placenta and the cervix are not seen clearly, or if it appears that the edge of the placenta is close to the cervix, vaginal ultrasound should be used liberally to clarify this relationship (Fig. 9.1).
■ For pregnancies greater than 16 weeks, if the placental edge ends 2 cm or more from the cervix, the placental location should be reported as normal.
■ Repeated ultrasound examinations should be performed until the placenta moves well away from the cervix or until it becomes clear that the previa will persist.

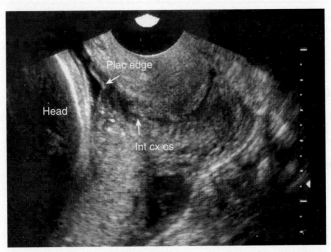

Fig. 9.1 Marginal placenta is clearly visible, and the edge of the placenta (Plac edge) extends 1.5 cm over the internal os (Int cx os). Calipers are not shown.

- The fetal mortality rate is high when vasa previa is not diagnosed before labor.
- Documentation of the cord insertion onto the placenta is good practice, and it is recommended when technically possible.
- A single umbilical artery is present in about 0.5% of all newborns. Because of the increased incidence of associated malformations, especially those that involve the kidneys and heart, this finding should prompt a detailed fetal survey.

UTERUS AND ADNEXA

- With any obstetric ultrasound, including those performed in the first trimester, the adnexal and uterine morphology should be evaluated. Multiple fibroids in the lower uterus can greatly complicate a low transverse cesarean delivery; ultrasound may help predict the need for a classical incision.
- Masses with features of malignancy—such as large size, multiple cystic cavities, thick septa, internal papillae, or solid areas—require careful evaluation and may require operative removal.

CERVIX

- The value of universal screening is unproven, and ACOG currently does not recommend this practice.[4]

ANATOMIC SURVEY

- Systematic evaluation of fetal anatomy is critical.
- All standard examinations (see Box 9.1) should include a full anatomic survey.

DOCUMENTATION

- AIUM guidelines in regard to record keeping state "Adequate documentation of the study is essential for high-quality patient care. This should include a permanent record of the sonographic images, incorporating whenever possible...measurement parameters and anatomic findings."[4]

Ultrasound for Determining Gestational Age

- It has become routine in developed countries to offer at least one ultrasound examination in the first half of pregnancy to accurately establish the gestational age.[4]

STANDARD MEASUREMENTS

- Because the fetus is often in a flexed position (Fig. 9.2), the CRL becomes less accurate after the first trimester and should not be used after it reaches 84 mm.

GESTATIONAL AGE DETERMINATION

- The measurement of the early embryo, either as the maximal embryo length or CRL, is commonly accepted as the best sonographic method for gestational age determination (see Fig. 9.2).

WHEN TO USE ULTRASOUND DATING

- In a 2014 reaffirmation of a 2009 ACOG practice bulletin,[4] it was suggested that ultrasound dates should take precedence over the menstrual dates if an ultrasound performed in the first trimester is more than 7 days different or an ultrasound exam before 20 weeks is discrepant by more than 10 days.
- Importantly, the committee opinion and the 2009 ACOG practice bulletin both note that in the third trimester aberrant growth is relatively common, so changing certain menstrual dates in favor of a late ultrasound date risks missing the presence of a significant growth disorder, and decisions about changing dates require careful consideration and close surveillance.[4]

Assessing Fetal Growth

- Because insufficient or excessive growth can be associated with significant fetal morbidity, recognition of growth abnormalities is one of the primary aims of prenatal care and is an important aspect of ultrasound examinations.

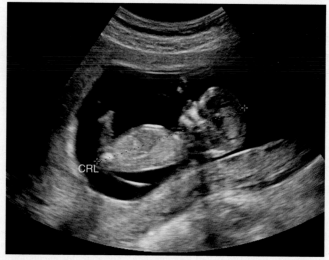

Fig. 9.2 Measurement of the crown-rump length (CRL). This is a sagittal view of the fetus with the crown of the head to the right and the rump to the left.

Estimating Fetal Weight

- All formulas incorporate the abdominal circumference because this is the standard measurement most susceptible to the variations in fetal soft tissue mass.
- It has been shown that the addition of measurements beyond the standard set does not significantly improve weight estimations. See Box 9.2 for a description of images for fetal biometry (Figs. 9.3 to 9.5).

BOX 9.2 ■ Description of Images for Fetal Biometry

Head
- Image is from side, not front or back.
- Head is oval rather than round.
- Midline structures are centered, not displaced to the side.
- Measure at the level of thalamus and cavum septum pellucidum.
- Image should not include the top of the orbits or any part of the brainstem or cerebellum.
- Measure outer edge of the proximal skull to the inner edge of the distal skull.
- Head circumference is measured at the level of the biparietal diameter, around the outer perimeter of the skull.

Abdomen
- Abdomen is nearly round, not oval or squashed.
- Obtain a true transverse image, not oblique.
- Images of ribs should be similar on both sides.
- Measure at the level where the umbilical vein joins the portal sinus.
- Calipers are all the way to the skin surface, not at the rib, liver, or spine edge.

Femur
- Femur should be perpendicular to direction of insonation.
- Ends should be sharply visible, not tapered or fuzzy.
- The measurement should exclude the distal epiphysis.

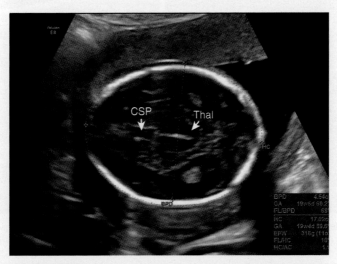

Fig. 9.3 Image of the fetal head for biparietal diameter and head circumference measurements. The cavum septum pellucidum (CSP) and the thalami (Thal) are indicated. Criteria for an appropriate image are listed in Box 9.2.

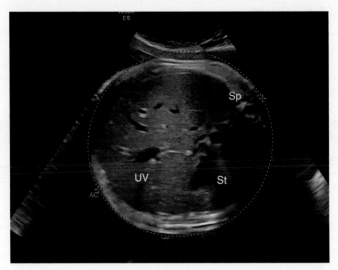

Fig. 9.4 Proper image for measurement of the abdominal circumference. Criteria for an appropriate image are listed in Box 9.2. The umbilical vein (UV) is seen at the level of the portal sinus. The stomach (St) and spine (Sp) are also labeled.

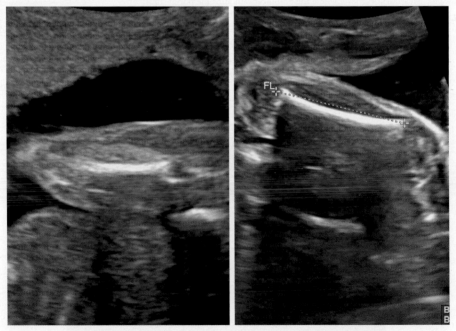

Fig. 9.5 In the left image, the entire diaphysis of the femur is not clearly shown. This will give an inappropriately short measurement. The ends should be distinct, as shown in the image on the right. FL, femur length.

Diagnosing Abnormal Growth

- If the estimated fetal weight is less than the 10th or greater than the 90th percentile, the fetus is said to be small or large for the gestational age.

Macrosomia

- The term *macrosomia* implies growth beyond a specific weight, usually 4000 or 4500 g.

Safety of Ultrasound

- Mechanical energy from the sound waves can cause the formation of microbubbles, resulting in a phenomenon called *cavitation*.

QUANTIFYING MACHINE POWER OUTPUT

- The thermal index denotes the potential for increasing the temperature of tissue being insonated with that power output.
- The AIUM propounds the "as low as reasonably achievable" principle. This means that the potential benefits and risks of each examination should be considered, and equipment controls should be adjusted to reduce as much as the possible the acoustic output from the transducer.

Ultrasound Diagnosis of Malformations

- Summarizing the results of large studies and systematic reviews, the Workshop on Fetal Imaging concluded that the range of detection rates for anomalies overall is wide, from 16% to 44% prior to 24 weeks of gestation, with a detection rate of 84% for major and lethal anomalies.[5] In the hands of a well-trained examiner, the detection rate of some anomalies should approach 100%.
- ACOG and the AIUM now recommend that attempts should be made to obtain these views in all second- and third-trimester scans.[4]

SCREENING FOR ANEUPLOIDY

First Trimester

- The most important sonographic component of first-trimester screening is the nuchal translucency measurement (Fig. 9.6). The presence or absence of a visible nasal bone is another important ultrasound finding.

Second Trimester

- "Soft markers" of Down syndrome include a thick nuchal fold, short nasal bone, cerebral ventriculomegaly, short femur or humerus, echogenic intracardiac focus, echogenic bowel, and pelviectasis.

"Entertainment" Ultrasound Examinations

- The use of ultrasound for nondiagnostic purposes has been condemned by the AIUM and the ACOG.

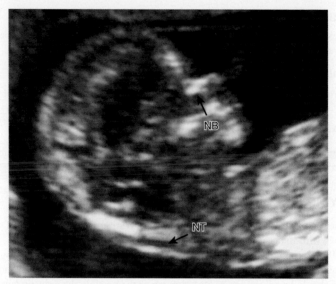

Fig. 9.6 Midsagittal view of a 12-week fetus showing the nuchal translucency (NT) and nasal bone (NB).

References for this chapter are available at ExpertConsult.com.

CHAPTER 10

Genetic Screening and Prenatal Genetic Diagnosis

Deborah A. Driscoll ■ Joe Leigh Simpson ■ Wolfgang Holzgreve ■ Lucas Otaño

KEY POINTS

- About 3% of liveborn infants have a major congenital anomaly due to a chromosome abnormality, single-gene mutation or multifactorial/polygenic inheritance, or exogenous factors (i.e., teratogens).

- Noninvasive screening tests for the common autosomal trisomies should be offered at any age, providing patient-specific aneuploidy risks. First-trimester screening using serum analytes (free hCG and pregnancy-associated plasma protein A) and an NT measurement has a detection rate of 85% to 87% with a false-positive rate of 5%. For women at high risk for trisomy 21, cfDNA analysis is available as early as 10 weeks' gestation, with a detection rate of greater than 99%; however, confirmatory invasive diagnostic testing is recommended.

- Second-trimester noninvasive screening with four analytes—hCG, AFP, uE_3, and inhibin A—has an 80% detection rate and can be performed in conjunction with first-trimester screening to yield a higher detection rate of 95%.

- Invasive prenatal diagnosis with chromosome microarrays allows comprehensive analysis of the entire genome at a finer resolution than a routine karyotype and is capable of detecting trisomies and unbalanced translocations as well as submicroscopic deletions and duplications of the genome (CNVs). It has several advantages over conventional cytogenetic testing, especially in the fetus with a structural malformation. Clinically significant CNVs were detected in 6% of the fetuses with a normal karyotype and suspected structural anomalies or growth abnormalities.

- Screening for carriers for β-thalassemia and α-thalassemia can be inexpensively performed on the basis of an MCV less than 80% followed by hemoglobin electrophoresis, once iron deficiency has been excluded.

- Cystic fibrosis (CF) is found in all ethnic groups, but the heterozygote frequency is higher in non-Hispanic whites of northern European (1 in 25) or Ashkenazi Jewish origin (1 in 24) than in other ethnic groups (black 1/61, Hispanic 1/58, Asian 1/94). More than 1500 mutations have been identified in the gene for CF, but carrier screening is obligatory only for a specified panel of 23 mutations. In northern European white and Ashkenazi Jewish individuals, the heterozygote detection rate using the specified panel is 88% and 94%, respectively. In other ethnic groups, detection rates are lower (64% in blacks, 72% in Hispanics, and 49% in Asian Americans).

- Most single-gene disorders can now be detected by molecular methods if fetal tissue is available, given that the location of the causative mutant gene is known for most disorders. Linkage analysis can be applied if the gene has been localized but not yet sequenced or if the mutation responsible for the disorder in a given family remains unknown despite sequencing.

- Amniocentesis (15 weeks or later) and CVS (10 to 13 weeks) are equivalent in safety (1 in 300 to 500 loss rate) and diagnostic accuracy. Amniocentesis before 13 weeks is not recommended because of an unacceptable risk for pregnancy loss and clubfoot (talipes equinovarus).
- Congenital malformations that involve a single organ system (e.g., spina bifida, facial clefts, cardiac defects) are considered multifactorial or polygenic. After the birth of one child with a birth defect that involves only one organ system, the recurrence risk in subsequent offspring is 1% to 5%. Many of these congenital anomalies can be diagnosed in utero using ultrasonography or fetal echocardiography.
- NTDs may be detected by either ultrasonography or MSAFP screening in the second trimester.
- PGD requires removal of one or more cells (polar body blastomere, trophectoderm) from the embryo. Diagnosis uses molecular techniques to detect single-gene disorders and either fluorescence in situ hybridization or chromosome array comparative genome hybridization to detect chromosome abnormalities (e.g., trisomy). PGD also allows for avoidance of clinical pregnancy termination, fetal (embryonic) diagnosis without disclosure of parental genotype (e.g., Huntington disease), and selection of human leukocyte antigen–compatible embryos.

Genetic History

- Obstetricians/gynecologists should attempt to take a thorough personal and family history to determine whether a woman, her partner, or a relative has a heritable disorder, birth defect, mental retardation, or psychiatric disorder that may increase their risk of having an affected offspring.
- A positive family history of a genetic disorder may warrant referral to a clinical geneticist or genetic counselor who can accurately assess the risk of having an affected offspring and review genetic screening and testing options.
- Data do not indicate that the risk of having aneuploid liveborns is increased based on paternal age.

Genetic Counseling

- Obstetricians should be able to counsel patients before performing screening tests for aneuploidy and neural tube defects (NTDs), carrier screening, and diagnostic procedures such as amniocentesis.

Chromosome Abnormalities

- The incidence of chromosome aberrations is 1 in 160 newborns. In addition, more than 50% of first-trimester spontaneous abortions and at least 5% of stillborn infants exhibit chromosome abnormalities.
- Autosomal trisomy can recur and has a recurrence risk of approximately 1% following either trisomy 18 or 21.

TRISOMY 21

- Trisomy 21, or Down syndrome, is the most frequent autosomal chromosome syndrome
- Translocations (sporadic or familial) most commonly associated with Down syndrome involve chromosomes 14 and 21.

AUTOSOMAL DELETIONS AND DUPLICATIONS

- Well-described genetic disorders have been associated with deletions or duplications of a number of chromosomes (Table 10.1). Although some of these may be diagnosed on a routine karyotype, most will only be detected by microarray analysis (MA) capable of detecting deletions and duplications smaller than 5 Mb (5 million base pairs).
- Most deletions and duplications occur sporadically because of nonallelic homologous recombination mediated by low-copy repetitive sequences of DNA during meiosis or mitosis and are not related to parental age. Hence, although the recurrence risk is low (<1%), it still may be elevated above baseline as a result of germline mosaicism.
- It is important to note that the phenotype of many deletion and duplication syndromes is highly variable, and even within the same family, this can range from mild to severe.

TABLE 10.1 ■ Common Deletion Syndromes

Chromosome Region	Syndrome	Clinical Features
4p16.3	Wolf-Hirschhorn	IUGR, failure to thrive, microcephaly, developmental delay, hypotonia, cognitive deficits, seizures, cardiac defects, GU abnormalities
5p15.2	Cri du chat	Microcephaly, SGA, hypotonia, catlike cry, cardiac defects
7q11.23	Williams	Supravalvular aortic stenosis, hypercalcemia, developmental delay, mild to moderate intellectual disability, social personality, attention-deficit disorder, female precocious puberty
15q11.2q13	Prader-Willi Angelman	*Prader-Willi:* Hypotonia, delayed development, short stature, small hands and feet, childhood obesity, learning disabilities, behavioral problems, delayed puberty *Angelman:* Developmental delay, intellectual disability, impaired speech, gait ataxia, happy personality, seizures, microcephaly
17p11.2	Smith-Magenis	Mild to moderate intellectual disability, delayed speech and language skills, behavioral problems, short stature, reduced sensitivity to pain and temperature, ear and eye abnormalities
20p12	Alagille	Bile duct paucity, peripheral pulmonary artery stenosis, cardiac defects, vertebral and GU anomalies
22q11.2	DiGeorge (velocardiofacial)	Cardiac defects, hypocalcemia, thymic hypoplasia, immune defect, renal and skeletal anomalies, delayed speech, learning difficulties, psychological and behavioral problems

GU, genitourinary; *IUGR,* intrauterine growth restriction; *SGA,* small for gestational age.

SEX CHROMOSOME ABNORMALITIES
Monosomy X (45,X)

- Monosomy X, or Turner syndrome, accounts for 10% of all first-trimester abortions; therefore it can be calculated that more than 99% of 45,X conceptuses are lost early in pregnancy.
- Common features include primary ovarian failure, absent pubertal development due to gonadal dysgenesis (streak gonads), and short stature (<150 cm).

Klinefelter Syndrome

- About 1 in 1000 males are born with Klinefelter syndrome, the result of two or more X chromosomes (47,XXY; 48,XXXY; and 49,XXXXY). Characteristic features include small testes, azoospermia, elevated follicle-stimulating hormone and luteinizing hormone levels, and decreased testosterone.

Polysomy X in Girls (47,XXX; 48,XXXX; 49,XXXX)

- About 1 in 800 liveborn girls has a 47,XXX complement.

Polysomy Y in Boys (47,XYY and 48,XXYY)

- 47,XYY boys are more likely than 46,XY boys to be tall and are at increased risk for learning disabilities, speech and language delay, and behavioral and emotional difficulties.

SCREENING FOR ANEUPLOIDY
First-Trimester Screening

- First-trimester screening can be performed between 11 and 14 weeks using a combination of biochemical markers, pregnancy-associated plasma protein A and free β–human chorionic gonadotropin (β-hCG), and ultrasound measurement of the nuchal translucency (NT), a sonolucent space present in all fetuses behind the fetal neck. The detection rate for trisomy 21 is greater than 80% with a false-positive rate of 5% compared with a 70% detection rate based on NT measurement alone.[1]
- First-trimester screening is comparable or superior to second-trimester screening alone and, most importantly, it provides parents with the option of earlier diagnostic testing in the event the screen indicates that the fetus is at high risk for aneuploidy.
- Women with an NT that exceeds 4 mm should be offered diagnostic testing without needing to undergo further analyte analysis.[2]
- A targeted ultrasound examination during the second trimester and fetal echocardiography are recommended when the NT measurement is 3.5 mm or greater and the fetal karyotype is normal.

Second-Trimester Serum Screening

- The most widely used second-trimester aneuploidy screening test is the so-called quad screen, which utilizes four biochemical analytes—alpha-fetoprotein (AFP), hCG, unconjugated estriol (uE$_3$), and dimeric inhibin A (INHA). Performed between 15 and 22 weeks' gestation, the detection rate for trisomy 21 is about 75% in women who are less than 35 years of age and over 80% in women 35 years or older, with a false-positive rate of 5%.
- Serum hCG and INHA levels are increased in women carrying fetuses with Down syndrome. Levels of AFP and uE$_3$ in maternal serum are lower in pregnancies affected with Down syndrome compared with unaffected pregnancies.

First- and Second-Trimester Screening

- Several approaches have been proposed using the combination of both first- and second-trimester screening to increase the detection rate over that achieved by screening in either trimester alone, with detection rates of 88% to 96% with false-positive rates of 5% reported.

Cell-Free DNA Analysis

- The newest screening test for aneuploidy uses maternal cell-free DNA (cfDNA).
- The American College of Obstetricians and Gynecologists (ACOG) and the American College of Medical Genetics (ACMG) recommend that women be offered aneuploidy screening, and both acknowledge that noninvasive prenatal testing is one of the screening options for women at increased risk for aneuploidy.[3,4]
- Patients need to be counseled that a negative cfDNA test does *not* ensure an unaffected pregnancy and cannot provide the diagnostic accuracy of an invasive prenatal diagnostic test, especially if fetal structural anomalies exist or with a family history of a genetic disorder.

Aneuploidy Screening in Multiple Gestation

- Down syndrome screening using multiple serum markers is less sensitive in twin pregnancies than in singleton pregnancies.

Ultrasound Screening for Aneuploidy

- There is a significant association between the thickness of the fetal nuchal skin fold and the presence of trisomy 21.
- Other markers commonly used in the genetic sonogram include the nasal bone length, short femur or humerus, echogenic intracardiac focus, echogenic bowel, and pyelectasis.
- Most of these markers perform poorly as individual predictors of Down syndrome and have a very low sensitivity and a high rate of false-positive results.[5]
- Women should be informed that the absence of markers does *not* rule out the possibility of Down syndrome or other chromosome abnormalities.

PRENATAL DIAGNOSTIC TESTING FOR CHROMOSOME ABNORMALITIES

Cytogenetic Testing

- The gold standard for prenatal cytogenetic testing has been the G-banded karyotype.
- ACOG recommends that women who desire an invasive prenatal diagnostic test be offered microarray (MA) as an option. Recent studies also support the use of MAs for the evaluation of the fetus with a structural malformation.
- Chromosome MAs allow comprehensive analysis of the entire genome at a finer resolution than a routine karyotype and are capable of detecting trisomies and submicroscopic deletions and duplications of the genome (copy number variants; CNVs).
- In addition, clinically significant CNVs were detected in 6% of fetuses with a normal karyotype and suspected structural anomalies or growth abnormalities.
- One of the major concerns with MA is the identification of variants of uncertain significance. One National Institute for Child Health and Human Development study detected variants of uncertain significance in 3.4% of cases with a normal karyotype.

Fluorescence in Situ Hybridization

- DNA sequences unique to the chromosome in question are labeled with a fluorochrome and are hybridized to a metaphase chromosome or interphase nuclei (Fig. 10.1).

Fig. 10.1 Fluorescence in situ hybridization (FISH) performed on interphase nuclei obtained from peripheral blood lymphocytes. Dual-color FISH has been performed using Vysis (Abbott Molecular) locus-specific probes for chromosome 13 (*green*) and chromosome 21 (*red*). Chromosomal DNA is stained with DAPI (*blue*). Two signals for each indicates disomy (normal numbers) for these two chromosomes. (Courtesy Helen Tempest, Florida International University, Miami.)

- Fluorescence in situ hybridization uses interphase cells and thus permits rapid or same-day diagnosis of aneuploidy.

Accuracy of Prenatal Cytogenetic Diagnosis

- Amniotic fluid analysis and chorionic villi analysis are highly accurate for the detection of numeric chromosome abnormalities.
- One vexing concern is that chromosome abnormalities detected in villi or amniotic fluid sometimes may not reflect fetal status.
- *True mosaicism* is more likely when the same abnormality is present in more than one clone or culture flask.
- Sometimes mosaicism is present in the placenta but not in the embryo; this is called *confined placental mosaicism* (CPM).
- Two potential adverse effects associated with CPM should be considered: intrauterine growth restriction (IUGR) and uniparental disomy.

Implications of De Novo Structural Abnormalities

- The risk for the fetus being abnormal has been tabulated at 6% for a de novo reciprocal inversion and 10% to 15% for a de novo translocation.
- Thus, when a de novo structural abnormality is present, an MA should be performed to determine whether a gain or loss has occurred at the breakpoint as a result of the abnormality.

Single-Gene or Mendelian Disorders

- Approximately 1% of liveborn infants are phenotypically abnormal as result of gene mutations.
- Carrier screening is performed to determine whether an individual has a mutation in one of two copies (heterozygous carrier) of the gene of interest.

TABLE 10.2 ■ **Genetic Screening in Various Ethnic Groups**

Ethnic Group	Disorder	Screening Test
All	Cystic fibrosis	DNA analysis of a selected panel of 23 CFTR mutations (alleles present in 0.1% of the general U.S. population)
Blacks	Sickle cell anemia	MCV <80%, followed by hemoglobin electrophoresis
Ashkenazi Jews	Tay-Sachs disease	Decreased serum Hexosaminidase-A or DNA analysis for selected alleles
	Canavan disease	DNA analysis for selected alleles
	Familial dysautonomia	DNA analysis for selected alleles
Cajuns	Tay-Sachs disease	DNA analysis for selected alleles
French-Canadians	Tay-Sachs disease	DNA analysis for selected alleles
Mediterranean (Italians, Greeks)	β-Thalassemia	MCV <80%, followed by hemoglobin electrophoresis if iron deficiency has been excluded
Southeast Asians (Filipino, Chinese, Vietnamese, Laotian, Cambodian) and Africans	α-Thalassemia	MCV <80%, followed by hemoglobin electrophoresis if iron deficiency has been excluded

CFTR, cystic fibrosis transmembrane conductance regulator; MCV, mean corpuscular volume.

- ACOG recommends population carrier screening for selected disorders in families amenable to prenatal diagnosis in which no previously affected individual has been born (Table 10.2).
- A cost-effective approach to carrier screening begins with testing the partner at risk (e.g., family history of the disease of interest) or the mother. However, it is also acceptable to test both concurrently. If one member of the couple has a mutation for an autosomal recessive disorder, the next step is to test the partner. When both parents are carriers for an autosomal recessive disorder, the risk of having an affected offspring is 25%.

ASHKENAZI JEWISH GENETIC DISEASES

- A number of genetic conditions are very prevalent among individuals of Ashkenazi Jewish ancestry (Table 10.3). Heterozygote or carrier detection rates for each condition are 95% to 99%.
- ACOG recommends carrier screening for Ashkenazi couples for Tay-Sachs, cystic fibrosis (CF), Canavan disease, and familial dysautonomia and also recommends that couples be made aware of the availability of carrier screening for other less prevalent and less severe diseases.[6] These disorders include mucolipidosis IV, Niemann-Pick disease type A, Fanconi anemia type C, Bloom syndrome, and Gaucher disease.

HEMOGLOBINOPATHIES

- Approximately 1 in 12 individuals with African ancestry are carriers of a single copy (heterozygous) of the mutation associated with sickle cell anemia and have sickle cell trait.

TABLE 10.3 ■ Genetic Screening for Selected Disorders in Ashkenazi Jews

Disorders	Carrier (Heterozygote) Frequency	Carrier (Heterozygote) Detection Rate (%)
Tay-Sachs	1/25	99
Canavan syndrome	1/40	97
Familial dysautonomia	1/35	99.5
Cystic fibrosis	1/25	96
Niemann-Pick disease	1/70	95
Fanconi anemia, type C	1/90	95
Bloom syndrome	1/100	95
Mucolipidosis type IV	1/125	96
Gaucher disease, type I	1/19	95

Hemoglobin electrophoresis is the recommended screening test because it can detect other abnormal forms of hemoglobin and thalassemia.

■ ACOG recommends a complete blood count (mean corpuscular volume [MCV]) and hemoglobin electrophoresis to detect thalassemia.[7] MCV values of less than 80% are indicative of either iron deficiency anemia or thalassemia heterozygosity; therefore it is necessary to test for iron deficiency. If a deficiency is not found, an elevated hemoglobin A_2 and hemoglobin F will confirm β-thalassemia. DNA-based testing is necessary to detect α-globin deletions, which cause α-thalassemia.[7]

CYSTIC FIBROSIS

■ Carrier screening for CF was initially recommended by ACOG and ACMG in 2001.[8,9] CF is more common in whites of Northern European and Ashkenazi Jewish ancestry.

■ CF may be diagnosed by the chloride sweat test or suspected on a newborn screening test, but mutation testing or DNA sequencing is used to confirm the diagnosis.

■ One mutation—ΔF508, a deletion of phenylalanine (F) at codon 508—accounts for about 75% of CF mutations in whites who are not Ashkenazi Jews. ACOG and ACMG recommend using a panethnic panel of 23 mutations as a screening test to identify CF carriers.[8]

NEWBORN SCREENING

■ The ACMG and the March of Dimes have recommended screening for a core panel of 31 conditions, including inborn errors of metabolism amenable to treatment such as phenylketonuria, galactosemia, and homocystinuria; endocrine conditions such as hypothyroidism and 21-hydroxylase deficiency; sickle cell anemia; and congenital hearing loss.

Multifactorial and Polygenic Disorders

■ It is postulated that some congenital malformations, especially those that involve a single organ system, are the result of the cumulative effects of more than one gene (polygenic) and gene-environment interactions (multifactorial).

■ After the birth of one child with a defect involving only one organ system, the recurrence risk in subsequent offspring is 1% to 5%.

SCREENING FOR NEURAL TUBE DEFECTS

- Maternal serum AFP (MSAFP) is a useful screening test for open NTDs.
- Approximately 3% to 5% of women have an elevated MSAFP depending on the threshold set and accuracy of pregnancy dating; most are false-positive results.
- MSAFP is greater than 2.5 MoM in 90% of pregnancies with anencephaly and in 80% with open spina bifida. With ultrasound alone, it is possible to achieve very high detection rates for NTDs (90% or higher in experienced centers), and this has led some centers to utilize ultrasonography as the primary screening test, acknowledging limitations that exist for the detection of small spinal defects.
- Ultrasound is recommended in twin gestations for assessment of NTDs.

Procedures for Prenatal Genetic Diagnosis

AMNIOCENTESIS

- Genetic amniocentesis is usually performed after 15 weeks' gestation. Early amniocentesis before 14 weeks' gestation, especially before 13 weeks' gestation, should be avoided because of higher rates of pregnancy loss, amniotic fluid leakage, and talipes equinovarus.
- The risk of amniocentesis is very low in experienced hands: approximately 1 in 300 to 500 procedure-related losses or less.

Amniocentesis in Twin Pregnancies

- In multiple gestations, amniocentesis can usually be performed on all fetuses. It is important to assess and record chorionicity, placental location, fetal viability, anatomy, and gender and to carefully identify each sac, should selective termination be desired at a later date. A simple and reliable technique to ensure that the same sac is not sampled twice is to inject 2 to 3 mL of indigo carmine following aspiration of amniotic fluid from the first sac, before the needle is withdrawn.

CHORIONIC VILLUS SAMPLING

- CVS is performed between 10 and 13 weeks' gestation by either a transcervical or transabdominal approach.
- CVS is a relatively safe procedure. Several studies, including randomized studies in the United States and Italy, reported that the risk for pregnancy loss is similar to that of second-trimester amniocentesis.
- The consensus of most studies is that limb reduction defects are not a major concern when CVS is performed at 10 to 13 weeks of gestation by experienced individuals.

FETAL BLOOD SAMPLING

- One of the most common indications for percutaneous umbilical blood sampling is a fetal malformation detected during the second and third trimesters. However, placental biopsy is a safer, easier, and faster alternative that has replaced fetal blood sampling in many centers.
- Collaborative data from 14 North American centers sampling 1600 patients at varying gestational ages for a variety of indications found an uncorrected fetal loss rate of 1.6%.[10]

Preimplantation Genetic Diagnosis

- At present, the preferred approach for PGD involves biopsy of the trophectoderm in the 5- to 6-day blastocyst.
- PGD is the only prenatal genetic diagnostic approach available for couples who wish to avoid an abnormal fetus yet are opposed to pregnancy termination for religious or other reasons.
- Viability is reduced by 10% when a single blastomere is removed.
- Available data indicate no increased rate of birth defects in liveborn infants who had been subjected as embryos to PGD.

References for this chapter are available at ExpertConsult.com.

CHAPTER 11

Antepartum Fetal Evaluation

Mara B. Greenberg ■ Maurice L. Druzin

KEY POINTS

- Although the PMR has fallen steadily in the United States since 1965, the number of fetal deaths has not changed substantially in the past decade.
- Perinatal events play an important role in infant mortality and long-term disability of survivors in addition to their contribution to fetal death.
- At least 20% of fetal deaths have no obvious fetal, placental, maternal, or obstetric etiology, and this percentage increases with advancing gestational age.
- The prevalence of an abnormal condition (i.e., fetal death) has great impact on the predictive value of antepartum fetal tests.
- Few of the antepartum tests commonly used in clinical practice today have been subjected to large-scale prospective and randomized evaluations that can speak to the true efficacy of testing.
- Fetal adaptation to hypoxemia is mediated by changes in heart rate and redistribution of cardiac output.
- The decrease in fetal movement with hypoxemia makes maternal assessment of fetal activity a potentially simple and widely applicable method of monitoring fetal well-being. However, prospective trials of this method for prevention of perinatal mortality have failed to conclusively show benefit.
- The CST has a low false-negative rate but a high false-positive rate and is cumbersome to perform and thus is used less frequently in common practice than other testing modalities.
- The observation that accelerations of the fetal heart rate in response to fetal activity, uterine contractions, or stimulation reflect fetal well-being is the basis for the NST.
- Use of VAS for a nonreactive NST or equivocal BPP does not increase the false-negative rate and may reduce the likelihood of unnecessary obstetric intervention.
- The NST has a low false-negative rate, although higher than that of CST, and a high false-positive rate.
- Fetal biophysical activities can be evaluated with real-time ultrasonography by BPP, and those fetal biophysical activities that are present earliest in fetal development are the last to disappear with fetal hypoxia.
- The mBPP performs comparably to the full BPP. Both modalities have a false-negative rate, or rate of fetal death within 1 week of a normal test, of 0.8 per 1000.
- Most amniotic fluid tests of fetal pulmonary maturation accurately predict pulmonary maturity, but results should be taken in context with anticipated total neonatal maturity as indicated by gestational age.
- Condition-specific testing involves modifying the frequency, type, and initiation of antenatal tests according to maternal high-risk conditions.
- Both costs and benefits should be considered when using a particular testing strategy, taking into account competing risks of fetal death and postnatal morbidity.

Defining the Problem of Perinatal Mortality

■ The National Center for Health Statistics provides two different definitions for perinatal mortality
■ Although the perinatal mortality rate (PMR) has fallen steadily in the United States since 1965, the number of fetal deaths has not changed substantially in the past decade (Fig. 11.1).

CHARACTERISTICS OF FETAL DEATH

■ Perinatal events play an important role in infant mortality.

CAUSES OF FETAL DEATH

■ In addition to declining frequency in PMR over time, the overall pattern of perinatal deaths in the United States has changed considerably during the past 40 years.
■ In summary, based on available data, about 30% of antepartum fetal deaths may be attributed to asphyxia (intrauterine growth restriction [IUGR], prolonged gestation), 30% to maternal complications (placental abruption, hypertension, preeclampsia, and diabetes mellitus), 15% to congenital malformations and chromosome abnormalities, and 5% to infection. At least 20% of fetal deaths have no obvious fetal, placental, maternal, or obstetric etiology, and this percentage increases with advancing gestational age.

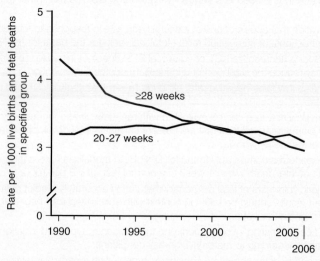

Fig. 11.1 U.S. trends in fetal mortality rates over time by period of gestation, 1990 through 2006. (Data from the Centers for Disease Control and Prevention/National Center for Health Statistics, National Vital Statistics System, August 2012.)

TIMING OF FETAL DEATH

- Antepartum fetal death is much more common than intrapartum fetal death, and unexplained fetal death occurs far more commonly than unexplained infant death.

IDENTIFYING THOSE AT RISK

- See Table 11.1.

TABLE 11.1 ■ Common Risk Factors for Fetal Death in the United States

Risk Factor	Prevalence (%)	Odds Ratio
All pregnancies	—	1.0
Low-risk pregnancies	80	0.86
Obesity:		
BMI 25-29.9	21-24	1.4-2.7
BMI >30	20-34	2.1-2.8
Nulliparity compared with second pregnancy	40	1.2-1.6
Fourth child or greater compared with second	11	2.2-2.3
Maternal age (reference: <35 y):		
35-39 y	15-18	1.8-2.2
≥40 y	2	1.8-3.3
Multiple gestation:		
Twins	2.7	1.0-2.2
Triplets or greater	0.14	2.8-3.7
Oligohydramnios	2	4.5
Assisted reproductive technologies (all)	1-3	1.2-3.0
Abnormal serum markers:		
First-trimester PAPP-A <5%	5	2.2-4.0
Two or more second-trimester markers	0.1-2	4.2-9.2
Intrahepatic cholestasis	<0.1	1.8-4.4
Renal disease	<1	2.2-30
Systemic lupus erythematosus	<1	6-20
Smoking	10-20	1.7-3.0
Alcohol use (any)	6-10	1.2-1.7
Illicit drug use	2-4	1.2-3.0
Low education and socioeconomic status	30	2.0-7.0
<4 antenatal visits*	6	2.7
Black (reference: white)	15	2.0-2.2
Hypertension	6-10	1.5-4.4
Diabetes	2-5	1.5-7.0
Large for gestational age (>97% without diabetes)	12	2.4
Fetal growth restriction (%):		
<3	3.0	4.8
3-10	7.5	2.8

Continued

TABLE 11.1 ■ Common Risk Factors for Fetal Death in the United States—cont'd

Risk Factor	Prevalence (%)	Odds Ratio
Previous growth-restricted infant	6.7	2.0-4.6
Previous preterm birth with growth restriction	2	4.0-8.0
Decreased fetal movement	4-8	4.0-12.0
Previous stillbirth	0.5	2.0-10.0
Previous cesarean section	22-25	1.0-1.5
Postterm pregnancy compared with 38-40 wk		2.0-3.0
41 wk	9	1.5
42 wk	5	2.0-3.0

Modified from Signore C, Freeman RK, Spong CY. Antenatal testing: a reevaluation. Executive Summary of a Eunice Kennedy Shriver National Institute of Child Health and Human Development Workshop. *Obstet Gynecol.* 2009;113:687-701; and Fretts RC. Stillbirth epidemiology, risk factors, and opportunities for stillbirth prevention. *Clin Obstet Gynecol.* 2010;53:588-596.
BMI, body mass index; *PAPP-A*, pregnancy associated plasma protein A.
*For stillbirths, 37 weeks' gestation.

MATERNAL CHARACTERISTICS
Maternal Age
- A J-shaped curve relationship exists between maternal age and fetal deaths, with the highest rates in teenagers and women older than 35 years.
- See Fig. 11.2.

Maternal Race
- Factors that contribute to increased rates of fetal death among black women compared with white women include disparities in socioeconomic status, access to health care, and preexisting medical conditions.

MATERNAL COMORBIDITIES
Obesity
- Prepregnancy obesity is associated with increased perinatal mortality especially in late gestation.

Diabetes Mellitus
- Although historically insulin-dependent diabetes has been a major risk factor for fetal death, the fetal death rate in women with optimal glycemic control now approaches that of women without diabetes.

Hypertensive Disorders
- Increased perinatal mortality is most often related to complicated hypertension with sequelae of placenta insufficiency and IUGR.

Thrombophilia
- No demonstrable link has been found between inherited thrombophilia and risk for fetal death. The presence of circulating maternal antiphospholipid antibodies has been associated with a variety of adverse pregnancy outcomes including fetal loss.

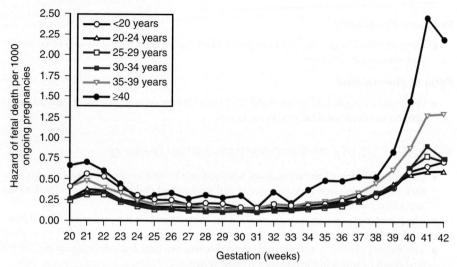

Fig. 11.2 Relationship of fetal death and maternal age across gestation. (From Reddy UM, Ko CW, Willinger M. Maternal age and the risk of stillbirth throughout pregnancy in the United States. Am J Obstet Gynecol. 2006;195:764-770.)

Intrahepatic Cholestasis

- The cause of fetal death in women with gestational cholestasis remains unknown, and timing and predictive features of impending fetal death remain unpredictable.

Renal Disease and Systemic Lupus Erythematosus

- With renal disease, fetal loss is often related to coexisting hypertension. In women with SLE, fetal loss is also related to coexisting hypertension as well as circulating autoantibodies.

Fertility History and Assisted Reproductive Technology

- An independent association between in vitro fertilization and fetal death exists.
- Nulliparity and high parity are both associated with fetal death.
- Increased perinatal mortality is related to complications unique to twins such as twin-twin transfusion syndrome as well as fetal growth restriction.

Early Pregnancy Markers

- First- and second-trimester serum markers for aneuploidy, when abnormally low or elevated, have been associated to varying degrees with adverse perinatal outcomes even in the absence of aneuploidy.

Amniotic Fluid Abnormalities

- The increased risk for fetal death is related to associations with other conditions such as diabetes and fetal growth restriction.

Fetal Growth Restriction

- Placenta malfunction is commonly implicated in nonmalformed and chromosomally normal IUGR fetuses.

Postterm Pregnancy

- The pathophysiology is related to impaired placental oxygen exchange and is often associated with oligohydramnios.

Fetal Malformations

- Pregnancies complicated by structural fetal anomalies are at increased risk of stillbirth independent of coexisting fetal growth restriction.

Potential Utility of Antepartum Fetal Testing

- Unfortunately, few of the antepartum tests commonly used in clinical practice today have been subjected to large-scale prospective and randomized evaluations that can speak to the true efficacy of testing.
- The prevalence of the abnormal condition has great impact on the predictive value of antenatal fetal tests.
- The number needed to evaluate and treat to prevent one fetal death decreases as the risk for fetal death increases in the population being tested.
- In interpreting the results of studies of antepartum testing, the obstetrician must consider the application of that test to his or her own population.

What Do These Tests Tell Us About the Fetus?

FETAL STATE

- Regarding fetal biophysical characteristics, it must be appreciated that during the third trimester, the normal fetus can exhibit marked changes in its neurologic state.
- Fetal adaptation to hypoxemia is mediated through changes in heart rate and redistribution of cardiac output.
- Fetal movement is a more indirect indicator of fetal oxygen status and central nervous system function, and decreased fetal movement is noted in response to hypoxemia.

Biophysical Techniques of Fetal Evaluation

MATERNAL ASSESSMENT OF FETAL ACTIVITY

- The decrease in fetal movement with hypoxemia makes maternal assessment of fetal activity a potentially simple and widely applicable method of monitoring fetal well-being. However, prospective trials of this method for prevention of perinatal mortality have failed to conclusively show benefit.
- About 80% of all mothers are able to comply with a program of counting fetal activity.
- See Fig. 11.3.

CONTRACTION STRESS TEST

- The *contraction stress test* (CST), also known as the *oxytocin challenge test*, was the first biophysical technique widely applied for antepartum fetal surveillance.
- An adequate CST requires uterine contractions of moderate intensity that last about 40 to 60 seconds with a frequency of 3 in 10 minutes. A positive CST demonstrates late decelerations with at least 50% of contractions. A negative CST includes no late or significant variable decelerations.

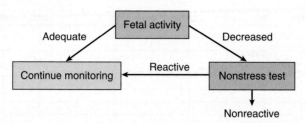

Fig. 11.3 Maternal assessment of fetal activity is a valuable screening test for fetal condition. Should the mother report decreased fetal activity, a nonstress test is performed. In this situation, most nonstress tests are reactive.

Predictive Value of the Contraction Stress Test

- A negative CST has been consistently associated with good fetal outcome.
- The CST, like most methods of antepartum fetal surveillance, cannot predict acute fetal compromise.
- The high incidence of false-positive CSTs is one of the greatest limitations of this test because such results could lead to unnecessary premature intervention.

NONSTRESS TEST

- Accelerations of the fetal heart rate in response to fetal activity, uterine contractions, or stimulation reflect fetal well-being formed the basis for the nonstress test (NST). A reactive NST is defined as a test with at least two accelerations with a peak of 15 beats/min and total duration of 15 seconds in a 20-minute window of monitoring (Fig. 11.4).

Fetal Heart Rate Patterns Observable on the Nonstress Test

- In summary, when accelerations of the baseline heart rate are seen during monitoring in the late second and early third trimesters, the NST has been associated with fetal well-being.
- Most fetuses that exhibit a nonreactive NST are not compromised but simply fail to exhibit heart rate reactivity during the 40-minute period of testing.
- In summary, vibroacoustic stimulation may be helpful in shortening the time required to perform an NST and may be especially useful in centers where large numbers of NSTs are done.

Other Nonstress Test Patterns or Findings

Sinusoidal Pattern

- This undulating pattern with virtually absent variability has been associated with fetal anemia and asphyxia as well as congenital malformations and certain narcotic medications.

Bradycardia

- If a bradycardia is observed, an ultrasound examination should be performed to assess amniotic fluid volume and to detect the presence of anomalies.

Tachycardia

- The most common etiology of fetal tachycardia is maternal-fetal fever secondary to maternal-fetal infection such as chorioamnionitis.

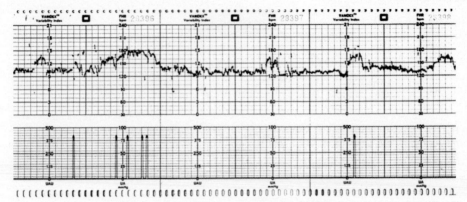

Fig. 11.4 A reactive nonstress test. Accelerations of the fetal heart greater than 15 beats/min and that last longer than 15 sec can be identified. When the patient appreciates a fetal movement, she presses an event marker on the monitor, which creates arrows on the lower portion of the tracing.

Arrhythmia
- Most arrhythmias are tachyarrhythmias (90%) representing either supraventricular tachycardia or atrial flutter. Fetal bradycardia with aventricular rate less than 100 beats/min may be due to atrioventricular block.

Deceleration
- In most cases, mild variable decelerations are not associated with poor perinatal outcome.

Predictive Value of the Nonstress Test

- The NST is most predictive when it is normal or reactive.
- In selected high-risk pregnancies, the false-negative rate associated with a weekly NST may be unacceptably high.

FETAL BIOPHYSICAL PROFILE

- See Table 11.2.
- The use of real-time ultrasonography to assess antepartum fetal condition has enabled the obstetrician to perform an in utero physical examination and evaluate dynamic functions that reflect the integrity of the fetal central nervous system.[1]
- Fetal biophysical activities that are present earliest in fetal development are the last to disappear with fetal hypoxia.
- The biophysical profile (BPP) correlates well with fetal acid-base status.

Predictive Value of the Biophysical Profile

- To summarize the results of multiple studies, the false-negative rate of a normal BPP is less than 0.1%, or less than 1 fetal death per 1000 within 1 week of a normal BPP.[2]

DOPPLER ULTRASOUND

- This method of fetal assessment has only been demonstrated to be of value in reducing perinatal mortality and unnecessary obstetric interventions in fetuses with suspected IUGR and possibly other disorders of uteroplacental blood flow.

TABLE 11.2 ■ **Management Based on Biophysical Profile**

Score	Interpretation	Management
10	Normal; low risk for chronic asphyxia	Repeat testing at weekly to twice-weekly intervals.
8	Normal; low risk for chronic asphyxia	Repeat testing at weekly to twice-weekly intervals.
6	Suspect chronic asphyxia	If ≥36-37 wk gestation or <36 wk with positive testing for fetal pulmonary maturity, consider delivery; if <36 wk and/or fetal pulmonary maturity testing is negative, repeat biophysical profile in 4-6 hr; deliver if oligohydramnios is present.
4	Suspect chronic asphyxia	If ≥36 wk gestation, deliver; if <32 wk gestation, repeat score.
0-2	Strongly suspect chronic asphyxia	Extend testing time to 120 min; if persistent score is 4 or less, deliver regardless of gestational age.

Modified from Manning FA, Harman CR, Morrison I, et al. Fetal assessment based on fetal biophysical profile scoring. *Am J Obstet Gynecol.* 1990;162:703; and Manning FA. Biophysical profile scoring. In Nijhuis J, ed: *Fetal behaviour.* New York, Oxford University Press; 1992:241.

Clinical Application of Tests of Fetal Well-Being

- Our ability to detect and prevent impending fetal death or injury depends not only on the predictive value of the tests used and the population selected for testing but also on our ability to respond to abnormal test results.
- The approach to prescribing testing modalities must take into account gestational age, medical comorbidities, and sociodemographic risk factors.
- The frequency with which to use specific tests will depend on a number of features, including the predictive value of the test and the underlying condition prompting the test.
- Initiating testing at 32 to 34 weeks of gestation has historically been prescribed for most high-risk pregnancies, with earlier testing recommended for cases with multiple comorbidities or particularly worrisome features.
- The basis for antepartum testing relies on the premise that the fetus whose oxygenation in utero is challenged will respond with a series of detectable physiologic adaptive or decompensatory signs as hypoxemia or frank metabolic academia develop.

EVIDENCE FOR CONDITION-SPECIFIC TESTING

- The authors acknowledge that no ideal single test or testing strategy exists for all high-risk pregnancies but that clinician judgment and logic, as well as evidence from observational trials, should guide testing strategies for each patient (Fig. 11.5).

🔗 *References for this chapter are available at ExpertConsult.com.*

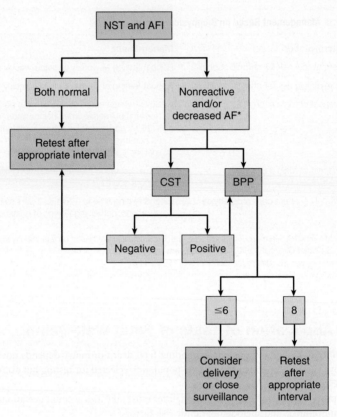

Fig. 11.5 Flow chart for antepartum fetal surveillance in which the nonstress test (NST) and amniotic fluid index (AFI) are used as the primary methods for fetal evaluation. A nonreactive NST and decreased AFI are further evaluated using either the contraction stress test (CST) or the biophysical profile (BPP). AF, amniotic fluid. *If the fetus is mature and amniotic fluid volume is reduced, delivery should be considered before further testing is undertaken. (Modified from Finberg HJ, Kurtz AB, Johnson RL, et al. The biophysical profile: a literature review and reassessment of its usefulness in the evaluation of fetal well-being. *J Ultrasound Med.* 1990;9:583.)

PART III

Intrapartum Care

CHAPTER 12

Normal Labor and Delivery

Sarah Kilpatrick ■ Etoi Garrison

KEY POINTS

- Labor is a clinical diagnosis that includes regular painful uterine contractions and progressive cervical effacement and dilation.
- Labor has three stages: the first stage is from labor onset until full dilation of the cervix, the second stage is from full cervical dilation until delivery of the baby, and the third stage begins with delivery of the baby and ends with delivery of the placenta. The first stage of labor is divided into two phases: the first is the *latent phase* and the second is the *active phase.*
- Active labor is diagnosed as the time when the slope of cervical change increases, which is more difficult to identify in nulliparas and may not occur until at least 6 cm dilation.
- The ability of the fetus to successfully negotiate the pelvis during labor and delivery is dependent on the complex interaction of three variables: uterine force, the fetus, and the maternal pelvis.
- Labor length is affected by many variables that include parity, epidural use, fetal position, fetal size, and maternal body mass index.
- Upright, rather than recumbent, positioning during labor is associated with a significantly shorter first stage of labor, less epidural use, and a reduction in the risk of cesarean delivery by 30%.
- The presence of a labor doula is associated with a significant reduction in the use of analgesia, oxytocin, and operative vaginal delivery or cesarean delivery and an increase in patient satisfaction.
- Routine midline episiotomy is associated with a significant increase in the incidence of severe perineal trauma and should be avoided.
- Active management of the third stage of labor is associated with a significant reduction in blood loss greater than1000 mL and therefore a lower risk of maternal anemia.
- Ultrasound may be a useful adjunct to the clinical examination in the peripartum period.

Overview

Labor: Definition and Physiology

- *Labor* is defined as the process by which the fetus is expelled from the uterus. More specifically, labor requires regular, effective contractions that lead to dilation and effacement of the cervix.
- The four phases of labor from quiescence to involution are outlined in Fig. 12.1.[1]

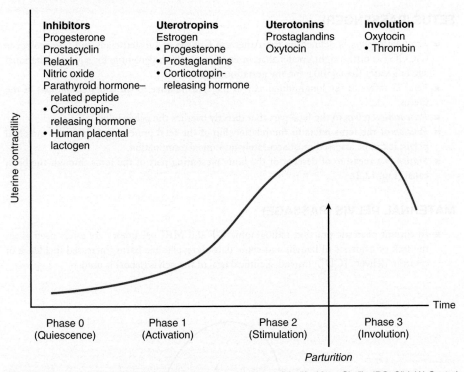

Fig. 12.1 Regulation of uterine activity during pregnancy and labor. (Modified from Challis JRG, Gibb W. Control of parturition. *Prenat Neonat Med.* 1996;1:283.)

Mechanics of Labor

■ Labor and delivery are not passive processes in which uterine contractions push a rigid object through a fixed aperture. The ability of the fetus to successfully negotiate the pelvis during labor and delivery depends on the complex interactions of three variables: uterine activity, the fetus, and the maternal pelvis. This complex relationship has been simplified in the mnemonic *powers, passenger, passage.*

UTERINE ACTIVITY (POWERS)

■ The *powers* refer to the forces generated by the uterine musculature. Uterine activity is characterized by the frequency, amplitude (intensity), and duration of contractions.
■ The most precise method for determination of uterine activity is the direct measurement of intrauterine pressure with an intrauterine pressure catheter.
■ Classically, three to five contractions in 10 minutes has been used to define adequate labor; this pattern has been observed in approximately 95% of women in spontaneous labor.
■ *Tachysystole* is defined as more than five contractions in 10 minutes averaged over 30 minutes. If tachysystole occurs, documentation should note the presence or absence of fetal heart rate decelerations. The term *hyperstimulation* should no longer be used.[2]

FETUS (PASSENGER)

- *Fetal macrosomia* is defined by the American College of Obstetricians and Gynecologists (ACOG) as birthweight greater than or equal to the 90th percentile for a given gestational age or greater than 4500 g for any gestational age.[3]
- Fetal *lie* refers to the longitudinal axis of the fetus relative to the longitudinal axis of the uterus.
- *Presentation* refers to the fetal part that directly overlies the pelvic inlet.
- *Position* of the fetus refers to the relationship of the fetal presenting part to the maternal pelvis; it can be assessed most accurately on vaginal examination.
- *Station* is a measure of descent of the bony presenting part of the fetus through the birth canal (Fig. 12.2).

MATERNAL PELVIS (PASSAGE)

- In current obstetric practice, radiographic CT and MRI pelvimetry are rarely used given the lack of evidence of benefit and some data show possible harm (increased incidence of cesarean delivery [CD]); instead, a clinical trial of the pelvis (labor) is used.

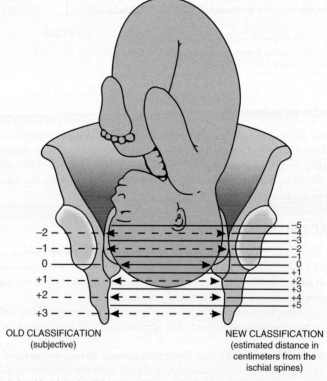

OLD CLASSIFICATION
(subjective)

NEW CLASSIFICATION
(estimated distance in
centimeters from the
ischial spines)

Fig. 12.2 The relationship of the leading edge of the presenting part of the fetus to the plane of the maternal ischial spines determines the station. Station +1/+3 (old classification), or +2/+5 (new classification), is illustrated.

- Clinical pelvimetry is currently the only method of assessing the shape and dimensions of the bony pelvis in labor.[4]
- An adequate trial of labor is the only definitive method to determine whether a fetus will be able to safely negotiate through the pelvis.

Cardinal Movements in Labor

- Although labor and birth comprise a continuous process, seven discrete cardinal movements are described: (1) engagement, (2) descent, (3) flexion, (4) internal rotation, (5) extension, (6) external rotation or restitution, and (7) expulsion (Fig. 12.3).

ENGAGEMENT

- *Engagement* refers to passage of the widest diameter of the presenting part to a level below the plane of the pelvic inlet (Fig. 12.4).
- With a cephalic presentation, engagement is achieved when the presenting part is at zero station on vaginal examination.

DESCENT

- *Descent* refers to the downward passage of the presenting part through the pelvis. Descent of the fetus is not continuous; the greatest rates of descent occur in the late active phase and during the second stage of labor.

FLEXION

- Flexion of the fetal head occurs passively as the head descends owing to the shape of the bony pelvis and the resistance offered by the soft tissues of the pelvic floor.
- The result of complete flexion is to present the smallest diameter of the fetal head (the suboccipitobregmatic diameter) for optimal passage through the pelvis.

INTERNAL ROTATION

- *Internal rotation* refers to rotation of the presenting part from its original position as it enters the pelvic inlet (usually occiput transverse) to the AP position as it passes through the pelvis.

EXTENSION

- Extension occurs once the fetus has descended to the level of the introitus.

EXTERNAL ROTATION

- External rotation, also known as *restitution*, refers to the return of the fetal head to the correct anatomic position in relation to the fetal torso.

EXPULSION

- *Expulsion* refers to delivery of the rest of the fetus.
- The anterior shoulder is delivered in much the same manner as the head, with rotation of the shoulder under the symphysis pubis.

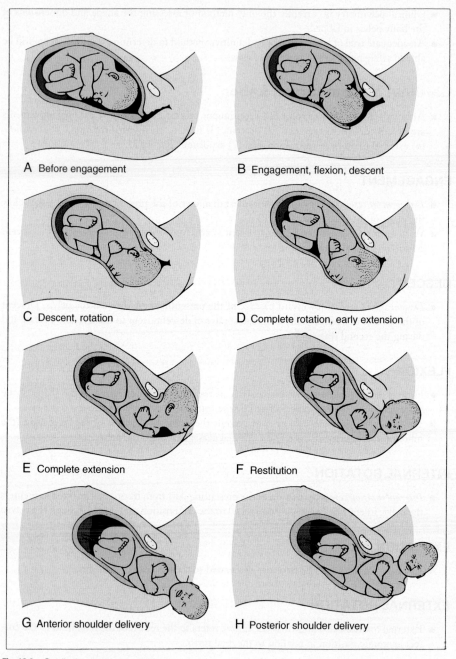

A Before engagement

B Engagement, flexion, descent

C Descent, rotation

D Complete rotation, early extension

E Complete extension

F Restitution

G Anterior shoulder delivery

H Posterior shoulder delivery

Fig. 12.3 Cardinal movements of labor.

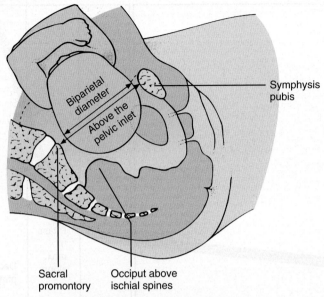

Biparietal diameter

Above the pelvic inlet

Symphysis pubis

Sacral promontory

Occiput above ischial spines

Fig. 12.4 Engagement of the fetal head.

Normal Progress of Labor

- Progress of labor is measured with multiple variables. With the onset of regular contractions, the fetus descends in the pelvis as the cervix both effaces and dilates. With each vaginal examination to judge labor progress, the clinician must assess not only cervical effacement and dilation but fetal station and position. This assessment depends on skilled digital palpation of the maternal cervix and the presenting part. As the cervix dilates in labor, it thins and shortens—or becomes more *effaced*—over time. Cervical *effacement* refers to the length of the remaining cervix and can be reported in length or as a percentage. If percentage is used, 0% effacement at term refers to at least a 2 cm long or a very thick cervix, and 100% effacement refers to no length remaining or a very thin cervix.

- Labor occurs in three stages: the *first stage* is from labor onset until full dilation of the cervix; the *second stage* is from full cervical dilation until delivery of the baby; and the *third stage* begins with delivery of the baby and ends with delivery of the placenta. The first stage of labor is divided into two phases: the first is the *latent phase,* and the second is the *active phase.*

- The *active phase* of labor is defined as the period in which the greatest rate of cervical dilation occurs.

- Recent analysis of contemporary labor from several studies challenges our understanding of the cervical dilation at which active labor occurs and suggests that the transition from the latent phase to the active phase of labor is a more gradual process.[5]

- Labor progress in nulliparous women who ultimately had a vaginal delivery is in fact slower than previously reported until 6 cm of cervical dilation.[6]

- It would be more appropriate to utilize a threshold of 6 cm cervical dilation to define active phase labor onset and that the rate of cervical dilation for nulliparas at the 95th percentile of normal may be greater than the 1 cm/h previously expected.

- A Cochrane meta-analysis of 11 randomized control trials (RCTs) did not identify a statistically significant difference in the mean length of the first stage of labor in women randomized to epidural analgesia compared with those who went without.

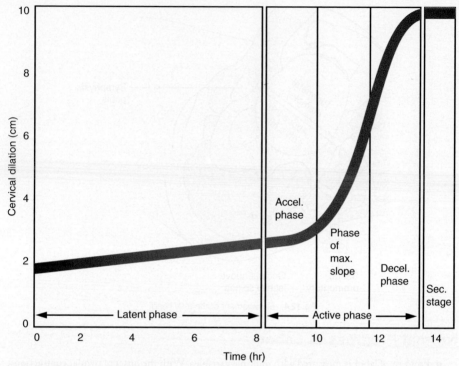

Fig. 12.5 Modern labor graph. Characteristics of the average cervical dilation curve for nulliparous labor. B, Zhang labor partogram. The 95th percentiles of cumulative duration of labor from admission among singleton term nulliparous women with spontaneous onset of labor. *Accel.,* acceleration; *Decel.,* deceleration; *Max.,* maximum; *Sec.,* seconds. (Modified from Friedman EA. *Labor: Clinical Evaluation and Management,* ed 2. Norwalk, CT: Appleton-Century-Crofts; 1978.)

- Factors significantly associated with a prolonged second stage include induced labor, chorioamnionitis, older maternal age, occiput posterior position, delayed pushing, nonblack ethnicity, epidural analgesia, and parity of five or more.[7,8]
- Epidural use significantly increases the mean duration of the second stage.
- An epidural was associated with an increase in the 95th percentile duration of the second stage in nulliparous women by 94 minutes.
- For multiparous women with a spontaneous vaginal delivery, an epidural increased the 95th percentile duration of the second stage by 102 minutes.
- In a case series of nearly 13,000 singleton vaginal deliveries at greater than 20 weeks' gestation, the median third-stage duration was 6 minutes and exceeded 30 minutes in only 3% of women.[9] However, third stages lasting greater than 30 minutes were associated with significant maternal morbidity that included an increased risk of blood loss greater than 500 mL, a decrease in postpartum hematocrit by greater than or equal to 10%, need for dilation and curettage, and a sixfold increased risk of postpartum hemorrhage.[9,10] These data suggest that if spontaneous separation does not occur, manual removal and/ or extraction of the placenta should be considered after 30 minutes to reduce the risk of maternal hemorrhage.

INTERVENTIONS THAT AFFECT NORMAL LABOR OUTCOMES

- A well-designed randomized trial[11] of over 1000 low-risk women in early labor at 3- to 5-cm cervical dilation compared ambulation with usual care and found no differences in the duration of the first stage, need for oxytocin, use of analgesia, neonatal outcomes, or route of delivery.
- Upright rather than recumbent positioning during labor was associated with a significantly shorter first stage of labor by 1 hour and 22 minutes.
- The presence of a labor doula was associated with a significant reduction in the use of analgesia, oxytocin, and operative vaginal delivery.
- Continuous labor support with a friend or family member should be encouraged.
- The available data suggest that IV fluid is beneficial in labor.

ACTIVE MANAGEMENT OF LABOR

- *Dystocia* refers to a lack of progress of labor for any reason, and it is the most common indication for CD in nulliparous women and the second most common indication for CD in multiparous women.
- Protocols for active management included (1) admission only when labor was established, evidenced by painful contractions and spontaneous rupture of membranes, 100% effacement, or passage of blood-stained mucus; (2) artificial rupture of membranes on diagnosis of labor; (3) aggressive oxytocin augmentation for labor progress of less than 1 cm/h with high-dose oxytocin (6 mIU/min initial dose, increased by 6 mIU/min every 15 minutes to a maximum of 40 mIU/min); and (4) patient education.[12]
- In a recent Cochrane review,[13] a meta-analysis of 11 trials (7753 women) concluded that early oxytocin augmentation in women with spontaneous labor was associated with a significant decrease in CD.
- Perhaps the most important factor in active management is delaying admission until active labor has been established.

SECOND STAGE OF LABOR

- Abnormal progress in fetal descent is the dystocia of the second stage.
- No specific threshold maximum second-stage duration exists beyond which all women should undergo operative vaginal delivery.[14] However, a direct correlation has been found between second-stage duration, adverse maternal outcomes (hemorrhage, infection, perineal lacerations), and the likelihood of a successful vaginal delivery.[15]
- Second-stage lengths of greater than 3 hours were associated with increased maternal and neonatal morbidity.[16]
- The benefits of vaginal delivery with second-stage prolongation must be weighed against possible small but significant increases in neonatal risk.[15] Although less frequent, adverse neonatal outcomes for multiparous women with a prolonged second-stage duration have also been reported.[15,17,18]
- Allow at least a 3- to 4-hour second-stage duration for nulliparous women and at least a 2- to 3-hour second-stage duration for multiparas, if maternal and fetal conditions permit.[14]
- A meta-analysis of 12 RCTs found that delayed pushing was associated with an increased rate of vaginal delivery. However, this benefit was not statistically significant among the quality studies reviewed.[19-23]

- Delayed pushing is not associated with fewer cesarean or operative deliveries and may have maternal risks. Additional studies are needed to determine whether delayed pushing is associated with increased neonatal risk.
- Nonrecumbent positioning in the second stage should be considered.

Spontaneous Vaginal Delivery

- When the fetal head crowns and delivery is imminent, gentle pressure should be used to maintain flexion of the fetal head and to control delivery, potentially protecting against perineal injury. Once the fetal head is delivered, external rotation (restitution) is allowed. If a shoulder dystocia is anticipated, it is appropriate to proceed directly with gentle downward traction of the fetal head before restitution occurs. During restitution, nuchal umbilical cord loops should be identified and reduced; in rare cases in which simple reduction is not possible, the cord can be doubly clamped and transected. The anterior shoulder should then be delivered by gentle downward traction in concert with maternal expulsive efforts; the posterior shoulder is delivered by upward traction. These movements should be performed with the minimal force possible to avoid perineal injury and traction injuries to the brachial plexus.
- No evidence shows that DeLee suction reduces the risk of meconium aspiration syndrome in the presence of meconium; thus this should not be performed.[24]
- The timing of cord clamping is usually dictated by convenience and is commonly performed immediately after delivery. However, an ongoing debate exists about the benefits and risks to the newborn of late cord clamping.
- In 2012, ACOG issued a committee opinion affirming the practice of delayed cord clamping for preterm infants in light of the up to 50% reduction in the risk of intraventicular hemorrhage reported for these infants when delayed cord clamping is performed.[25] However, for term infants, ACOG determined that evidence was insufficient to either confirm or refute the benefits of delayed cord clamping.
- Keeping the infant warm is particularly important, and because heat is lost quickly from the head, placing a hat on the infant is appropriate.
- Immediate or early skin-to-skin contact increases the likelihood of breastfeeding initiation at 1 to 4 months.
- There is a significant reduction in neonatal mortality, nosocomial infection and sepsis, and hypothermia as well as improvements in measures of infant growth, breastfeeding, and mother-infant attachment with kangaroo care compared with conventional methods for low-birthweight infants.[26]

Delivery of the Placenta and Fetal Membranes

- Placental separation is heralded by lengthening of the umbilical cord and a gush of blood from the vagina, signifying separation of the placenta from the uterine wall.
- Implementation of active management strategies in the third stage of labor can significantly decrease the risk of postpartum hemorrhage.
- Routine manual exploration of the uterus after delivery is unnecessary unless retained products of conception or a postpartum hemorrhage is suspected.

Episiotomy and Perineal Injury and Repair

- Following delivery of the placenta, the vagina and perineum should be carefully examined for evidence of injury.
- A *first-degree tear* is defined as a superficial tear confined to the epithelial layer; it may or may not need to be repaired depending on size, location, and amount of bleeding.

A *second-degree tear* extends into the perineal body but not into the external anal sphincter. A *third-degree tear* involves superficial or deep injury to the external anal sphincter, whereas a *fourth-degree tear* extends completely through the sphincter and the rectal mucosa. All second-, third-, and fourth-degree tears should be repaired.

- A recent Cochrane review of eight RCTs that compared restrictive to routine use of episiotomy showed a significant reduction of severe perineal tears, suturing, and healing complications in the restrictive group.[27]
- Based on the lack of consistent evidence that episiotomy is of benefit, routine episiotomy has no role in modern obstetrics.[27–31] In fact, a recent evidence-based review recommended that episiotomy should be avoided if possible, based on U.S. Preventive Task Force quality of evidence.[32]
- The relationship of episiotomy to subsequent pelvic relaxation and incontinence has been evaluated, and no studies suggest that episiotomy reduces risk of incontinence.
- No data suggest that episiotomy protects the woman from later incontinence; therefore avoidance of fourth-degree tearing should be a priority.

Ultrasound in Labor and Delivery

- Ultrasound is a useful adjunct to the clinical examination in the peripartum period.
- The association between sonographic cervical length at term and labor outcome has also been studied.
- An association has been found between cervical parameters at term and successful labor induction.[33–35]
- Fetal head position and station during labor are best determined by careful digital pelvic examination.

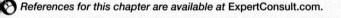 *References for this chapter are available at ExpertConsult.com.*

CHAPTER 13

Abnormal Labor and Induction of Labor

Lili Sheibani ■ Deborah A. Wing

KEY POINTS

- *Labor* is a clinical diagnosis defined as uterine contractions that result in progressive cervical effacement and dilation.
- The most common causes of protraction or arrest disorders are inadequate uterine activity and abnormal positioning of the fetal presenting part.
- Under new guidelines, neither a protracted active phase nor arrest of dilation should be diagnosed in a nullipara before 6 cm cervical dilation.
- Before a diagnosis of active-phase arrest is made, rupture of membranes should have occurred and the cervix must be dilated at least 6 cm, with either 4 hours or more of adequate contractions (e.g., more than 200 Montevideo units) or 6 hours or more of inadequate contractions and no cervical change.
- Induction of labor should be undertaken when the benefits of delivery to either mother or fetus outweigh the risks of pregnancy continuation.
- Studies have demonstrated that routine induction of labor at 41 weeks' gestation is not associated with an increased risk of cesarean delivery regardless of parity, state of the cervix, or method of induction.
- If elective induction is undertaken for nonmedical reasons, women should have pregnancies of 39 weeks' gestation or more.
- Induction of labor with IV oxytocin, intravaginal prostaglandin compounds, and expectant management (with defined time limits) are all reasonable options for women and their infants in the face of premature rupture of the membranes at term because they result in similar rates of neonatal infection and cesarean delivery.

Diagnosis

ABNORMAL LABOR AT TERM

■ The diagnosis of labor protraction and arrest should be considered based on the level of cervical dilation (Table 13.1).

DISORDERS OF THE LATENT PHASE

■ Because the duration of latent labor is highly variable, even in the setting of a prolonged latent phase, expectant management is appropriate because most women will ultimately enter the active phase.

TABLE 13.1 ■ Labor at Term (Zhang)

Cervical Dilation (cm)	Parity 0	Parity 1	Parity 2+
From 3 to 4	1.2 (6.6)		
From 4 to 5	0.9 (4.5)	0.7 (3.3)	0.7 (3.5)
From 5 to 6	0.6 (2.6)	0.4 (1.6)	0.4 (1.6)
From 6 to 7	0.5 (1.8)	0.4 (1.2)	0.3 (1.2)
From 7 to 8	0.4 (1.4)	0.3 (0.8)	0.3 (0.7)
From 8 to 9	0.4 (1.3)	0.3 (0.7)	0.2 (0.6)
From 9 to 10	0.4 (1.2)	0.2 (0.5)	0.2 (0.5)
From 4 to 10	3.7 (16.7)	2.4 (13.8)	2.2 (14.2)

Data from Zhang J, Troendle J, Mikolajczyk R, et al. The natural history of the normal first stage of labor. *Obstet Gynecol.* 2010;115(4):705.
Data presented in hours as median (95th percentile).

DISORDERS OF THE ACTIVE PHASE

- Based on Friedman's work, the active phase begins once cervical dilation progresses at a minimum rate of 1.2 cm/h for nulliparous women and 1.5 cm/h for multiparous women.
- The threshold for the active phase of labor is now cervical dilation of 6 cm.
- The diagnosis of arrest (i.e., no cervical change) in the first stage of labor should be reserved for women at or beyond 6 cm cervical dilation with membrane rupture and one of the following: 4 hours or more of adequate contractions (e.g., more than 200 Montevideo units) or 6 hours or more of inadequate contractions.[1]
- The most common cause of a protraction disorder is inadequate uterine activity.
- An intrauterine pressure catheter is frequently used when inadequate uterine activity is suspected owing to a protraction or arrest disorder. It can also be used to titrate oxytocin augmentation of labor to the desired effect, particularly when an external monitor cannot effectively record contractions.

DISORDERS OF THE SECOND STAGE

- Evidence shows that maternal morbidities—including perineal trauma, chorioamnionitis, instrumental delivery, and postpartum hemorrhage—increase with second stages that last greater than 2 hours.
- Nevertheless, a specific absolute maximum length of time spent in the second stage of labor beyond which all women should undergo operative delivery has not been identified.

DISORDERS OF THE THIRD STAGE

- The interval between delivery of the infant and delivery of the placenta and fetal membranes is usually less than 10 minutes and is complete within 15 minutes in 95% of deliveries.
- Because of the associated increased incidence of hemorrhage after 30 minutes, most practitioners diagnose retained placenta after this time interval has elapsed.
- Compared with expectant management of the third stage, active management has been associated with a reduced risk of postpartum hemorrhage.

Induction of Labor

ELECTIVE INDUCTION OF LABOR

- *Elective induction of labor* refers to the initiation of labor for convenience in an individual with a term pregnancy who is free of medical or obstetric indications.

FAILED INDUCTION

- No universal standard exists for what constitutes a failed induction.
- Membrane rupture and oxytocin administration should in most cases be a prerequisite before diagnosis of failed induction of labor. Additionally, experts have proposed waiting at least 24 hours in the setting of both oxytocin and ruptured membranes before diagnosing failed induction of labor.[2]

Techniques for Cervical Ripening and Labor Induction

OXYTOCIN

- The plasma half-life of oxytocin is estimated at 3 to 6 minutes, and steady-state concentrations are reached within 30 to 40 minutes of initiation or dose change.
- At this time, no one oxytocin protocol has demonstrated its superiority in both efficacy and safety over another.

PROSTAGLANDINS

- Local administration of prostaglandin E2 is effective in enhancing cervical effacement and dilation thus shortening the induction-to-delivery interval, and reducing oxytocin use and cesarean delivery for failure to progress.
- Administration of prostaglandin E1 for preinduction cervical ripening is considered a safe and effective off-label use by ACOG.[3]

TRANSCERVICAL BALLOON CATHETER

- Use of a transcervical balloon catheter has been shown to be as effective as prostaglandins for cervical ripening.

CHAPTER 14

Operative Vaginal Delivery

Peter E. Nielsen ■ Shad H. Deering ■ Henry L. Galan

KEY POINTS

- Rates of cesarean delivery have risen in the United States, reaching a rate of approximately 25% of all deliveries, whereas rates of forceps deliveries have declined from 17.7% in 1980 to 4% in 2000.
- Treat the vacuum extractor with the same respect as the forceps. The prerequisites for application of forceps or vacuum extractor are identical.
- When using vacuum extraction, descent of the fetal head should occur with each pull. If no descent occurs after three pulls, the operative attempt should be stopped.
- The risks of fetal injury associated with operative vaginal delivery are generally instrument specific: vacuum deliveries account for higher rates of cephalohematoma and subgaleal and retinal hemorrhages, and forceps deliveries account for a nonsignificantly higher rate of scalp and facial injuries.
- The sequential use of vacuum extraction and forceps increases the likelihood of adverse maternal and neonatal outcomes more than the sum of the relative risks of each instrument.

Operative Vaginal Delivery

CLASSIFICATION, PREREQUISITES, AND INDICATIONS

- In 1988, ACOG revised the classification[1] of forceps operations to address two significant shortcomings of the previous system: that *midforceps* was too widely defined and *outlet forceps* was too narrowly defined.
- Investigators validated the 1988 ACOG classification scheme by demonstrating that the higher station and more complex deliveries carried a greater risk of maternal and fetal injury compared with those that were more straightforward.
- The prerequisites for application of either forceps or vacuum extractor are listed in Box 14.1.
- When these prerequisites have been met, the following indications are appropriate for consideration of either forceps delivery or vacuum extraction: (1) prolonged second stage, (2) suspicion of immediate or potential fetal compromise, or (3) shortening of the second stage of labor for maternal benefit (i.e., maternal exhaustion, maternal cardiopulmonary or cerebrovascular disease).

Operative Vaginal Delivery Instruments

FORCEPS INSTRUMENTS

- Except when used at cesarean delivery, forceps are paired instruments and are broadly categorized according to their intended use as *classic forceps, rotational forceps,* and *specialized forceps* designed to assist vaginal breech deliveries.

BOX 14.1 ■ Prerequisites for Forceps or Vacuum Extractor Application

- Fetal vertex is engaged.
- Membranes have ruptured.
- Cervix is fully dilated.
- Position is precisely known.
- Assessment of maternal pelvis reveals adequacy for the estimated fetal weight.
- Adequate maternal analgesia is available.
- Bladder is drained.
- Operator is knowledgeable.
- Operator is willing to abandon the procedure if necessary.
- Informed consent has been obtained.
- Necessary support personnel and equipment are present.

- Classic forceps instruments are typically used when rotation of the vertex is not required for delivery.
- Forceps instruments used for rotation are characterized as having a cephalic curve amenable to application to the molded vertex and either only a slight pelvic curve or none at all. The absence of a pelvic curve in these instruments facilitates rotation of the vertex without moving the handles of the instrument through a wide arc, as is necessary when using one of the classic instruments to accomplish rotation.
- Forceps to assist with delivery of the aftercoming head during vaginal breech delivery (Piper forceps) have a cephalic curve, a reverse pelvic curve, long parallel shanks, and an English lock (see Fig. 14.1).

VACUUM EXTRACTION DEVICES

- A vacuum extractor is essentially a cup connected to a handle grip with tubing that connects them both to a vacuum source (Fig. 14.2). The vacuum generated through this tubing attaches the fetal scalp to the cup and allows traction on the vertex. The vacuum force can be generated either from wall suction or by a handheld device with a pumping mechanism.
- Data are limited to provide evidence-based support for the maximum duration of safe vacuum application, the maximum number of pulls required before delivery of the fetal head, and the maximum number of pop-offs or cup detachments before abandonment of the procedure. There is a general consensus, however, that descent of the fetal bony vertex should occur with each pull, and if no descent occurs after three pulls, the operative attempt should be stopped.

Risks of Operative Vaginal Delivery

- The sequential use of vacuum and forceps requires particular attention because use in this manner is associated with a maternal and neonatal risk that is greater than the sum of the individual risks of these instruments.

MATERNAL RISKS

- The focus of recent attention regarding operative vaginal delivery has been the risk of perineal trauma and subsequent pelvic floor dysfunction. The principal risks appear to be those of urinary and fecal incontinence. However, the difficulty in establishing the precise risks of this dysfunction in patients who have had an operative vaginal delivery compared with those

TYPES OF FORCEPS

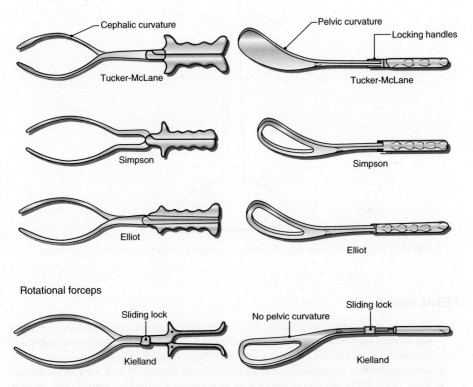

Classical forceps

Cephalic curvature

Tucker-McLane

Pelvic curvature

Locking handles

Tucker-McLane

Simpson

Simpson

Elliot

Elliot

Rotational forceps

Sliding lock

Kielland

No pelvic curvature

Sliding lock

Kielland

Forceps for delivery of aftercoming head of the breech

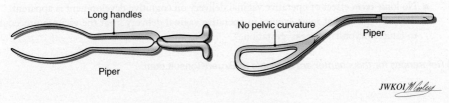

Long handles

Piper

No pelvic curvature

Piper

JWKOL/MCorley

Fig. 14.1 Classification of forceps.

who have not is confounded by many factors, including the indication for the operative delivery, number of deliveries, maternal weight, neonatal birthweight and head circumference, perineal body length, episiotomy, and the effects of maternal aging.

- The precise association between mode of vaginal delivery (spontaneous, forceps, or vacuum) and urinary incontinence remains unclear at this time.
- Overall rates of anal sphincter injury noted at the time of vaginal delivery in nulliparous patients are reported to be between 7% and 11.5%. Operative vaginal delivery has been associated with an increased risk of perineal injury, specifically third- and fourth-degree lacerations.

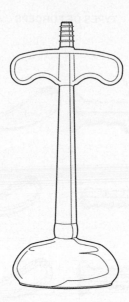

Fig. 14.2 M-style mushroom vacuum extractor cup with a centrally located stem and handle.

FETAL RISKS

- The risks of fetal injury are generally instrument specific, and vacuum deliveries account for significantly higher rates of cephalohematoma and subgaleal and retinal hemorrhages, and forceps deliveries account for a nonsignificantly higher rate of scalp and facial injuries.
- Data suggest that subgaleal hemorrhage occurs nearly exclusively with the vacuum device.
- Rates of clinically significant intracranial hemorrhage for vacuum, forceps, and cesarean delivery during labor are similar (1/860, 1/664, and 1/907, respectively) but are higher than those for cesarean delivery without labor (1/2750) and for spontaneous vaginal delivery (1/1900).[2]
- No long-term effect of operative vaginal delivery on cognitive development is apparent.
- ACOG reports that most experts in operative vaginal delivery limit the vacuum procedure to fetuses beyond 34 weeks' gestation.[3]

🔘 *References for this chapter are available at ExpertConsult.com.*

CHAPTER 15

Intrapartum Fetal Evaluation

David Arthur Miller

- The goal of intrapartum FHR monitoring is to assess the adequacy of fetal oxygenation during labor so that timely and appropriate steps can be taken when necessary to avoid fetal hypoxic injury.
- Fetal oxygenation involves the transfer of oxygen from the environment to the fetus. Oxygen is transported by maternal and fetal blood along the oxygen pathway, which includes the maternal lungs, heart, vasculature, uterus, placenta, and umbilical cord.
- The consequences of interruption of fetal oxygenation can lead sequentially to fetal hypoxemia (low oxygen content in the blood), fetal hypoxia (low oxygen content in the tissues), metabolic acidosis (accumulation of lactic acid in the tissues), metabolic acidemia (accumulation of lactic acid in the blood), and eventually injury or death.
- The FHR monitor provides reliable information regarding interruption of the oxygen pathway. The observation of an FHR deceleration that reaches its nadir in less than 30 seconds (variable deceleration) suggests compression of the umbilical cord. However, the mere fact that a deceleration reaches its nadir in less than 30 seconds does not exclude interruption of the oxygen pathway at other points, such as the lungs (hypoxemia), heart (poor cardiac output), vasculature (acute hypotension), uterus (uterine rupture, uterine contraction), or placenta (placental abruption). A late deceleration, by definition, reaches its nadir in 30 seconds or more. Historically, late decelerations have been attributed to uteroplacental insufficiency, which suggests interruption of the oxygen pathway at the level of the uterus or placenta. However, the fact that a deceleration takes 30 seconds to reach its nadir does not exclude the possibility of interruption of the oxygen pathway at other points, such as the maternal lungs (hypoxemia), heart (poor cardiac output), or vasculature (hypotension). A prolonged deceleration can result from interruption of the oxygen pathway at any point. For the purposes of practical FHR interpretation, all clinically significant FHR decelerations that have any potential impact on fetal oxygenation (variable, late, or prolonged decelerations) have the same common trigger: interruption of the oxygen pathway *at one or more points*. This unifying concept helps reduce conflict and controversy and offers the additional benefits of standardization, simplicity, factual accuracy, and ease of articulation.
- In addition to providing practical information regarding interruption of the oxygen pathway, the FHR monitor provides useful information regarding the adequacy of fetal oxygenation. Moderate FHR variability or accelerations reliably exclude fetal hypoxic injury at the time they are observed; however, the converse is not true. The absence of moderate variability and/or accelerations does not indicate the presence of hypoxic injury.
- The negative predictive value of electronic FHR monitoring is excellent. A normal test virtually precludes fetal hypoxic injury at the time it is observed.
- The positive predictive value of electronic FHR monitoring is poor. Abnormal FHR monitoring accurately predicts CP approximately one time out of 500, yielding a false-positive rate above 99%. Except in extreme cases, no FHR pattern or combination of

patterns has been demonstrated to predict hypoxic neurologic injury with a meaningful degree of accuracy.

- Even in the setting of abnormal FHR monitoring, the pathway from intrapartum hypoxic-ischemic injury to subsequent CP must progress through neonatal encephalopathy. The absence of neonatal encephalopathy is inconsistent with hypoxic-ischemic neurologic injury near the time of delivery.

- No randomized controlled trials, cohort studies, case-control studies, or other peer-reviewed studies in the literature support the hypothesis that fetal head compression caused by uterine contractions or maternal pushing efforts can cause local cerebral ischemia and hypoxic-ischemic injury in the absence of the established mechanism of global hypoxia. Similarly, no predictors of perinatal ischemic stroke are known upon which to base prevention strategies, and no known relationship exists between FHR monitoring and local cerebral hypoxic injury or stroke that can be used to identify, predict, or prevent such injuries.

- In the United States, standard FHR terminology has been proposed by the NICHD and is endorsed by virtually all major organizations that represent providers of obstetric care. Consistent use of standard terminology helps to ensure effective communication and optimize outcomes.

Direct Fetal Heart Rate and Uterine Activity Monitoring

▪ An appropriately calibrated intrauterine pressure catheter permits accurate assessment of the frequency, duration, and intensity of uterine contractions as well as the baseline uterine tone between contractions.

Indirect Fetal Heart Rate and Uterine Activity Monitoring

▪ When properly positioned on the maternal abdomen, the external tocodynamometer permits assessment of the relative frequency and duration of uterine contractions. However, it does not directly measure intrauterine pressure and therefore does not provide a reliable assessment of uterine contraction intensity or resting tone between contractions.

Physiologic Basis for Electronic Fetal Heart Rate Monitoring

TRANSFER OF OXYGEN FROM THE ENVIRONMENT TO THE FETUS

▪ Oxygen is transferred from the environment to the fetus by maternal and fetal blood along a pathway that includes the maternal lungs, heart, vasculature, uterus, placenta, and umbilical cord (Fig. 15.1).

EXTERNAL ENVIRONMENT

▪ By the time oxygen reaches fetal umbilical venous blood, the partial pressure may be as low as 30 mm Hg. After oxygen is delivered to fetal tissues, the Po_2 of deoxygenated blood in the umbilical arteries returning to the placenta is approximately 15 to 25 mm Hg.[1-3]

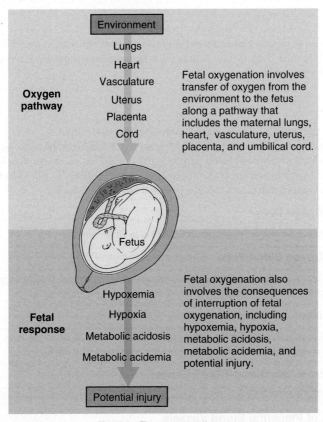

Fig. 15.1 The oxygen pathway.

MATERNAL LUNGS

■ Inspiration carries oxygenated air to the distal lung (alveoli) where the alveolar Po_2 is approximately 100 to 105 mm Hg.

MATERNAL BLOOD

■ In general, the tendency for hemoglobin to release oxygen is increased by factors that signal an increased requirement for oxygen.

MATERNAL HEART

■ In a healthy obstetric patient, the most common cause of reduced cardiac output is reduced preload resulting from hypovolemia or compression of the inferior vena cava by the gravid uterus.

MATERNAL VASCULATURE

■ Interruption of oxygen transfer from the environment to the fetus at the level of the maternal vasculature commonly results from hypotension caused by regional anesthesia, hypovolemia, impaired venous return, impaired cardiac output, or medication.

UTERUS

- Interruption of oxygen transfer from the environment to the fetus at the level of the uterus commonly results from uterine contractions that compress intramural blood vessels and impede the flow of blood.

PLACENTA

- At term, the umbilical arteries receive 40% of fetal cardiac output.
- Oxygen is transferred from the intervillous space to the fetal blood by a process that depends upon the Pao_2 of maternal blood perfusing the intervillous space, the flow of oxygenated maternal blood into and out of the intervillous space, the chorionic villous surface area, and the rate of oxygen diffusion across the placental blood-blood barrier.

Intervillous Space Pao_2

- The average intervillous space Pao_2 is in the range of 45 mm Hg.

Intervillous Space Blood Flow

- At term uterine perfusion accounts for 10% to 15% of maternal cardiac output or 700 to 800 mL/min.

Chorionic Villous Surface Area

- This area may be limited by conditions that affect placenta architecture such as infarction, thrombosis, inflammation, infection or insufficient placental growth.

Diffusion Across the Blood-Blood Barrier

- At term, the placental blood-blood barrier is very thin, and the diffusion distance is short.

Interruption of Placental Blood Vessels

- Damaged chorionic vessels can allow leakage of fetal blood into the intervillous space, leading to fetal maternal hemorrhage.

Summary of Placental Causes of Interrupted Oxygenation

FETAL BLOOD

- Although fetal Po_2 and hemoglobin saturation values are low in comparison to adult values, adequate delivery of oxygen to the fetal tissues is maintained by a number of compensatory mechanisms such as greater hemoglobin concentration in the fetus as well as affinity for oxygen.

UMBILICAL CORD

- Interruption of the transfer of oxygen from the environment to the fetus at the level of the umbilical cord can result from simple mechanical compression.

Fetal Response to Interrupted Oxygen Transfer

- When oxygen is in short supply, tissues may be forced to switch from aerobic to anaerobic metabolism, which generates energy less efficiently and results in the production of lactic acid. Accumulation of lactic acid in the tissues results in metabolic acidosis.

- It is critical to distinguish between *respiratory acidemia*, caused by accumulation of CO_2, and *metabolic acidemia*, caused by accumulation of lactic acid in excess of buffering capacity. Respiratory acidemia is relatively common and clinically benign.

MECHANISMS OF INJURY

Injury Threshold

- It has become apparent that most cases of cerebral palsy (CP) are unrelated to intrapartum events and therefore cannot be prevented by modification of intrapartum management, including fetal heart rate (FHR) monitoring.
- It is important to recognize that even when significant metabolic acidemia is present, neonatal encephalopathy and fetal neurologic injury are uncommon.
- Conditions such as epilepsy, mental retardation, and attention-deficit/hyperactivity disorder do not result from intrapartum fetal hypoxia in the absence of CP.
- A 2014 report further concluded that "unless the newborn has accumulated significant metabolic acidemia, the likelihood of subsequent neurologic and cardiovascular morbidities attributable to perinatal events is low," and "in a fetus exhibiting either moderate variability or accelerations of the FHR, damaging degrees of hypoxia-induced metabolic acidemia can reliably be excluded."

Pattern Recognition and Interpretation

- The clinical application of electronic FHR monitoring consists of three independent elements: (1) definition, (2) interpretation, and (3) management.

2008 National Institute of Child Health and Human Development Consensus Report (Table 15.1)

PHYSIOLOGY

- The 2008 NICHD consensus report concluded that moderate variability reliably predicts the absence of fetal metabolic acidemia at the time it is observed. However, the converse is not true; minimal or absent variability does *not* confirm the presence of fetal metabolic acidemia or ongoing hypoxic injury.
- The 2014 Neonatal Encephalopathy Task Force consensus report[4] identified moderate variability as one of the features of the FHR tracing that reliably excludes "damaging degrees of hypoxia-induced metabolic acidemia."
- The NICHD report concluded that accelerations reliably predict the absence of fetal metabolic acidemia. However, the converse is not true. The absence of accelerations does *not* confirm the presence of fetal metabolic acidemia or ongoing hypoxic injury.
- The 2014 Neonatal Encephalopathy Task Force concluded that the presence of FHR accelerations reliably excludes "damaging degrees of hypoxia-induced metabolic acidemia."
- Accelerations can be provoked with a variety of methods that include vibroacoustic stimulation, transabdominal halogen light stimulation, and direct fetal scalp stimulation. Accelerations provoked by external stimuli have the same clinical significance as spontaneous accelerations.
- *Early decelerations are not associated with interruption of fetal oxygenation or adverse neonatal outcome and are considered clinically benign.*
- A *late deceleration* is a reflex fetal response to transient hypoxemia during a uterine contraction.

TABLE 15.1 ■ **Standard Fetal Heart Rate Definitions**

Pattern	Definition
Baseline	Mean FHR rounded to increments of 5 beats/min in a 10-min window, excluding accelerations, decelerations, and periods of marked FHR variability (>25 beats/min). There must be at least 2 min of identifiable baseline segments (not necessarily contiguous) in any 10-min window or the baseline for that period is indeterminate. • Normal baseline FHR range 110 to 160 beats/min • *Tachycardia* is defined as an FHR baseline >160 beats/min • *Bradycardia* is defined as an FHR baseline <110 beats/min
Variability	Fluctuations in the FHR baseline are irregular in amplitude and frequency and are visually quantitated as the amplitude of the peak to the trough in beats per minute. • Absent—amplitude range undetectable • Minimal—amplitude range detectable but ≤5 beats/min • Moderate (normal)—amplitude range 6 to 25 beats/min • Marked—amplitude range >25 beats/min
Accelerations	Abrupt increase (onset to peak <30 sec) in the FHR from the most recently calculated baseline. At ≥32 weeks, an acceleration peaks ≥15 beats/min above baseline and lasts ≥15 sec but <2 min. At <32 weeks, acceleration peaks ≥10 beats/min above baseline and lasts ≥10 sec but <2 min. Prolonged acceleration lasts ≥2 min but <10 min. Acceleration ≥10 min is a baseline change.
Early	Gradual (onset to nadir ≥30 sec) decrease in FHR during a uterine contraction. Onset, nadir, and recovery of the deceleration occur at the same time as the beginning, peak, and end of the contraction, respectively.
Late	Decrease in FHR is gradual (onset to nadir ≥30 sec) during a uterine contraction. Onset, nadir, and recovery of the deceleration occur after the beginning, peak, and end of the contraction, respectively.
Variable	Decrease in the FHR is abrupt (onset to nadir <30 sec) and ≥15 beats/min below the baseline and lasting ≥15 sec but less than 2 min.
Prolonged	Deceleration is ≥15 beats/min below baseline and lasts ≥2 min or more but <10 min. Deceleration ≥10 min is a baseline change.
Sinusoidal pattern	Pattern in FHR baseline is smooth, sine wave–like, and undulating with a cycle frequency of 3 to 5/min that persists for at least 20 min.

FHR, fetal heart rate.

- If interruption of fetal oxygenation is sufficient to result in metabolic acidemia, a late deceleration may result from direct hypoxic myocardial depression during a contraction,
- *Regardless of the underlying mechanism, all late decelerations reflect interruption of oxygen transfer from the environment to the fetus at one or more points along the oxygen pathway.*
- Variable decelerations represent a fetal autonomic reflex response to transient mechanical compression or stretch of the umbilical cord.
- For the purposes of standardized FHR interpretation, a prolonged deceleration reflects interruption of oxygen transfer from the environment to the fetus at one or more points along the oxygen pathway.
- Although the pathophysiologic mechanism of a sinusoidal pattern is unknown, this pattern is classically associated with severe fetal anemia.

A STANDARDIZED "ABCD" APPROACH TO FETAL HEART RATE MANAGEMENT

Assess the Oxygen Pathway

■ Initial assessment of the maternal lungs, heart, and vasculature usually is accomplished by reviewing the vital signs, including respiratory rate, heart rate, and blood pressure. Uterine activity is assessed by palpation or by review of the information provided by a tocodynamometer or intrauterine pressure catheter. Suspected uterine rupture or placental abruption requires immediate attention and targeted evaluation. Finally, umbilical cord prolapse usually can be excluded by visualization or examination. If rapid evaluation of these steps suggests that further investigation is warranted, it should be undertaken as necessary.

Begin Corrective Measures as Indicated

■ The choice of appropriate corrective measures is based on interpretation of the FHR tracing as a whole. Selection of the most appropriate corrective measures can be refined by acknowledging some specific associations. For example, in the setting of variable decelerations, initial attention may focus on umbilical cord compression or prolapse. In the setting of late decelerations, initial attention may focus on maternal cardiac output, blood pressure, and uterine activity.

■ Conservative corrective measures may include supplemental oxygen, maternal position changes, IV fluid administration, reduction of uterine activity, and amnioinfusion.

■ During the second stage of labor maternal expulsive efforts can be associated with FHR decelerations. Open glottis rather than Valsalva-style pushing may be implemented or pushing less frequently may be helpful as a corrective measure.

Reevaluate the Fetal Heart Rate Tracing

■ The tracing should be reevaluated after corrective measures. The decision to perform routine or heightened surveillance is based on clinical judgment. If the FHR progresses to category 3, despite corrective measures, delivery is expedited as quickly as possible. Tracings that remain in category 2 warrant additional evaluation (Fig. 15.2).

Clear Obstacles to Rapid Delivery

■ This does not constitute a commitment to a particular time or method of delivery. Instead, this step serves as a forcing function to systematically address common sources of unnecessary delay so that important factors are not overlooked and decisions are made in a timely manner. This is accomplished by considering information relevant to the next action and communicating proactively with other members of the team.

Determine Decision-to-Delivery Time

■ After appropriate conservative measures have been implemented, it is reasonable to make a good-faith estimate of the time needed to accomplish delivery in the event of a sudden deterioration of the FHR. This step can be facilitated by systematically considering individual characteristics of the facility, staff, mother, fetus, and labor.

EXPECTANT MANAGEMENT VERSUS DELIVERY

■ The decision balances the likelihood of safe vaginal delivery against the potential for fetal hypoxic injury. In 2013, Clark and colleagues proposed a standardized approach to the management of persistent category 2 FHR tracings. As illustrated in Fig. 15.2, the algorithm emphasizes the reliability of moderate variability or accelerations to exclude ongoing hypoxic injury.

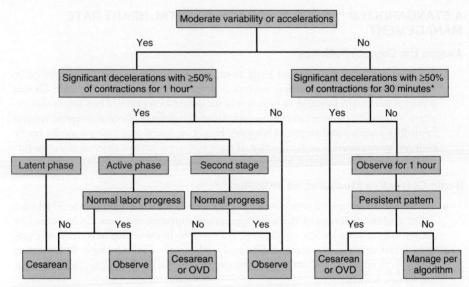

Fig. 15.2 Algorithm for management of category II fetal heart rate tracings.
*Have not resolved with appropriate conservative corrective measures, which may include supplemental oxygen, maternal position changes, intravenous fluid administration, correction of hypotension, reduction or discontinuation of uterine stimulation, administration of uterine relaxant, amnioinfusion, and/or changes in second-stage breathing and pushing techniques. OVD, operative vaginal delivery. (*Clark SL, Nageotte MP, Garite TJ, et al. Intrapartum management of category II fetal heart rate tracings: towards standardization of care. Am J Obstet Gynecol. 2013;209[2]:89-97.*)

- Recommended management of prolonged decelerations includes discontinuation of the algorithm and initiation of appropriate corrective measures. In the setting of moderate variability or accelerations and normal progress in the active phase or second stage of labor, the algorithm permits continued expectant management with close observation in most cases, regardless of the presence of decelerations. One exception is the scenario in which conservative measures fail to correct recurrent significant decelerations remote from delivery. Another is the setting in which vaginal bleeding and/or previous cesarean section introduces the risks of placental abruption or uterine rupture. In such situations, further evaluation may be necessary, and adherence to the algorithm should be individualized.

UMBILICAL CORD BLOOD GAS DETERMINATION

- **No contraindications exist to obtaining cord gases. The ACOG Committee on Obstetric Practice recommends that physicians should attempt to obtain umbilical venous and arterial blood samples in the following situations:** cesarean delivery for fetal compromise, low 5-minute Apgar, severe intrauterine growth restriction, abnormal FHR tracing, maternal thyroid disease, intrapartum fever, and multiple gestations.
- A much lower pH (7.0) has been defined as the threshold of potential injury. Acidemia is categorized as respiratory, metabolic, or mixed. Isolated *respiratory acidemia* is diagnosed when the umbilical artery pH is less than 7.20, the Pco_2 is elevated, and the base deficit is less than 12 mmol/L. This reflects interrupted exchange of blood gases, usually as a transient phenomenon related to umbilical cord compression. Isolated respiratory acidemia is not associated with fetal neurologic injury. Isolated *metabolic acidemia* is diagnosed when the

pH is less than 7.20, the Pco_2 is normal, and the base deficit is at least 12 mmol/L. Metabolic acidemia can result from recurrent or prolonged interruption of fetal oxygenation that has progressed to the stage of peripheral tissue hypoxia, anaerobic metabolism, and lactic acid production in excess of buffering capacity.

■ *Mixed acidemia* (respiratory and metabolic) is diagnosed when the pH is below 7.20, the Pco_2 is elevated, and the base deficit is 12 mmol/L or greater. The clinical significance of mixed acidemia is similar to that of isolated metabolic academia.

Benefits of Electronic Fetal Monitoring

■ Nonrandomized studies in the 1970s reported significantly lower perinatal mortality rates in *electronically* monitored women. In subsequent years, only one randomized controlled trial was able to replicate these observations. In appropriately selected patients, electronic FHR monitoring and intermittent auscultation can be expected to perform similarly with respect to maternal and perinatal morbidity and mortality.

Limitations of Electronic Fetal Monitoring

■ Electronic FHR monitoring is not a diagnostic test for hypoxic neurologic injury, but instead is a screening test that detects *transient* intrapartum interruption of fetal oxygenation, which may be a precursor to hypoxic neurologic injury.

⊗ *References for this chapter are available at* ExpertConsult.com.

CHAPTER 16

Obstetric Anesthesia

Joy L. Hawkins ▪ Brenda A. Bucklin

Personnel

■ A communication system should be in place to encourage contact between obstetric providers, anesthesiologists, and other members of the multidisciplinary team.[1]

Pain Pathways

■ During cesarean delivery anesthesia is required to the level of thoracic spinal nerve 4 (T4) to completely block peritoneal discomfort.

Effects of Pain and Stress

■ Animal studies indicate that both epinephrine and norepinephrine can decrease uterine blood flow in the absence of maternal heart rate and blood pressure changes, which contributes to occult fetal asphyxia.

Analgesia for Labor

SYSTEMIC OPIOID ANALGESIA

■ All opioids provide sedation and a sense of euphoria, but their analgesic effect in labor is limited, and their primary mechanism of action is sedation.
■ All opioids freely cross the placenta to the newborn and decrease beat-to-beat variability in the fetal heart rate.
■ An important and significant disadvantage of opioid analgesia is the prolonged effect of these agents on maternal gastric emptying.

Patient-Controlled Analgesia

■ IV patient-controlled analgesia is often used for women who have a contraindication to neuraxial analgesia (e.g., severe thrombocytopenia).
■ Fentanyl, remifentanil,[2] and meperidine are the opioids most commonly used.
■ Normeperidine is an active metabolite of meperidine and potentiates meperidine's depressant effects in the newborn.

SEDATIVES

■ Sedatives such as barbiturates, phenothiazines, and benzodiazepines do not possess analgesic qualities. All sedatives and hypnotics cross the placenta freely.
■ Two major disadvantages of benzodiazepines are that they cause undesirable maternal amnesia and may disrupt thermoregulation in newborns.

INHALED NITROUS OXIDE

■ Nitrous oxide is safe for the mother and the fetus and does not diminish uterine contractility; the main side effects are nausea and dizziness. It can also be used for short painful procedures such as perineal repair or manual removal of the placenta.[3]

PLACENTAL TRANSFER

■ Essentially, all analgesic and anesthetic agents except highly ionized muscle relaxants cross the placenta freely.

NEURAXIAL ANALGESIC AND ANESTHETIC TECHNIQUES

- Neuraxial analgesic and anesthetic techniques—spinal, epidural, or a combination—use local anesthetics to provide sensory blockade.

Lumbar Epidural Analgesia/Anesthesia

- Epidural analgesia offers the most effective form of pain relief[4] and is used by the majority of women in the United States.

Complications of Neuraxial Blocks

Hypotension

- Treatment of hypotension begins with prophylaxis.
- Hypotension is corrected by increasing the rate of IV fluid infusion and left uterine displacement. If these simple measures do not suffice, a vasopressor is indicated.
- Phenylephrine may be given to safely treat hypotension during neuraxial anesthesia for cesarean delivery and leads to higher umbilical artery pH values.

Local Anesthetic Toxicity

- Local anesthetic reactions have two components: central nervous system and cardiovascular.
- Resuscitation of patients who receive an intravascular injection of bupivacaine is extremely challenging.
- Bupivacaine and all local anesthetics should be administered by slow, incremental injection.
- IV lipid emulsion may be an effective therapy for cardiotoxic effects of lipid-soluble local anesthetics such as bupivacaine or ropivacaine.

Allergy to Local Anesthetics

- A true allergic reaction to an amide-type local anesthetic is extremely rare.

High Spinal or "Total Spinal" Anesthesia

- This complication occurs when the level of anesthesia rises dangerously high and results in paralysis of the respiratory muscles, including the diaphragm (C3-C5).
- Numbness and weakness of the fingers and hands indicates that the anesthesia has reached the cervical level (C6-C8).

Nerve Injury

- The incidence of claims for nerve injury has increased and is now the most common cause of liability in obstetric anesthesia.[5]
- When nerve damage follows neuraxial analgesia during obstetric or surgical procedures, the anesthetic technique must be suspected, although causation is rare. Other potential etiologies include incorrectly positioned stirrups, difficult forceps applications, or abnormal fetal presentations.
- The risks of epidural hematoma and epidural abscess are 1 case per 168,000 women and 1 per 145,000 respectively.

Spinal Headache

- Spinal headache usually occurs when, during the process of administering an epidural block, the dura is punctured with a large-bore needle ("wet tap").
- A spinal headache is more severe in the upright position and is relieved by the supine position. The epidural blood patch is remarkably effective and nearly complication free, despite the fact that it is an iatrogenic epidural hematoma.

Back Pain
- The incidence of back pain after childbirth is the same whether women had neuraxial analgesia for their delivery or not.

Effects on Labor and Method of Delivery
- Neuraxial techniques are the most effective and least depressant treatments for labor pain. Epidural analgesia does not increase the risks of cesarean delivery. [6]

Progress of Labor and Cesarean Delivery Rate
- Epidural analgesia is associated with a significant increase in the use of oxytocin after the initiation of epidural analgesia.
- Effective neuraxial analgesia prolongs the second stage of labor by 15 to 30 minutes.[7]
- Potential strategies for decreasing the risk of instrument-assisted delivery include reduced density of neuraxial analgesia during the second stage, delayed pushing, and avoiding arbitrary definitions of a prolonged second stage.

PARACERVICAL BLOCK
- Paracervical block should be used cautiously and should not be used in the presence of non-reassuring fetal heart rate monitoring or suspected uteroplacental insufficiency.

Anesthesia for Instrumented Vaginal Delivery or Perineal Repair
LOCAL ANESTHESIA
- In the form of perineal infiltration, local anesthesia is widely used and very safe.

PUDENDAL NERVE BLOCK
- The potential for local anesthetic toxicity is higher with pudendal block, compared with perineal infiltration, because of large vessels proximal to the injection site.

MONITORED ANESTHESIA CARE WITH SEDATION
- For urgent or unanticipated instrumented deliveries, an anesthesiologist, anesthesiologist assistant, or nurse anesthetist may administer nitrous oxide or IV analgesia while maintaining protective laryngeal and cough reflexes. The obstetrician should add local infiltration or a pudendal block.

SPINAL (SUBARACHNOID) BLOCK
- A saddle block is a spinal block in which the level of anesthesia is limited to little more than the perineum.

Anesthesia for Cesarean Delivery
- In the United States, general anesthesia is used for about 10% of cesarean births (depending on the size of the hospital), and spinal, epidural, or combined spinal-epidural anesthetics are used for approximately 90% of these deliveries.

ASPIRATION AND ASPIRATION PROPHYLAXIS

- Aspiration of partially digested food produces the most severe physiologic and histologic alterations.
- Use of a clear antacid is considered routine for all parturients prior to surgery. Additional aspiration prophylaxis using an H_2-receptor blocking agent and metoclopramide may be given to parturients with risk factors such as morbid obesity, diabetes mellitus, or a difficult airway or for those who have previously received opioids.

LEFT UTERINE DISPLACEMENT

- Aortocaval compression is detrimental to both mother and fetus.

GENERAL ANESTHESIA

- The term *balanced general anesthesia* refers to a combination of various agents.

Preoxygenation

- Preoxygenation is especially important in pregnant patients.

Induction

- Induction agents that may be used are propofol, etomidate, and ketamine.
- Pressure on the cricoid compresses the esophagus and is extremely important.

Intubation

- In approximately 1 in 533 obstetric patients, intubation is difficult, delayed, or impossible.
- When the obstetrician recognizes airway abnormalities, patients should be referred for an early preoperative evaluation by the anesthesiologist.

Failed Intubation

- Rarely, in situations of dire fetal compromise, the anesthesiologist and obstetrician may jointly decide to proceed with cesarean delivery while the anesthesiologist provides oxygenation, ventilation, and anesthesia by face mask ventilation or laryngeal mask airway, with an additional person maintaining continuous cricoid pressure.

Agents
Nitrous Oxide and Oxygen

- These agents are usually added to provide analgesia and amnesia.

Volatile Halogenated Agent

- Uterine relaxation does not result from low concentrations of these agents, and bleeding should not be increased secondary to their addition.

Extubation

- To prevent aspiration, the patient must be awake and conscious.

NEURAXIAL ANESTHESIA

- If the fetal status permits and no maternal contraindications exist, neuraxial anesthesia is preferred for cesarean delivery (Box 16.1).

BOX 16.1 ■ Advantages and Disadvantages of Neuraxial Anesthesia

Advantages

- The patient is awake and can participate in the birth of her child.
- There is little risk of drug depression or aspiration and no intubation difficulties.
- Newborns generally have good neurobehavioral scores.
- The father is more likely to be allowed in the operating room.
- Postoperative pain control using neuraxial opioids may be superior to intravenous patient-controlled anesthesia.

Disadvantages

- Patients may prefer not to be awake during major surgery.
- A block that provides inadequate anesthesia may result.
- Hypotension, perhaps the most common complication of neuraxial anesthesia, occurs during 25% to 85% of spinal or epidural anesthetics.
- Total spinal anesthesia may occur, which necessitates airway management.
- Local anesthetic toxicity may occur.
- Although extremely rare, permanent neurologic sequelae may occur.
- Several contraindications exist.

POSTOPERATIVE CARE

- The addition of nonsteroidal antiinflammatory drugs significantly improves pain scores with neuraxial morphine and reduces use of patient-controlled opioids.

References for this chapter are available at ExpertConsult.com.

CHAPTER 17

Malpresentations

Susan M. Lanni ■ Robert Gherman ■ Bernard Gonik

KEY POINTS

- *Fetal lie* refers to the orientation of the fetal spine relative to that of the mother. Normal fetal lie is longitudinal and by itself does not connote whether the presentation is cephalic or breech.
- Fetal malpresentation requires timely diagnostic exclusion of major fetal or uterine malformations and/or abnormal placentation.
- A closely monitored labor and vaginal delivery is a safe possibility with face or brow malpresentations. However, cesarean delivery is the only acceptable alternative if normal progress toward spontaneous vaginal delivery is not observed.
- External cephalic version of the infant in breech presentation near term is a safe and often successful management option. Use of tocolytics and epidural anesthesia may improve success.
- Appropriate training and experience is a prerequisite to the safe vaginal delivery of selected infants in breech presentation.
- In experienced hands, women with twins presenting vertex/nonvertex can undergo a trial of labor because this management has maternal and perinatal outcomes similar to a planned cesarean delivery.
- A simple compound presentation may be permitted a trial of labor as long as labor progresses normally with reassuring fetal status. However, compression or reduction of the fetal part may result in injury.

Overview

- The word *malpresentation* suggests the possibility of adverse consequences, and malpresentation is often associated with increased risk to both the mother and the fetus.
- In contemporary practice, cesarean delivery has become the recommended mode of delivery in the malpresenting fetus.

Clinical Circumstances Associated With Malpresentation

- Generally, factors associated with malpresentation include (1) diminished vertical polarity of the uterine cavity, (2) increased or decreased fetal mobility, (3) obstructed pelvic inlet, (4) fetal malformation, and (5) prematurity.

Abnormal Axial Lie

- The fetal *lie* indicates the orientation of the fetal spine relative to the spine of the mother. The normal fetal lie is longitudinal and by itself does not indicate whether the presentation is cephalic or breech.

- Great parity, prematurity, contraction or deformity of the maternal pelvis, and abnormal placentation are the most commonly reported clinical factors associated with abnormal lie.
- The sensitivity of Leopold maneuvers for the detection of malpresentation is only 28%, and the positive predictive value was only 24% compared with immediate ultrasound verification.
- The ready availability of ultrasound in most clinical settings is of benefit, and its use can obviate the vagaries of the abdominal palpation techniques. In all situations, early diagnosis of malpresentation is of benefit.
- Cord prolapse occurs 20 times as often with abnormal lie as it does with a cephalic presentation.

Management of a Singleton Gestation

- External cephalic version (ECV) is recommended at 36 to 37 weeks to help diminish the risk of adverse outcome.
- ECV has been found to be safe and relatively efficacious.[1]
- A low transverse (Kerr) uterine incision has many surgical advantages and is generally the preferred approach for cesarean delivery for an abnormal lie (see Chapter 19).
- In the uncommon case of a transverse or oblique lie with a poorly developed lower uterine segment, when a transverse incision is deemed unfeasible or inadequate, a vertical incision (low vertical or classical) may be a reasonable alternative.

Face Presentation

- A face presentation is characterized by a longitudinal lie and full extension of the fetal neck and head with the occiput against the upper back (Fig. 17.1). The fetal chin (mentum) is chosen as the point of designation during vaginal examination.

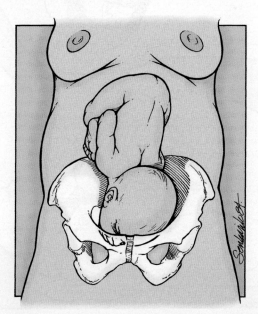

Fig. 17.1 This fetus with the vertex completely extended on the neck enters the maternal pelvis in a face presentation. The cephalic prominence would be palpable on the same side of the maternal abdomen as the fetal spine.

- All clinical factors known to increase the general rate of malpresentation have been implicated in face presentation; many infants with a face presentation have malformations.
- Face presentation is more often discovered by vaginal examination.

MECHANISM OF LABOR

- The labor of a face presentation must include engagement, descent, internal rotation generally to a mentum anterior position, and delivery by flexion as the chin passes under the symphysis (Fig. 17.2).
- The prognosis for labor with a face presentation depends on the orientation of the fetal chin.
- Persistence of the mentum posterior position with an infant of normal size, however, makes safe vaginal delivery less likely. Overall, 70% to 80% of infants with a face presenting can be delivered vaginally, either spontaneously or by low forceps in the hands of a skilled operator, whereas 12% to 30% require cesarean delivery.

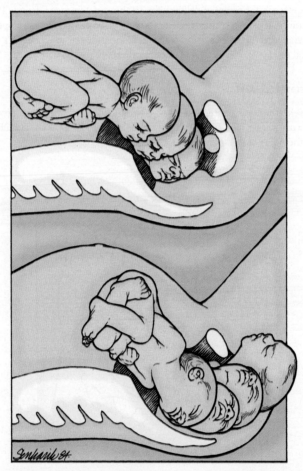

Fig. 17.2 Engagement, descent, and internal rotation remain cardinal elements of vaginal delivery in the case of a face presentation, but successful vaginal delivery of a term-size fetus presenting a face generally requires delivery by flexion under the symphysis from a mentum anterior position, as illustrated here.

- Prolonged labor is a common feature of face presentation and has been associated with an increased number of intrapartum deaths.
- There is a tenfold increase in fetal compromise with face presentation.
- If external Doppler heart rate monitoring is inadequate and an internal electrode is recommended, placement of the electrode on the fetal chin is often preferred.
- Fetal laryngeal and tracheal edema that results from the pressure of the birth process might require immediate nasotracheal intubation.

Brow Presentation

- A fetus in a brow presentation occupies a longitudinal axis with a partially deflexed cephalic attitude midway between full flexion and full extension (Fig. 17.3). The frontal bones are the point of designation.
- Fewer than 50% of brow presentations are detected before the second stage of labor, and most of the remainder are undiagnosed until delivery.
- Most brow presentations convert spontaneously by flexion or further extension to either a vertex or a face presentation and are then managed accordingly.

Compound Presentation

- Whenever an extremity, most commonly an upper extremity, is found prolapsed beside the main presenting fetal part, the situation is referred to as a *compound presentation* (Fig. 17.4). The combination of an upper extremity and the vertex is the most common.
- When intervention is necessary, cesarean delivery appears to be the only safe choice.
- Cord prolapse occurs in 11% to 20% of cases, and it is the most frequent complication of this malpresentation.
- The prolapsed extremity should not be manipulated. However, it may spontaneously retract as the major presenting part descends.
- Cesarean delivery is the only appropriate clinical intervention for cord prolapse and nonreassuring fetal heart rate (FHR) patterns because both version extraction and repositioning the prolapsed extremity are associated with adverse outcome and should be avoided.

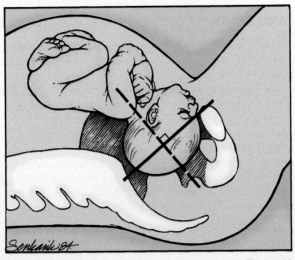

Fig. 17.3 This fetus is in a brow presentation in a frontum anterior position. The head is in an intermediate deflexion attitude.

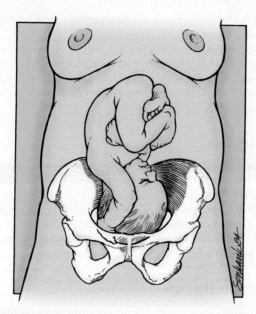

Fig. 17.4 The compound presentation of an upper extremity and the vertex illustrated here most often spontaneously resolves with further labor and descent.

■ Persistent compound presentation with parts other than the vertex and hand in combination in a term-sized infant has a poor prognosis for safe vaginal delivery, and cesarean delivery is usually necessary.

Breech Presentation

■ Prematurity, fetal malformation, müllerian anomalies, and polar placentation are commonly observed causative factors.

MECHANISM AND CONDUCT OF LABOR AND VAGINAL DELIVERY

■ The two most important elements for the safe conduct of vaginal breech delivery are continuous electronic FHR monitoring and noninterference until spontaneous delivery of the breech to the umbilicus has occurred.
■ Engagement has occurred when the bitrochanteric diameter of the fetus has progressed beyond the plane of the pelvic inlet, although by vaginal examination, the presenting part may be palpated only at a station of –2 to –4 (out of 5).
■ The point of designation in a breech labor is the fetal sacrum.
■ Premature or aggressive intervention may adversely affect the delivery in at least two ways. First, complete cervical dilation must be sustained for sufficient duration to retard retraction of the cervix and entrapment of the aftercoming fetal head. Rushing the delivery of the trunk may result in cervical retraction. Second, the safe descent and delivery of the breech infant must be the result of uterine and maternal expulsive forces only in order to maintain neck flexion. Any traction by the provider in an effort to speed delivery would encourage deflexion of the neck and result in the presentation of the larger occipitofrontal fetal cranial profile to the pelvic inlet (Fig. 17.5). Such an event could be catastrophic. Rushed delivery

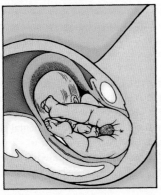 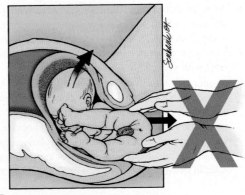

A Spontaneous expulsion   B Undesired deflexion

Fig. 17.5 The fetus emerges spontaneously **(A)**, whereas uterine contractions maintain cephalic flexion. Premature aggressive traction **(B)** encourages deflexion of the fetal vertex and increases the risk of head entrapment or nuchal arm entrapment.

also increases the risk of a nuchal arm, with one or both arms trapped behind the head above the pelvic inlet.

- Primary cesarean delivery is often advocated for nonfrank breech presentations.

CONTEMPORARY MANAGEMENT OF THE TERM BREECH

- The practical reality today is that intentional vaginal breech delivery is rare.

FURTHER DISCUSSION OF DELIVERY FOR THE TERM FRANK OR COMPLETE BREECH

- Breech outcomes relate to degree of prematurity, maternal pregnancy complications, and fetal malformations as well as to birth trauma or asphyxia.
- Breech-presenting fetuses are at increased risk for neurologic adversity, even when controlled for birth order, prematurity, smallness for gestational age, assisted reproduction, sex, and route of delivery.
- In no case should a woman with an infant presenting as a breech be allowed to labor unless (1) anesthesia coverage is immediately available, (2) cesarean delivery can be undertaken promptly, (3) continuous FHR monitoring is used, and (4) the delivery is attended by a pediatrician and two obstetricians, of whom at least one is experienced with vaginal breech birth.

Term Breech Trial

- One of the most influential publications was the multicenter prospective study known as the Term Breech Trial.
- For countries with both low and high perinatal mortality rates (PMRs), the occurrence of perinatal mortality or serious neonatal morbidity (defined within the report) was significantly lower in the planned cesarean delivery group than in the planned vaginal delivery group (relative risk, 0.33; 95% confidence interval [CI], 0.19 to 0.56; $P < .0001$). In countries with an already low PMR, a proportionately greater risk reduction in PMR was found in the planned cesarean delivery. No differences existed in maternal mortality or serious maternal morbidity between the groups.[2]

- Mode of delivery and birthweight were both significantly associated with adverse fetal outcome without a significant degree of interaction of these variables. Essentially, smaller infants (less than 2800 g) were at greatest risk (odds ratio, 2.13; 95% CI, 1.2 to 3.8; P = .01).
- A prelabor cesarean delivery is associated with the lowest rates of adverse outcome compared with vaginal breech delivery.[3]
- To summarize the Term Breech Trial, if a trial of labor is attempted and is successful, infants born by planned vaginal delivery have a small but significant risk of dying or sustaining a debilitating insult in the short term compared with a planned cesarean delivery. If they survive, no difference is seen in the mortality rate or in the presence of developmental delay when compared with children born by planned cesarean delivery.
- Currently, 17% of cesarean deliveries are performed for breech.[4] In the United States, the cesarean delivery rate for breech presentation increased from 11.6% to 85% as of 2003.[5-7]

SPECIAL CLINICAL CIRCUMSTANCES AND RISKS: PRETERM BREECH, HYPEREXTENDED HEAD, AND FOOTLING BREECH

- The premature breech, the breech with a hyperextended head, and the footling breech are categories that have high rates of fetal morbidity or mortality. Complications associated with incomplete dilation and cephalic entrapment may be more frequent. For these three breech situations, in general, cesarean delivery appears to optimize fetal outcome and is therefore recommended.
- Hyperextension of the fetal head during vaginal breech delivery has been consistently associated with a high (21%) risk of spinal cord injury.
- The footling breech carries a prohibitively high (16% to 19%) risk of cord prolapse during labor.

BREECH SECOND TWIN

- Approximately one-third of all twin gestations present as cephalic/breech—that is, first twin is a cephalic presentation and the second is a breech (see also Chapter 32). The management alternatives in the case of the cephalic/breech twin pregnancy in labor include cesarean delivery, vaginal delivery of the first twin, and either attempted ECV or internal podalic version (IPV) and breech extraction of the second twin.
- The Twin Birth Study,[8] a multicenter randomized trial, showed that cesarean delivery of twins demonstrated neither a decrease nor an increase in the rate of fetal or neonatal death or morbidity compared with vaginal delivery. The authors of this study advocate that patients seek out providers who are skilled in the vaginal birth of the second twin.
- If internal podalic version/extraction of the second twin is to be performed, it can be facilitated by ultrasonic guidance.
- A uterine relaxing agent may be used, with nitroglycerin 50 to 200 μg intravenously being one of the fastest acting, safest agents in appropriately selected patients.

EXTERNAL CEPHALIC VERSION

- ECV is recommended for the breech fetus at 36 to 37 weeks' gestation.[1,9]
- Reported success with ECV varies from 60% to 75%, and a similar percentage of these remain vertex at the time of labor.[1]
- Outcomes of pregnancies after ECV prove that it is a safe and effective intervention.[1]
- Gentle, constant pressure applied in a relaxed patient with frequent FHR assessments are elements of success stressed by all investigators.[9]

- Terbutaline before ECV is recommended.
- Regional anesthesia *in combination with tocolysis* demonstrated more successful ECVs than the tocolytic drug alone (relative risk, 0.67; 95% CI, 0.51 to 0.89), but no difference was noted in either the rate of cesarean delivery or cephalic presentation in labor, and no difference in the occurrence of fetal bradycardia was observed. Data were insufficient to determine the efficacy of vibroacoustic stimulation, amnioinfusion, opioids, nitric oxide donors, or calcium channel blockers for improving ECV success rate.[10]
- Rh-negative unsensitized women should receive RhD immune globulin.

Shoulder Dystocia

- Shoulder dystocia occurs when the fetal shoulders are obstructed at the level of the pelvic inlet. Shoulder dystocia results from a size discrepancy between the fetal shoulders and the pelvic inlet, which may be absolute or relative, because of malposition.
- The percentage of deliveries complicated by shoulder dystocia for unassisted births not complicated by diabetes was 5.2% for infants weighing 4000 to 4250 g, 9.1% for those between 4250 and 4500 g, 14.3% for those 4500 and 4750 g, and 21.1% for those 4750 to 5000 g.[11] It must be remembered that approximately 50% to 60% of shoulder dystocias occur in infants who weigh less than 4000 g. Moreover, even if the birthweight of the infant is over 4000 g, shoulder dystocia will complicate only 3.3% of the deliveries.[12]
- Recurrence risks for shoulder dystocia have been reported to range from approximately 10% to 25%.[13]
- The American College of Obstetricians and Gynecologists recommends that planned cesarean delivery *may be considered* with estimated fetal weights that exceed 5000 g in women without diabetes and 4500 g in women with diabetes.[14]
- Unilateral brachial plexus palsies are the most common neurologic injury sustained by the neonate.
- Approximately one-third of brachial plexus palsies will be associated with a concomitant bone fracture, most commonly of the clavicle (94%).[15]
- In addition to research within the obstetric community, the pediatric, orthopedic, and neurologic literature now stresses that the existence of brachial plexus paralysis does not constitute a priori proof that exogenous forces were the cause of the injury.[16]
- Clinical diagnosis of shoulder dystocia results from failure of delivery of the fetal shoulder(s) after an initial traction attempt.
- When shoulder dystocia is clinically diagnosed, the first order of business should be to stop all endogenous and exogenous forces until an attempt is made to alleviate the obstruction.
- Whenever extraction (exogenous) forces are applied by the delivering clinician, the fetal head should be maintained in an axial position, and rotation of the head should be avoided.
- The McRoberts maneuver is a simple, logical, and effective measure and is typically considered as the first-line treatment for shoulder dystocia.
- It is reasonable to consider performing delivery of the posterior shoulder/arm as the next maneuver in this sequence (Fig. 17.6).
- Posterior arm delivery required the least exogenous force to effect delivery and resulted in the lowest brachial plexus stretch.
- Delivery of the posterior shoulder was the most successful maneuver (84.4%) to alleviate shoulder dystocia, and the Woods maneuver (72%), Rubin maneuver (66%), and suprapubic pressure (62.2%) also showed high rates of delivery.
- Rotational maneuvers routinely performed include the Rubin or Woods corkscrew maneuvers.

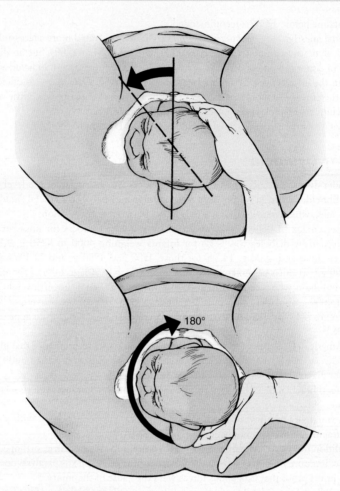

Alternative method

Fig. 17.6 Rotation of the anterior shoulder forward through a small arc or of the posterior shoulder forward through a larger one will often lead to descent and delivery of the shoulders. Forward rotation is preferred, because it tends to compress and diminish the size of the shoulder girdle, whereas backward rotation would open the shoulder girdle and increase its size.

- The need for cutting a generous episiotomy must be based on clinical circumstances, such as a narrow vaginal fourchette in a nulliparous patient. Episiotomy can allow for greater access to the vagina for the performance of the internal manipulations necessary for the rotational maneuvers or for delivery of the posterior shoulder.[17]
- Contemporaneous documentation of the management of shoulder dystocia is recommended to record significant facts, findings, and observations about the shoulder dystocia event and its sequelae. Although no standard has been defined as to what exactly should be documented, a useful guideline is the ACOG Patient Safety Checklist.[18]

⊗ *References for this chapter are available at ExpertConsult.com.*

Bibliography

Face Presentation

Browne ADH, Carney D. Management of malpresentations in obstetrics. *BMJ*. 1964;5393:1295.

Duff P. Diagnosis and management of face presentation. *Obstet Gynecol*. 1981;57:105.

Mechanism of Labor

Lansford A, Arias D, Smith BE. Respiratory obstruction associated with face presentation. *Am J Dis Child*. 1968;116:318.

Salzmann B, Soled M, Gilmour T. Face presentation. *Obstet Gynecol*. 1960;16:106.

Brow Presentation

Levy DL. Persistent brow presentation—a new approach to management. *South Med J*. 1976;69:191.

Mechanism and Conduct of Labor and Vaginal Delivery

Brown L, Karrison T, Cibils L. Mode of delivery and perinatal results in breech presentation. *Am J Obstet Gynecol*. 1994;171:28.

Contemporary Management of the Term Breech

NIH consensus development statement on cesarean childbirth. *Obstet Gynecol*. 1981;57:537.

Further Discussion of Delivery for the Term Frank or Complete Breech

Badr I, Thomas SM, Cotterill AD, et al. X-ray pelvimetry—which is the best technique? *Clin Radiol*. 1997;52:136.

Mansani FE, Cerutti M. The risk in breech delivery. *Contrib Gynecol Obstet*. 1977;3:86.

Mark 3rd C, Roberts PH. Breech scoring index. *Am J Obstet Gynecol*. 1968;101:572.

Seitchik J. Discussion of "breech delivery—evaluation of the method of delivery on perinatal results and maternal morbidity" by Bowes et al. *Am J Obstet Gynecol*. 1979;135:970.

Thomas SM, Bees NR, Adam EJ. Trends in the use of pelvimetry techniques. *Clin Radiol*. 1998;53:293.

Wolter DF. Patterns of management with breech presentation. *Am J Obstet Gynecol*. 1976;125:733.

Zatuchni GI, Andros GJ. Prognostic index for vaginal delivery in breech presentation at term. *Am J Obstet Gynecol*. 1967;98:854.

The Term Breech Trial

Anderson G, Strong C. The premature breech: caesarean section or trial of labour? *J Med Ethics*. 1988;14:18.

Ballas S, Toaff R, Jaffa AJ. Deflexion of the fetal head in breech presentation. *Obstet Gynecol*. 1978;52:653.

Blickstein I, Schwartz-Shoham Z, Lancet M. Vaginal delivery of the second twin in breech presentation. *Obstet Gynecol*. 1987;69:774.

Cox C, Kendall AC, Hommers M. Changed prognosis of breech-presenting low birthweight infants. *Br J Obstet Gynaecol*. 1982;89:881.

Cruikshank DP. Premature breech [letter to the editor]. *Am J Obstet Gynecol*. 1978;130:500.

Graves WK. Breech delivery in twenty years of practice. *Am J Obstet Gynecol*. 1980;137:229.

Martin JA, Brady EH, Sutton PD, et al. Births: final data for 2007. *National Center for Health Statistics*. 2010;58:24.

Martin JA, Hamilton BE, Sutton PD, et al. *National Vital Statistics Reports*. vol. 52. No 10. Centers for Disease Control and Prevention, National Center for Health Statistics, National Vital Statistics System; 2003.

Niswander KR. Discussion of "The randomized management of term frank breech presentation—vaginal delivery versus cesarean section" by Collea et al. *Am J Obstet Gynecol*. 1978;131:193.

Rabinovici J, Reichman B, Serr DM, et al. Internal podalic version with unruptured membranes for the second twin in transverse lie. *Obstet Gynecol*. 1988;71:428.

Tejani N, Verma U, Shiffman R, et al. Effect of route of delivery on periventricular/intraventricular hemorrhage in the low birthweight fetus with a breech presentation. *J Reprod Med*. 1987;32:911.

Vas J, Aranda JM, Nishishiny B. Correction of nonvertex presentation with moxibustion: a systematic review and meta-analysis. *Am J Obstet Gynecol*. 2009;201:241.

Ventura SJ, Martin JA, Curtin SC, et al. *National Vital Statistics Reports*. vol. 48. No 3. Centers for Disease Control and Prevention, National Center for Health Statistics, National Vital Statistics System; 2000.

Weissman A, Blazer S, Zimmer EZ, et al. Low birthweight breech infant: short-term and long-term outcome by method of delivery. *Am J Perinatol*. 1988;5:289.

Shoulder Dystocia

Acker DB, Gregory KD, Sachs BP, et al. Risk factors for Erb-Duchenne palsy. *Obstet Gynecol.* 1988;71:389.

ACOG practice bulletin clinical management guidelines for obstetrician-gynecologists. *Obstet Gynecol.* 2002;100:1045.

Chauhan SP, Grobman WA, Gherman RA, et al. Suspicion and treatment of the macrosomic fetus: a review. *Am J Obstet Gynecol.* 2005;193:332.

Gherman RB. Shoulder dystocia: prevention and management. *Obstet Gynecol Clin North Am.* 2005;32:297.

Gonik B, Walker A, Grimm M. Mathematical modeling of forces associated with shoulder dystocia: the use of a mathematic dynamic model. *Am J Obstet Gynecol.* 2000;182:689.

Lewis DF, Edwards MS, Asrat T, et al. Can shoulder dystocia be predicted? *J Reprod Med.* 1998;43:654.

Modanlou HD, Dorchester WL, Thorosian A, et al. Macrosomia—maternal, fetal, and neonatal implications. *Obstet Gynecol.* 1980;55:420.

Parks DG, Ziel HK. Macrosomia—a proposed indication for primary cesarean section. *Obstet Gynecol.* 1978;52:407.

Pecorari D. A guest editorial from abroad: meditations on a nightmare of modern midwifery: shoulder dystocia. *Obstet Gynecol Surv.* 1999;54:353.

Sandmire HF, DeMott RK. Erb's palsy: concepts and causation. *Obstet Gynecol.* 2000;95:940.

CHAPTER 18

Antepartum and Postpartum Hemorrhage

Karrie E. Francois ■ Michael R. Foley

KEY POINTS

- Understanding the hemodynamic changes of pregnancy and the physiologic responses that occur with hemorrhage assists in appropriate management. Clinicians should recognize the four classes of hemorrhage to allow for rapid intervention.
- Placental abruption is diagnosed primarily by clinical findings and is confirmed by radiographic, laboratory, and pathologic studies. Management of placental abruption is dependent on the severity, gestational age, and maternal-fetal status.
- Placenta previa is typically diagnosed with sonography. Placenta previa remote from term can be expectantly managed, and outpatient management is possible in selected cases.
- Placenta previa in association with a prior cesarean delivery is a major risk factor for placenta accreta.
- Placenta accreta is best managed with a multidisciplinary approach. Scheduled preterm delivery at 34 to 35 weeks of gestation is recommended.
- Antenatal detection of vasa previa is possible with sonography and significantly improves perinatal outcomes.
- Postpartum hemorrhage complicates 1 in 20 to 1 in 100 deliveries. Every obstetrician and birth attendant needs to have a thorough understanding of normal delivery-related blood loss in order to recognize postpartum hemorrhage.
- Management of uterine atony should follow a rapidly initiated sequenced protocol that may include bimanual massage, uterotonic therapy, uterine tamponade, selective arterial embolization, or surgical intervention.
- Coagulopathy mandates treatment of the initiating event and rapid replacement of consumed blood products. Transfusion of blood components should not be delayed, and replacement protocols should be followed.

Pregnancy-Related Hemodynamic Changes

■ Pregnancy is associated with five significant hemodynamic changes: plasma volume expansion, increase in red blood cell mass, increased maternal cardiac output, fall in systemic vascular resistance, and an increase in fibrinogen and the majority of procoagulant blood factors.

Physiologic Adaptation to Hemorrhage

■ There is a defined sequence of physiologic adaptations that occurs with hemorrhage (Fig. 18.1).

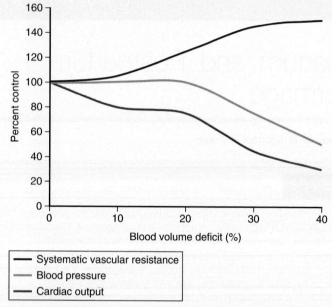

Fig. 18.1 Relationships among systemic vascular resistance, blood pressure, and cardiac output in the face of progressive blood volume deficit.

TABLE 18.1 ■ **Hemorrhage Classification and Physiologic Response**

Class	Acute Blood Loss (mL)	% Lost	Physiologic Response
1	1000	15	Dizziness, palpitations, minimal blood pressure change
2	1500	20-25	Tachycardia, tachypnea, sweating, weakness, narrowed pulse pressure
3	2000	30-35	Significant tachycardia and tachypnea, restlessness, pallor, cool extremities
4	≥2500	40	Shock, air hunger, oliguria or anuria

Modified from Baker RJ. Evaluation and management of critically ill patients. *Obstet Gynecol Annu.* 1977;6:295; and Bonnar J. Massive obstetric haemorrhage. *Baillieres Best Pract Res Clin Obstet Gynaecol.* 2000;14:1.

Classification of Hemorrhage

- See Table 18.1.
- Understanding the physiologic responses that accompany varying degrees of volume deficit can assist the clinician when caring for hemorrhaging patients.
- The average 70-kg pregnant woman maintains a blood volume of 6000 mL by 30 weeks of gestation (85 mL/kg).
- *Class 1 hemorrhage* corresponds to approximately 1000 mL of blood loss (15% volume deficit).
- *Class 2 hemorrhage* is characterized by 1500 mL of blood loss, or a 20% to 25% volume deficit. Tachypnea and tachycardia are present as well as often a narrowing of pulse pressure. Orthostatic hypotension is present.

- *Class 3 hemorrhage* is defined as a blood loss of 2000 mL and corresponds to a volume deficit of 30% to 35%. Signs include tachycardia and tachypnea as well as overt hypotension, pallor, and cool extremities.
- *Class 4 hemorrhage* is characterized by more than 2500 mL of blood loss (40% of blood volume). It is accompanied by absent distal pulses, shock, air hunger, and oliguria.

Antepartum Hemorrhage

PLACENTAL ABRUPTION

Definition and Pathogenesis

- *Placental abruption,* or *abruptio placentae,* refers to the premature separation of a normally implanted placenta from the uterus prior to delivery of the fetus.
- Whereas some placental abruptions may occur acutely after a sudden mechanical event (e.g., blunt trauma, sudden uterine decompression, or motor vehicle accident), most cases result from more chronic processes.

Incidence

- The overall incidence of placental abruption is approximately 1 in 100 births.
- About one-third of all antepartum bleeding can be attributed to placental abruption, which peaks in the third trimester; 40% to 60% of abruptions occur prior to 37 weeks of gestation.

Clinical Manifestations

- Several factors determine the clinical manifestations of placental abruption, including temporal nature of the process and severity.
- The amount of vaginal bleeding correlates poorly with the extent of placental separation and its potential for fetal compromise. Concealed abruption occurs in 10% to 20% of cases.
- Chronic abruption may be insidious in its presentation and is often associated with ischemic placental disease.

Risk Factors

- Increasing parity and maternal age
- Maternal substance abuse (e.g., cigarette smoking, cocaine use)
- Blunt or penetrating trauma
- Maternal diseases (e.g., hypertension)
- Preterm premature rupture of membranes
- Rapid uterine decompression associated with multiple gestations and polyhydramnios
- Uterine and placental factors (e.g., uterine anomalies, synechiae, fibroids, cesarean scars)
- Prior abruption (recurrence risk is 5% to 15%)

Diagnosis

- Clinical diagnosis is supported by radiographic, laboratory, and pathologic studies.

Radiology

- Ultrasound.
- Three predominant locations for placental abruption (subchorionic, retroplacental, and prepalcental).
- See Fig. 18.2.
- Retroplacental hematomas are associated with a worse prognosis for fetal survival than subchorionic hemorrhage.

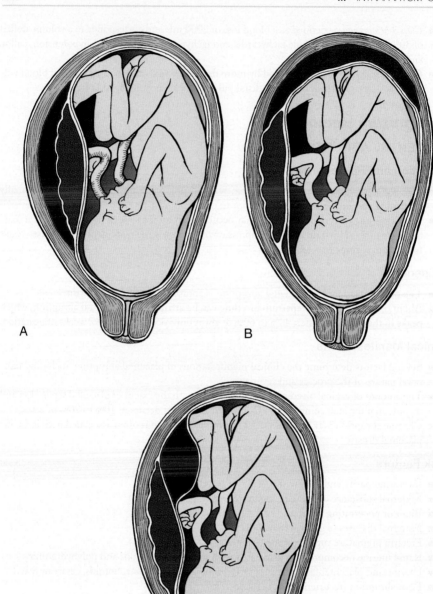

Fig. 18.2 The classification system of placental abruption. **A,** Retroplacental abruption. The bright red area represents a blood collection behind the placenta (*dark red*). **B,** Subchorionic abruption. The bright red area represents subchorionic bleeding, which is observed to dissect along the chorion. **C,** Preplacental abruption. The bright red area represents a blood collection anterior to the placenta within the amnion and chorion (subamniotic). (*Modified from Trop I, Levine D. Hemorrhage during pregnancy: sonography and MR imaging. AJR Am J Roentgenol. 2001;176:607.*)

Laboratory Findings

- Hypofibrinogenemia and evidence of consumptive coagulopathy may accompany severe abruption.

Management

- Both maternal and fetal complications may occur with placental abruption. Maternal complications include blood loss, consumptive coagulopathy, need for transfusion, end-organ damage, cesarean delivery, and death. Fetal complications include intrauterine growth restriction, oligohydramnios, prematurity, hypoxemia, and stillbirth.
- Typically, management of placental abruption depends on the severity, gestational age, and maternal-fetal status.
- Management consists of insuring availability of blood products, serial laboratory assessment (complete blood cell count, and coagulation studies), continuous fetal heart rate and contraction monitoring, and communication with operating room and neonatal personnel.
- Small placental abruptions remote from term (<34 weeks) may be managed expectantly.
- Women who present at or near term with a placental abruption should undergo delivery. Induction or augmentation of labor is not contraindicated in the setting of an abruption; however, close surveillance for any evidence of maternal or fetal compromise is advised.

Neonatal Outcome

- Tenfold increased risk for perinatal death.
- Greater risk for adverse long-term neurobehavioral outcomes.
- Hypoxia-associated periventricular leukomalacia and sudden infant death syndrome are more common in newborns delivered after placental abruptions.

PLACENTA PREVIA

Definition and Pathogenesis

- *Placenta previa* is defined as the presence of placental tissue over or adjacent to the cervical os.
- Recent revised classification of placenta previa consists of two variations: true *placenta previa,* in which the internal cervical os is covered by placental tissue, and *low-lying placenta,* in which the placenta lies within 2 cm of the cervical os but does not cover it.

Incidence

- The overall reported incidence of placenta previa at delivery is 1 in 200 births. In the second trimester, placenta previa may occur in up to 6% of pregnancies. The term *placental migration* has been used to explain this "resolution" of placenta previa that is noted near term.

Clinical Manifestations

- Placenta previa typically presents as painless vaginal bleeding in the second or third trimester.
- 70% to 80% of patients with placenta previa will have at least one bleeding episode.

Risk Factors

- Increasing parity, age, and race
- Cigarette smoking and cocaine use
- Prior placenta previa
- Prior uterine surgery and prior cesarean delivery

TABLE 18.2 ■ Potential for Placenta Previa at Term by Gestational Age at Diagnosis

Gestational Age at Diagnosis (wk)	Previa at Term (%)
15-19	12
20-23	34
24-27	49
28-31	62
32-35	73

From Dashe JS, McIntire DD, Ramus RM, et al. Persistence of placenta previa according to gestational age at ultrasound detection. Obstet Gynecol. 2002;99:692.

Diagnosis

- Most cases are detected antenatally with ultrasound.

Radiology

- Transabdominal and transvaginal ultrasound provide the best means for diagnosing placenta previa.
- If a placenta previa or low-lying placenta is diagnosed in the second trimester, repeat sonography should be obtained in the early third trimester at 32 weeks. More than 90% of the cases of placenta previa diagnosed in the second trimester resolve by term.
- See Table 18.2.

Management

- Serial ultrasounds to assess placental location and fetal growth, avoidance of cervical examinations and intercourse, activity restrictions, counseling regarding labor symptoms and vaginal bleeding, and early medical attention if any vaginal bleeding occurs.

Asymptomatic Placenta Previa

- Asymptomatic women with placenta previa may be managed expectantly as outpatients.
- Candidates for outpatient management must (1) be compliant, (2) live within a short commute from the hospital, (3) have 24-hour emergency transportation to the hospital.

Bleeding Placenta Previa

- Acute vaginal bleeding requires hospitalization and immediate evaluation to assess maternal-fetal stability.
- Antenatal corticosteroids (less than 34 weeks).
- Tocolysis may be used if the vaginal bleeding is preceded by or associated with uterine contractions.
- RhO(D) immune globulin should be given to all Rh-negative unsensitized women with third-trimester bleeding from placenta previa.

Delivery

- Cesarean delivery is indicated for all women with sonographic evidence of placenta previa and most women with low-lying placenta. Blood should be available for transfusion.

- Cesarean delivery of asymptomatic placenta previa should occur between $36^{0/7}$ and $37^{0/7}$ weeks of gestation. In cases of complicated placenta previa (bleeding associated with non-reassuring fetal heart pattern, life-threatening hemorrhage), delivery should occur immediately regardless of gestational age.

PLACENTA ACCRETA

Definition and Pathogenesis

- Placenta accreta represents the abnormal attachment of the placenta to the uterine lining due to an absence of the decidua basalis and an incomplete development of the fibrinoid layer.

Incidence and Risk Factors

- The overall incidence of placenta accreta or one of its variations is 3 per 1000 deliveries.
- Significant risk factors are placenta previa and prior cesarean delivery.
- Increasing parity and maternal age, submucosal uterine fibroids, prior uterine surgery, cesarean scar, and endometrial defects are other risk factors.[1,2]

Clinical Manifestations

- Profuse bleeding usually follows attempted manual placental separation. Hematuria can be a feature of placenta percreta with bladder invasion.

Diagnosis

- Most cases of placenta accreta are diagnosed antenatally by advanced radiographic techniques (ultrasound is the preferred technique).
- MRI can be used in conjunction with sonography to assess abnormal placental invasion.
- Placenta accreta is confirmed by the pathologic examination of a hysterectomy specimen.

Management

- Placenta accreta accounts for a large percentage of peripartum hysterectomies.[3] A multidisciplinary team approach is the ideal way to manage these cases.
- Delivery recommended at $34^{0/7}$ to $35^{6/7}$ weeks.
- Adequate IV access with two large-bore catheters and ample blood product availability are mandatory.
- It is recommended that the uterus be incised above the placental attachment site and that the placenta be left in situ after clamping the cord because disruption of the implantation site may result in rapid blood loss.

VASA PREVIA

Definition and Pathogenesis

- Vasa previa is defined as the presence of fetal vessels over the cervical os.
- Velamentous cord insertion may occur without vasa previa and can occasionally exist as fetal vessels that run between a bilobed or succenturiate-lobed placenta.

Incidence and Risk Factors

- The overall incidence of vasa previa is 1 in 2500 deliveries.
- Bilobed and succenturiate-lobed placentas, pregnancies that result from assisted reproductive technology, multiple gestations, and history of second-trimester placenta previa or low-lying placenta are risk factors.[4-6]

Clinical Manifestations

- Acute onset of vaginal bleeding from a lacerated fetal vessel following artificial rupture of membranes.

Diagnosis

- The diagnosis is confirmed by documenting umbilical vessels over the cervical os using color and pulsed Doppler imaging.

Management

- When diagnosed antenatally, vasa previa should be managed similarly to placenta previa.
- Cesarean delivery is recommended between $34^{0/7}$ to $36^{0/7}$ weeks of gestation.[7,8]

POSTPARTUM HEMORRHAGE

- Postpartum hemorrhage is an obstetric emergency that complicates between 1 in 20 and 1 in 100 deliveries.

Normal Blood Loss and Postpartum Hemorrhage

- Postpartum hemorrhage is defined as blood loss in excess of 500 mL for vaginal delivery and 1000 mL for a cesarean delivery.

Etiologies

- The etiologies of postpartum hemorrhage can be categorized as primary (early or within 24 hours of delivery) or secondary (late or more than 24 hours and up to 12 weeks postpartum).

UTERINE ATONY

Definition and Pathogenesis

- Uterine atony is the most common cause of primary postpartum hemorrhage.

Incidence and Risk Factors

- Uterine atony complicates 1 in 20 deliveries and is responsible for 80% of postpartum hemorrhage cases.
- Uterine overdistention, labor induction, rapid or prolonged labor, grand multiparity, uterine infection, uterine inversion, retained products of conception, abnormal placentation, and use of uterine-relaxing agents are risk factors.

Clinical Manifestations and Diagnosis

- Rapid uterine bleeding associated with a lack of myometrial tone and an absence of other etiologies for postpartum hemorrhage.

Prevention and Management

- Three preventive methods for atonic postpartum hemorrhage are (1) active management of the third stage of labor, (2) spontaneous placental separation during cesarean delivery, and (3) prolonged postpartum oxytocin infusion.

Bimanual Uterine Massage
- The uterus should be compressed between the external, fundally placed hand and the internal, intravaginal hand.

Uterotonic Therapy
- See Table 18.3.
- The genital tract should be carefully inspected for lacerations before proceeding with therapeutic measures.

Uterine Tamponade
- Uterine packing is a safe, simple, and effective way to control postpartum hemorrhage. Various balloon catheters may be placed in the uterus to tamponade bleeding.

Selective Arterial Embolization
- Selective arterial embolization is an option for hemodynamically stable patients with postpartum hemorrhage (success rates 90% to 97%).

Surgical Intervention
- The goal of arterial ligation is to decrease uterine perfusion and subsequent bleeding.
- Bakri has described a newer technique for bilateral uterine artery ligation in combination with tamponade balloon placement.

Bilateral Looped Uterine Vessel Sutures
- Uterine compression sutures include B-Lynch suture, Hayman vertical sutures, Pereira transverse and vertical sutures, and multiple square sutures.[9,10]
- Hysterectomy is used for refractory bleeding,

GENITAL TRACT LACERATIONS

Definition and Pathogenesis
- Genital tract lacerations may occur with both vaginal and cesarean deliveries.
- The most common lower genital tract lacerations are perineal, vulvar, vaginal, and cervical. Upper genital tract lacerations are typically associated with broad ligament and retroperitoneal hematomas.

Incidence and Risk Factors
- Genital tract lacerations are a leading cause of postpartum hemorrhage. Risk factors include instrumented vaginal delivery, fetal malpresentation or macrosomia, episiotomy, precipitous delivery, prior cerclage placement, Dührssen incisions, and shoulder dystocia.

Clinical Manifestations and Diagnosis
- For diagnosis, it is best to evaluate the lower genital tract superiorly from the cervix and to progress inferiorly to the vagina, perineum, and vulva.

Management
- Once a genital tract laceration is identified, management depends on its severity and location.

Vulvar Hematoma
- Vulvar hematomas usually result from lacerated vessels in the superficial fascia of the anterior or posterior pelvic triangle.
- Surgical drainage is the primary treatment for most vulvar hematomas.

Vaginal Hematoma
- Vaginal hematomas result from delivery-related soft tissue damage.

TABLE 18.3 ■ Uterotonic Therapies

Agent	Dose	Route	Dosing Interval	Side Effects	Contraindications
Oxytocin (Pitocin)	10-80U in 500-1000 mL crystalloid solution	First line: IV Second line: IM or IU	Continuous	Nausea, emesis, water intoxication	None
Misoprostol (Cytotec)	600-1000 µg	First line: PR Second line: PO or SL	Single dose	Nausea, emesis, diarrhea, fever, chills	None
Methylergonovine (Methergine)	0.2 mg	First line: IM Second line: IU or PO	Every 2-4 h	Hypertension, hypotension, nausea, emesis	Hypertension, migraines, scleroderma, Raynaud syndrome
Prostaglandin F$_{2\alpha}$ (Hemabate)	0.25 mg	First line: IM Second line: IU	Every 15-90 min (maximum of 8 doses)	Nausea, emesis, diarrhea, flushing, chills	Active cardiac, pulmonary, renal, or hepatic disease
Prostaglandin E$_2$ (Dinoprostone)	20 mg	PR	Every 2 h	Nausea, emesis, diarrhea, fever, chills, headache	Hypotension

IM, intramuscular; *IU*, intrauterine; *IV*, intravenous; *PO*, per os; *PR*, per rectum; *SL*, sublingual.

- Vaginal hematomas may or may not require surgical drainage.
- Selective arterial embolization may be considered.

Retroperitoneal Hematoma
- Retroperitoneal hematomas are the most serious and life-threatening.
- These hematomas usually occur after a vessel laceration from the internal iliac (hypogastric) arterial tre
- Treatment of a retroperitoneal hematoma typically involves laparotomy, hematoma evacuation, and arterial ligation. In some situations, selective arterial embolization may be used as a primary or adjunctive treatment.

RETAINED PRODUCTS OF CONCEPTION

Definition and Pathogenesis
- Retained products of conception—namely, placental tissue and amniotic membranes—can inhibit the uterus from adequate contraction and can result in hemorrhage.

Incidence and Risk Factors
- Retained products of conception complicate 0.5% to 1% of deliveries. Risk factors include midtrimester delivery, chorioamnionitis, and accessory placental lobes.

Clinical Manifestations and Diagnosis
- Retained products of conception typically present with uterine bleeding and associated atony.
- Transabdominal or transvaginal ultrasound may be used for diagnosis.

Management
- Manual extraction and uterine curettage are used.

UTERINE RUPTURE

Definition and Pathogenesis
- Uterine rupture refers to the complete nonsurgical disruption of all uterine layers—endometrium, myometrium, and serosa.

Incidence and Risk Factors
- The overall incidence of uterine rupture (scarred and unscarred uterus) is 1 in 2000 deliveries. Uterine rupture is most common in women with a scarred uterus, including those with prior cesarean delivery and myomectomy.
- Risk factors for women undergoing a trial of labor after cesarean section may include multiple prior cesarean deliveries, no previous vaginal delivery, induced or augmented labor, term gestation, thin uterine scar identified by ultrasound, multiple gestation, fetal macrosomia, postcesarean delivery infection, single-layer closure of hysterotomy incision, and short interpregnancy interval.

Clinical Manifestations and Diagnosis
- Uterine rupture is associated with both fetal and maternal clinical manifestations.
- Fetal bradycardia with or without preceding variable or late decelerations.
- Loss of fetal station in labor.
- Acute vaginal bleeding, constant abdominal pain or uterine tenderness, change in uterine shape, cessation of contractions, hematuria.

- Signs of hemodynamic instability.
- Uterine rupture is suspected clinically but confirmed surgically.

Management

- Site of rupture should be assessed to determine whether it can be repaired.

UTERINE INVERSION

Definition and Pathogenesis

- Uterine inversion refers to the collapse of the fundus into the uterine cavity and is classified by degree and timing. With regard to degree, uterine inversion may be first degree (incomplete), second degree (complete), third degree (prolapsed), or fourth degree.
- The two most commonly proposed etiologies for uterine inversion include excessive umbilical cord traction with a fundally attached placenta and fundal pressure in the setting of a relaxed uterus.

Incidence and Risk Factors

- Uterine inversion is a rare event that complicates about 1 in 1200 to 1 in 57,000 deliveries.[11]
- Risk factors include uterine overdistention, fetal macrosomia, rapid labor and delivery, congenital uterine malformations, uterine fibroids, invasive placentation, retained placenta, short umbilical cord, use of uterine-relaxing agents, nulliparity, manual placental extraction, and Ehlers-Danlos syndrome.

Clinical Manifestations and Diagnosis

- Brisk vaginal bleeding, inability to palpate the fundus abdominally, and maternal hemodynamic instability.

Management

- Once diagnosed, uterine inversion requires rapid intervention to restore maternal hemodynamic stability and control hemorrhage.

COAGULOPATHY

Definition and Pathogenesis

- Coagulopathy represents an imbalance between the clotting and fibrinolytic systems.
- See Fig. 18.3.

Incidence and Risk Factors

- Massive antepartum or postpartum hemorrhage; sepsis; severe preeclampsia; hemolysis, elevated liver enzymes, low platelets syndrome; amniotic fluid embolism; fetal demise; placental abruption; septic abortion; and acute fatty liver of pregnancy.

Clinical Manifestations and Diagnosis

- The primary clinical manifestations of consumptive coagulopathy include bleeding, hypotension out of proportion to blood loss, microangiopathic hemolytic anemia, acute lung injury, acute renal failure, and ischemic end-organ tissue damage.
- Consumptive coagulopathy is a clinical diagnosis that is confirmed with laboratory data.

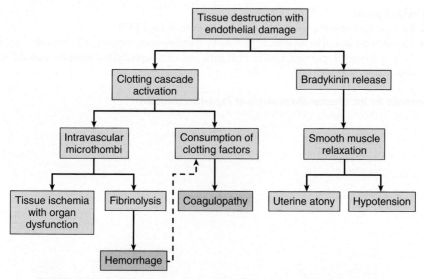

Fig. 18.3 Pathophysiology and clinical manifestations of consumptive coagulopathy.

Management

- The most important factor in the successful treatment of coagulopathy is identifying and correcting the underlying etiology.
- Delivery of the fetus initiates resolution of the coagulopathy.
- Have two large-bore IV catheters for fluid and blood component therapy; laboratory studies should be drawn serially every 4 hours until resolution.
- Maintain adequate oxygenation and normothermia.
- Vitamin K, recombinant activated factor VII, human recombinant factor VIIa for consumptive coagulopathy, and hemostatic agents may be used in individual cases.

Fluid Resuscitation and Transfusion

Volume Resuscitation

- Warmed crystalloid solution in a 3:1 ratio to the estimated blood loss should be rapidly infused.

Packed Red Blood Cells

- Each packed red blood cell (RBC) unit contains approximately 300 mL of volume (250 mL RBCs and 50 mL of plasma). In a 70-kg patient, one unit of packed RBCs will raise the hemoglobin by 1 g/dL and the hematocrit by 3%.

Platelet Concentrates

- Transfusion of platelets should be considered when the platelet count is less than 20,000/mm^3 after a vaginal delivery or less than 50,000/mm^3 after a cesarean delivery, or when coagulopathy is evident.

Fresh Frozen Plasma

- Each unit contains approximately 250 mL.
- Fresh frozen plasma (FFP) should raise the fibrinogen level by 5 to 10 mg/dL.

Cryoprecipitate
- Cryoprecipitate is the precipitate that results from thawed FFP.
- Cryoprecipitate can be measured clinically by the fibrinogen response, which should increase by 5 to 10 mg/dL per unit. Unlike FFP, each unit of cryoprecipitate provides minimal volume (10 to 15 mL).

References for this chapter are available at ExpertConsult.com.

CHAPTER 19

Cesarean Delivery

Vincenzo Berghella ■ A. Dhanya Mackeen ■ Eric R.M. Jauniaux

KEY POINTS

- In 1970, the CD rate was about 5%. By 2008, it had reached 32.8%, the highest rate ever recorded in the United States. The rates of vaginal births after cesarean delivery have plummeted, from a peak of 28.3% in 1996 to 8.5% in 2008, contributing to the rise in CD. Most recently, CD rates have stabilized around 32% to 33% in the United States.

- Factors that have contributed to the rise in CD during the past decades include (1) continued increase in primary CDs for dystocia, failed induction, and abnormal presentation; (2) an increase in the proportion of women with obesity, diabetes mellitus, and multiple gestations; (3) increased use of planned CD; and (4) limited use of TOLAC because of both safety and medicolegal concerns.

- Single-dose, preoperative prophylactic antibiotics are of clear benefit in reducing the frequency of postcesarean endomyometritis and wound infection.

- Mechanical prophylaxis with graduated compression stockings or a pneumatic compression device during and after all cesarean deliveries should be considered.

- Horizontal skin incision is preferred because vertical skin incision is associated with long-term postoperative complications, such as wound dehiscence and abdominal incisional hernia, and it is also cosmetically less pleasing.

- A low transverse uterine incision is preferred for almost all CDs.

- Blunt uterine extension is associated with decreased blood loss and is therefore preferred.

- Delayed cord clamping should be done for 30 to 120 seconds for all infants delivered at less than 37 weeks' gestation.

- IV oxytocin, 10 to 80 IU in 1 L crystalloid, should be given prophylactically after the infant is delivered in all CDs.

- Several randomized controlled trials have demonstrated greater blood loss and a higher rate of endometritis with manual extraction of the placenta at CD. Thus spontaneous expulsion of the placenta with gentle cord traction is preferred.

- The uterine incision can be repaired in a single layer if the patient has completed childbearing, such as a bilateral tubal ligation performed concurrently with CD. Consider double-layer closure otherwise.

- When closing the abdomen after a CD, the subcutaneous tissue is closed if its thickness exceeds 2 cm. This approach significantly reduces the risk for wound disruption.

- The skin should be closed with sutures, not staples.

- Postcesarean endomyometritis remains the most common complication of CD. With the use of appropriate prophylactic antibiotics as described previously, its frequency is usually less than 5%.

Incidence

- Cesarean delivery (CD) rates have risen in the United States in a dramatic fashion from less than 5% in the 1960s to 32.7% by 2013, with stable rates around 32% to 33% in the past 5 years.[1]
- Among the reasons for this increase are (1) a continued increase in primary CDs for dystocia, failed induction, and malpresentation; (2) an increase in the proportion of women with obesity, diabetes mellitus, and multiple gestation, which predispose to CD; (3) increased practice of CD on maternal request; and (4) limited use of a trial of labor after cesarean (TOLAC) delivery due to both safety and medicolegal concerns.
- The World Health Organization has proposed an incidence of CD between 10% and 15% as a target to optimize maternal and perinatal health.
- Maternal and perinatal morbidity and mortality should be the outcomes monitored to ensure best quality of care.
- Instead of setting goals or limits for overall CD rates, it is most important to monitor maternal and perinatal health outcomes.
- Two populations often targeted for comparison include nulliparous women with a singleton vertex gestation at 37 weeks or greater without other complications and women with one prior low transverse CD delivering a single vertex fetus at 37 weeks or greater without other complications.[2]

Indications for Cesarean Delivery

MATERNAL-FETAL INDICATIONS

- The suggestions for definitions of *arrest* of labor in the first and second stage and *failed induction,* shown in Box 19.1, should be followed for management as long as maternal and fetal conditions are reassuring.

FETAL INDICATIONS

- Fetal indications are primarily recognized by nonreassuring FHR testing with the potential for long-term consequences of metabolic acidosis.

MATERNAL INDICATIONS

- Maternal indications for CD are relatively few and can be considered as medical or mechanical in nature (see Box 19.2).

CESAREAN DELIVERY ON MATERNAL REQUEST

- The lack of specificity of the term "elective" suggests the most reasonable and prudent course of action is to not use it, but rather to document the specific indication—whether medical or nonmedical—for the intervention or procedure (i.e., CD on maternal request).[3]
- Women who desire several children should be advised against non–medically indicated CD because of the direct association with an increasing number of CDs and increasing life-threatening complications such as placenta previa, placenta accreta, and the need for cesarean hysterectomy.[4]

BOX 19.1 ■ Safe Prevention of Cesarean Delivery

First Stage of Labor

- A prolonged latent phase (>20 h in NP women and >14 h in MP women) should not be an indication for CD. (Grade 1B)
- Slow but progressive labor in the first stage rarely should be an indication for CD. (Grade 1B)
- As long as fetal and maternal status are reassuring, cervical dilation of 6 cm should be considered the threshold for the active phase in most laboring women. Thus before 6 cm of dilation is achieved, standards of active-phase progress should not be applied. (Grade 1B)
- CD for active-phase arrest in the first stage of labor should be reserved for women at or beyond 6 cm of dilation with ruptured membranes who fail to progress despite 4 h of adequate uterine activity or at least 6 h of oxytocin administration with inadequate uterine activity and no cervical change. (Grade 1B)

Second Stage of Labor

- A specific absolute maximum length of the second stage of labor above which all women should be delivered operatively has not been identified. (Grade 1C)
- Before diagnosing arrest of labor in the second stage, if the maternal and fetal conditions permit, allow for the following:
  - At least 2 h of pushing in MP women (Grade 1B)
  - At least 3 h of pushing in NP women (Grade 1B)

Longer durations may be appropriate on an individualized basis (e.g., with the use of epidural analgesia or with fetal malposition) as long as progress is being documented. (Grade 1B)

- Operative vaginal delivery in the second stage of labor should be considered an acceptable alternative to CD. Training in, and ongoing maintenance of, practical skills related to operative vaginal delivery should be encouraged. (Grade 1B)
- Manual rotation of the fetal occiput in the setting of fetal malposition in the second stage of labor is a reasonable alternative to operative vaginal delivery or CD. To safely prevent CD in the setting of malposition, it is important to assess fetal position throughout the second stage of labor. (Grade 1B)

Fetal Heart Rate Monitoring

- Amnioinfusion for repetitive variable fetal heart rate decelerations may safely reduce the CD rate. (Grade 1A)
- Scalp stimulation can be used as a means of assessing fetal acid-base status when abnormal or indeterminate (*nonreassuring*) fetal heart patterns (e.g., minimal variability) are present, and it is a safe alternative to CD in this setting. (Grade 1C)

Induction of Labor

- Induction of labor generally should be performed based on maternal and fetal medical indications and after informed consent is obtained and documented. Inductions at $41^{0/7}$ weeks of gestation and beyond should be performed to reduce the risk of CD and the risk of perinatal morbidity and mortality. (Grade 1A)
- Cervical ripening methods should be used when labor is induced in women with an unfavorable cervix. (Grade 1B)
- If the maternal and fetal status allow, CDs for failed induction of labor in the latent phase can be avoided by allowing longer durations of the latent phase (up to 24 h or longer) and requiring that oxytocin be administered for at least 18 h after membrane rupture before deeming the induction a failure. (Grade 1B)

Fetal Malpresentation

- Fetal presentation should be assessed and documented beginning at $36^{0/7}$ weeks of gestation to allow for external cephalic version to be offered. (Grade 1C)

Continued

BOX 19.1 ■ Safe Prevention of Cesarean Delivery—cont'd

Suspected Fetal Macrosomia

- CD to avoid potential birth trauma should be limited to estimated fetal weights of at least 5000 g in women without diabetes and at least 4500 g in women with diabetes. The prevalence of birthweight of 5000 g or more is rare, and patients should be counseled that estimates of fetal weight, particularly late in gestation, are imprecise. (Grade 2C)
- Women should be counseled about the IOM maternal weight guidelines in an attempt to avoid excessive weight gain. (Grade 1B)

Twin Gestations

- Perinatal outcomes for twin gestations in which the first twin is in cephalic presentation are not improved by CD. Thus women with either cephalic/cephalic-presenting twins or cephalic/noncephalic-presenting twins should be counseled to attempt vaginal delivery. (Grade 1B)

Other

- Individuals, organizations, and governing bodies should work to ensure that research is conducted to provide a better knowledge base to guide decisions regarding CD and to encourage policy changes that safely lower the rate of primary CD. (Grade 1C)

CD, cesarean delivery; *IOM,* Institute of Medicine; *MP,* multiparous; *NP,* nulliparous.
Modified from the American College of Obstetricians and Gynecologists, Society for Maternal-Fetal Medicine, Caughey AB, Cahill AG, Guise JM, Rouse DJ. Safe prevention of the primary cesarean delivery. *Am J Obstet Gynecol.* 2014;210(3):179-193.

BOX 19.2 ■ Selected Indications for Cesarean Delivery by Category

Maternal-Fetal

Cephalopelvic disproportion
Placental abruption
Placenta previa
Repeat cesarean delivery
Cesarean delivery on maternal request

Maternal

Specific cardiac disease (e.g., Marfan syndrome with dilated aortic root)

Fetal

Nonreassuring fetal status
Breech or transverse lie
Maternal herpes

- Perinatal mortality has been reported to be several times lower with a planned CD compared with labor and vaginal birth.
- CD also presents a risk for future placental abnormalities, including placenta previa and placenta accreta. These risks increase with the increasing number of CDs performed for each woman and are substantial with more than three operations. Thus the decision to undergo CD on request must include thoughtful consideration of future childbearing plans.

Technique of Cesarean Delivery

PRECESAREAN ANTIBIOTICS

- Prophylactic preoperative antibiotics are of clear benefit in reducing the frequency of post-cesarean endomyometritis and wound infection in both laboring and nonlaboring CDs.[5]
- For women with clinical chorioamnionitis, treatment with combination antibiotic therapy is recommended.

PRECESAREAN THROMBOPROPHYLAXIS

- Because venous thromboembolism is the leading cause of maternal mortality in developed countries, and CD increases this risk, thromboprophylaxis should be considered in all CDs.
- Urinary bladder catheterization for CD is prudent until evidence can delineate that eliminating this practice will not result in an increase in bladder or ureteral injury.

SITE PREPARATION

- Hair does not have to be removed from the operative site.
- Incision-site preparation is accomplished in the operating room through application of a surgical scrub. CD wounds are considered to be clean contaminated. Chlorhexidine-alcohol scrub has been associated with a lower incidence of wound infection compared with povidone-iodine scrub.[6]
- Drapes should not be adhesive.

ABDOMINAL SKIN INCISION AND ABDOMINAL ENTRY

- The surgeon has a choice of a transverse or vertical skin incision, with the transverse Pfannenstiel being the most common incision type in the United States. Factors that influence the type of incision include the urgency of the delivery, placental disorders such as anterior complete placenta previa and placenta accreta, prior incision type, and the potential need to explore the upper abdomen for nonobstetric pathology. Although some still prefer a vertical incision in emergency situations, a Pfannenstiel incision actually adds only 1 minute of extra operative time in primary and 2 minutes in repeat cesareans, differences that are not associated with improved neonatal outcome compared with that of a vertical incision.[7]
- The Joel-Cohen and the Pfannenstiel are the recommended cesarean technique skin incisions.

BLADDER FLAP

- Creation of a bladder flap versus a direct uterine incision above the bladder fold has been compared in four randomized trials of 581 women.[8] Bladder flap development was associated with a longer incision-to-delivery interval of 1.27 minutes without any differences in bladder injury, total operating time, blood loss, or hospital length of stay.[8] It is important to note that emergency CDs were excluded from the studies, and the majority of pregnancies were over 32 weeks' gestation.

UTERINE INCISION

- The low transverse incision is preferred to a vertical incision because it is associated with less blood loss, is easier to perform and repair, and provides for the option of subsequent

TOLAC because the rate of subsequent rupture is lower than with incisions that incorporate the upper uterine segment.[9]

- A vertical uterine incision may need to be performed if the lower uterine segment is poorly developed or if the fetus is in a back-down transverse lie; in cases of an anterior placenta previa or accreta, often in combination with a hysterectomy (Chapter 21); or if leiomyomas obstruct the lower segment.

DELIVERY OF THE FETUS

- When the vertex is wedged in the maternal pelvis, usually in advanced second-stage arrest, reverse breech extraction (the "pull" method) has been associated with shorter operating time, less extension of the uterine incision, and postpartum endometritis compared with vaginal displacement of the presenting part upward.[10]
- Delayed cord clamping is recommended for all CDs done before 37 weeks.

PREVENTION OF POSTPARTUM HEMORRHAGE

- Studies suggest that 10 to 80 IU of oxytocin in 1 L crystalloid infused over 4 to 8 hours significantly prevents uterine atony and postpartum hemorrhage.[11]

PLACENTAL EXTRACTION

- Removal of the placenta by spontaneous expulsion with gentle cord traction has been shown by several randomized controlled trials to be associated with less blood loss and a lower rate of endometritis than manual extraction.[12-14] Therefore spontaneous expulsion with gentle cord traction and uterine massage should be performed for delivery of the placenta. Intraoperative glove change has not been shown to decrease the risk of endometritis after CD.[13]

UTERINE REPAIR

- The first layer of uterine closure is performed using continuous suturing. This technique is associated with less operating time and reduced blood loss compared with interrupted sutures.[15] The locking of the primary layer of closure facilitates hemostasis but may not be necessary if the incision is fairly hemostatic before closure. Size 1-0 or 0-0 synthetic suture is used. Full-thickness repair that includes the endometrial layer is associated with improved healing as evidenced by ultrasound 6 weeks after CD.[16,17]

ABDOMINAL CLOSURE

- The subcutaneous tissue is closed if it will facilitate skin closure or if the fat thickness is at least 2 cm. Closure of the subcutaneous tissue of at least 2 cm with sutures is associated with fewer wound complications—such as a hematoma, seroma, wound infection, or wound separation—compared with no closure.[18]
- The transverse cesarean skin incision should be closed with subcuticular suture, rather than staples, because suture closure significantly decreases by 57% the risks of wound complications (from 10.6% to 4.9%) and specifically wound separation (from 7.4% to 1.6%).[19,20] Staple closure is approximately 7 minutes faster than suture closure.[21] Evidence is insufficient to make a recommendation for closure method for CDs performed using vertical skin incisions.[19,20]

Complications of Cesarean Delivery

INTRAOPERATIVE COMPLICATIONS

Uterine Lacerations

- Most lacerations are myometrial extensions that can be closed with a running locking suture independently or in conjunction with closure of the primary uterine incision. High lateral extensions may require unilateral ascending uterine artery branch ligation.

Bladder Injury

- Bladder dome lacerations are generally repaired with a double-layer closure technique using 2-0 or 3-0 Vicryl suture. The mucosa may be avoided with closure, although this is not imperative.

Ureteral Injury

- Most ureteral injuries follow attempts to control bleeding from lateral extensions into the broad ligament. Opening the broad ligament before suture placement may reduce the risk for this complication.

Maternal Mortality

- Similar rates of maternal death have been reported among women delivered by CD versus those delivered vaginally when adjusting for maternal age and the presence of severe preeclampsia.

MATERNAL POSTOPERATIVE MORBIDITY

Endomyometritis

- Postcesarean endomyometritis remains the most common complication of CD. With the use of appropriate prophylactic antibiotics as described previously, its frequency is usually less than 5%,[22,23] much reduced from preantibiotic times.
- The diagnosis of postpartum endomyometritis is based on fever with either fundal tenderness or foul-smelling discharge in the absence of any other source.
- A regimen of clindamycin and an aminoglycoside such as gentamicin is associated with better safety and efficacy compared with other regimens.

Wound Infection

- Wound infection complicates about 1% to 5% of cesarean deliveries.[24] Most CD wounds are considered clean contaminated owing to the interface with the lower reproductive tract. Emergent CDs and those associated with chorioamnionitis are considered contaminated and have higher wound infection rates.
- Extreme wound discoloration, extensive infection, gangrene, bullae, or anesthesia of the surrounding tissue should prompt consideration of necrotizing fasciitis, a life-threatening surgical emergency that has been reported to develop in 1 in 2500 women undergoing primary CD.

Thromboembolic Disease

- The incidence of deep vein thrombosis was reported at 0.17%, and that of pulmonary embolism at 0.12%, in women undergoing CD.

Septic Pelvic Thrombophlebitis

- Septic pelvic thrombophlebitis is most often a diagnosis of exclusion established in refractory cases of women being treated for endomyometritis. A pelvic CT scan may aid in the diagnosis, although the sensitivity and specificity of this technique are clearly difficult to establish.

Tubal Sterilization

MODIFIED POMEROY

- The Pomeroy technique as originally described included grasping the fallopian tube at its midportion, creating a small knuckle, and then ligating the loop of tube with a double strand of catgut suture.

References for this chapter are available at ExpertConsult.com.

CHAPTER 20

Vaginal Birth After Cesarean Delivery

Mark B. Landon ■ William A. Grobman

KEY POINTS

- VBAC rates have plummeted from a peak of approximately 30% in 1996 to 5% in 2010.
- Two-thirds of women with a prior low transverse CD are candidates for TOLAC and should be counseled about and offered this option.
- The success rate for TOLAC is influenced by prior indication for cesarean delivery, history of vaginal delivery, demographic characteristics such as maternal age and body mass index, the occurrence of spontaneous labor, and cervical status at admission.
- Oxytocin may be used for induction, as well as augmentation, of labor in women undergoing TOLAC.
- The use of misoprostol for cervical ripening is contraindicated in women undergoing TOLAC.
- The most consistent sign associated with uterine rupture is fetal heart rate abnormalities that include prolonged variable decelerations and bradycardia.

Trends

- It has been suggested that about two-thirds of women with a prior cesarean delivery (CD) are actually candidates for a trial of labor after cesarean (TOLAC) delivery and most planned repeat operations are influenced by physician discretion and patient choice.
- Despite two recent large-scale contemporary multicenter studies that attest to their relative safety,[1,2] there is restriction of a women's access to TOLAC or vaginal birth after cesarean (VBAC) delivery, The National Institutes of Health held a consensus development conference concerning VBAC in 2010. The panel at that conference concluded that TOLAC is a reasonable birth option for many women with a previous CD. The panel also found that existing practice guidelines and the medical liability climate were restricting access to TOLAC-VBAC and that these factors need to be addressed.[3]

CANDIDATES FOR TOLAC

The following are selection criteria suggested by ACOG[4] for identifying candidates for TOLAC:
- One or two previous low-transverse CDs
- Clinically adequate pelvis
- No other uterine scars or previous rupture
- Physicians immediately available throughout active labor capable of monitoring labor and performing an emergency cesarean delivery
- A TOLAC should *not* be attempted in the following circumstances:
  - Previous classical or T-shaped incision, or extensive transfundal uterine surgery
  - Previous uterine rupture
  - Medical or obstetrical complications that preclude vaginal delivery

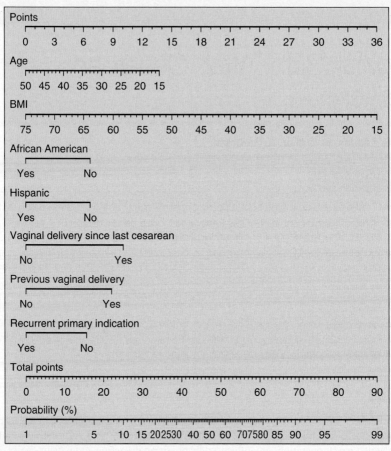

Fig. 20.1 Graphic nomogram used to predict probability of vaginal birth after cesarean (VBAC). The nomogram is used by locating each patient characteristic and finding the number of points on the uppermost scale to which that characteristic corresponds. The sum of total points predicts the probability of VBAC on the lower scale. BMI, body mass index. (*Modified from Grobman WA, Lai Y, Landon MB, et al, for the National Institute of Child Health and Human Development [NICHD] Maternal Fetal Medicine Units Network [MFMU]. Development of a nomogram for prediction of vaginal birth after cesarean delivery. Obstet Gynecol. 2007;109:806-812.*)

SUCCESS RATES FOR TOLAC

- The overall success rate for a population of women undergoing TOLAC appears to be in the 60% to 80% range.[4]
- Several authors have developed models for predicting VBAC (Fig. 20.1).

Maternal Demographics

- Race, age, body mass index, and insurance status have all been demonstrated to be associated with the success of TOLAC.[5]

Prior Indication for Cesarean Delivery

- Prior cesarean delivery for cephalopelvic disproportion or failure to progress has been associated with success rates that range from 50% to 67%.

Prior Vaginal Delivery

- Women with a prior vaginal delivery had an 87% TOLAC success rate, compared with a 61% success rate in women without a prior vaginal delivery.

Birthweight

- Birthweight greater than 4000 g in particular is associated with a higher risk for failed VBAC.[6]

Labor Status and Cervical Examinations

- An 86% success rate in women who presented in labor with cervical dilation greater than 4 cm. Conversely, the VBAC success rate dropped to 67% if the cervix was dilated less than 4 cm on admission.
- A 67.4% success rate in women who underwent induction versus 80.5% in those who underwent spontaneous labor.[7]

Previous or Unknown Incision Type

- Women whose previous incision type is unknown have VBAC success rates similar to those of women with documented prior low transverse incisions.[5] Similarly, women with previous low vertical incisions do not appear to have lower VBAC success rates.[8]

Multiple Prior Cesarean Deliveries

- Women with more than one prior CD have been demonstrated to have a lower likelihood of achieving VBAC.

Postterm Pregnancy

- TOLAC success rates may be lower for women at or beyond 40 weeks of gestation when compared with those who are prior to 40 weeks of gestation.

Twin Gestation

- Success rates for women undergoing TOLAC with twins are not different than for those with singleton gestations.[2,5]

Risks Associated With a Trial of Labor After Cesarean

UTERINE RUPTURE

- It is important to differentiate between *uterine rupture* and *uterine scar dehiscence*. This distinction is clinically relevant because dehiscence most often represents an occult scar separation observed at laparotomy in women with a prior CD.
- The large multicenter MFMU Network Study[1] reported a 0.69% frequency of uterine rupture, with 124 symptomatic ruptures occurring in 17,898 women undergoing TOLAC.
- Women with a prior low vertical uterine incision are not at significantly increased risk for rupture compared with women with a prior low transverse incision.
- In counseling women with an unknown scar, the physician should attempt to understand whether a prior CD had been performed under circumstances in which it was more likely that a different type of incision had been used.
- An overall rate of rupture-related perinatal death of 0.11 per 1000 TOLACs.

Risk Factors For Uterine Rupture

- Rates of uterine rupture vary significantly depending on a variety of associated risk factors. In addition to the type of uterine scar, characteristics of the obstetric history that include the number of prior cesarean and vaginal deliveries, the interdelivery interval, and the uterine closure technique have been reported to be associated with the risk for uterine rupture.

TABLE 20.1 ■ Risk for Uterine Rupture Following Multiple Prior Cesarean Deliveries

| | | Rupture Rate | | |
Study	N	Single Prior (%)	Multiple Prior (%)	RR (CI)
Miller et al[13]	3728	0.6	1.7	3.1 (1.9-4.8)
Caughey et al[14]	134	0.8	3.7	4.5 (1.2-11.5)
Macones et al[15]	1082	0.9	1.8	2.3 (1.4-3.9)
Landon et al[16]	975	0.7	0.9	1.4 (0.7-2.7)

CI, confidence interval; *N,* number of women with multiple prior cesarean sections attempting vaginal birth after cesarean; *RR,* relative risk.

Number of Prior Cesarean Deliveries

- It thus appears that even if having had more than one prior cesarean section is associated with an increased risk for uterine rupture, the magnitude of any additional risk is fairly small (Table 20.1). ACOG considers it reasonable to offer TOLAC to women with more than one prior CD and to counsel such women based on the combination of other factors that affect their probability of achieving a successful VBAC.[4]

Prior Vaginal Delivery

- Prior vaginal delivery, either before or after a prior CD, appears to be highly protective against uterine rupture in the setting of TOLAC.

Uterine Closure Technique

- No association between the number of layers closed and uterine rupture has been found.[9] Thus it remains unclear whether the single-layer closure technique increases the risk for rupture.

Interpregnancy Interval

- No increased risk for uterine rupture with an interdelivery interval of less than 18 months.[10]

Induction Of Labor

- The risk for uterine rupture for women undergoing induction is elevated nearly threefold. Although the attributable risk of rupture related to labor induction is relatively small (1.0% vs. 0.4%), those with only one prior low transverse cesarean delivery showed an increase in uterine rupture compared with those undergoing induction who had no prior vaginal delivery. There is no increased risk of uterine rupture with labor induction among women who had a TOLAC with a history of prior vaginal delivery.
- The need for cervical ripening does seem to affect the frequency of uterine rupture. However, it remains unclear whether induction increases the risk for uterine rupture in comparison to expectant management—the clinical alternative for women who desire a TOLAC.
- Conflicting data have also been reported concerning whether various induction methods increase the risk for uterine rupture (Table 20.2). At present, based on the limited data that do exist, ACOG suggests that misoprostol (prostaglandin E_1) not be used for third-trimester cervical ripening or labor induction in women who have had a CD and that sequential use of prostaglandin E_2 and oxytocin be avoided in women undergoing TOLAC.

TABLE 20.2 ■ Risk for Uterine Rupture After Labor Induction

| | Study | | |
	Lydon-Rochelle et al[17]	Landon et al[1]	Dekker et al[18]
All inductions	24/2326 (1.0)	48/4708 (1.0)	16/1867 (0.9)
Spontaneous	56/10,789 (0.5)	24/6685 (0.4)	16/8221 (0.2)
Prostaglandins	9/366 (2.5)	0/227 (0.0)	4/586 (0.7)
Prostaglandin and oxytocin	—	13/926 (1.4)	4/226 (1.8)

Labor Augmentation

- Data as to whether oxytocin used for labor augmentation during TOLAC in contemporary obstetric practice is associated with an increased risk of uterine rupture are conflicting.
- There is a possible dose-response relationship between maximal oxytocin dose and the risk for rupture among women who attempt TOLAC. Thus oxytocin may be used in women undergoing TOLAC, although higher infusion rates should be used with caution.

Sonographic Evaluation of the Uterine Scar

- Ultrasound measurement of the thickness of residual myometrium in the lower uterine segment as well as the width, depth, and length of the hypoechoic interface at the site of the prior cesarean have been assessed but appear to be no value in clinical practice to predict the integrity of the uterine scar during labor.

Other Risks Associated With a Trial of Labor After Cesarean Delivery

- Maternal death attributable to uterine rupture is exceedingly rare, and in the population of the MFMU Cesarean Registry, maternal death was not significantly more common with planned repeat cesarean delivery.[1] However, the study was not powered to detect a difference between this group and women attempting a TOLAC.

MANAGEMENT OF A TRIAL OF LABOR AFTER CESAREAN

- The optimal management of labor in women undergoing a TOLAC is based on not randomized trials but primarily on opinion.
- Continuous electronic fetal monitoring is recommended and studies that have examined fetal heart rate patterns before uterine rupture consistently report that nonreassuring signs, particularly prolonged decelerations or bradycardia, are the most common finding accompanying uterine rupture.[11, 12]
- Epidural analgesia is not a contraindicated in the setting of TOLAC and does not appear to affect success rates.[5]
- Because uterine rupture may be a catastrophic event, ACOG continues to recommend that it is optimal to attempt TOLAC in institutions equipped to respond to emergencies, with physicians immediately available to provide emergency care.

COUNSELING FOR TOLAC

- Regardless of the approach to delivery, a pregnant woman with a previous CD is at risk for both maternal and perinatal complications. Complications associated with both procedures should be discussed, and an attempt should be made to include an individualized risk assessment for the likelihood of successful VBAC (Box 20.1).

BOX 20.1 ■ Risks Associated With Trial of Labor After Cesarean Delivery

Uterine Rupture and Related Morbidity

Uterine rupture (0.5-1.0/100)
Perinatal death and/or encephalopathy (0.5/1000)
Hysterectomy (0.3/1000)

Increased Maternal Morbidity With Failed TOLAC

Transfusion
Endometritis
Length of stay

Other Risks With TOLAC

Potential risk for perinatal asphyxia with labor (cord prolapse, abruption)
Potential risk for antepartum stillbirth beyond 39 weeks' gestation

---

TOLAC, trial of labor after cesarean.

- It is essential to make an effort to obtain records of the prior CD to ascertain the previous uterine incision type. This is particularly relevant to cases in which it is more likely that a non–low transverse uterine incision was used.
- Based on the available evidence, TOLAC should continue to remain an option for most women with a prior CD, particularly when the low absolute risks that accompany TOLAC are considered. The attributable risk for a serious adverse perinatal outcome (perinatal death or hypoxic-ischemic encephalopathy) at term appears to be about 1 per 2000 TOLACs.
- Combining an independent risk for hysterectomy attributable to uterine rupture at term with the risk for newborn HIE indicates the chance of one of these adverse events occurring to be about 1 in 1250 cases.
- Following informed consent detailing the most relevant risks and benefits for the individual woman, the delivery plan should be formulated using a shared decision-making process by both the patient and physician. There should be clear recognition that this plan may change depending on clinical circumstances including events during the labor process.

Cost-Effectiveness of TOLAC

- TOLAC was found to be cost effective over a wide variety of circumstances, even when women had a probability of VBAC as low as 43%.

🔵 *References for this chapter are available at ExpertConsult.com.*

CHAPTER 21

Placenta Accreta

Eric R.M. Jauniaux ■ Amar Bhide ■ Jason D. Wright

KEY POINTS

- Prior CD is the most important factor associated with PA, and the risk of PA increases with the number of prior CDs.
- Suspected PA on prenatal imaging allows planned management of the condition and has been associated with a reduced rate of maternal morbidity.
- Ultrasound imaging is superior to MRI for routine screening of PA in at-risk women, but the degree of invasion to adjacent pelvic tissues and organs may be better ascertained with MRI.
- The optimum time for planned delivery for a woman with suspected PA and placenta previa is approximately 34 weeks, following a course of corticosteroid injections.
- When a PA is suspected, it is best to avoid disturbing the placenta and to leave it attached at the time of cesarean delivery.
- The role of interventional radiology at the time of primary caesarean delivery and hysterectomy remains uncertain.
- A pregnancy following a previous PA that was treated with conservative management is at increased risk for adverse maternal outcomes such as recurrent PA, uterine rupture, PPH, and peripartum hysterectomy.

Overview

- The term *placenta increta* is used to describe deep myometrial invasion by trophoblast villi; *placenta percreta* refers to villi perforating through the full thickness of the myometrium and uterine serosa with possible involvement of adjacent organs. The difference between placenta accreta, increta, and percreta is related to the extent of invasion, and the umbrella term *disorders of invasive placentation* is used to encompass all three (Fig. 21.1).
- When placenta accreta (PA) is present, the failure of the entire placenta to separate normally from the uterine wall after delivery is typically accompanied by severe postpartum hemorrhage.

Pathogenesis

- Total or partial absence of decidua is the characteristic histologic feature of PA and is relatively clear-cut in cases of implantation on a uterine scar. This results in the absence of the normal plane of cleavage above the decidua basalis, thus preventing placental separation after delivery.

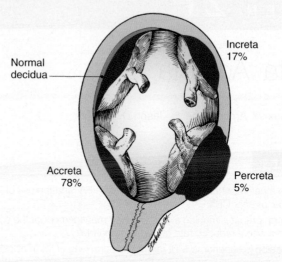

Fig. 21.1 Uteroplacental relationships found with invasive placentation.

BOX 21.1 ■ Primary and Secondary Uterine Pathologies Associated With Placenta Accreta

Primary Uterine Pathology

  Major uterine anomalies
  Adenomyosis
  Submucous uterine fibroids
  Myotonic dystrophy

Secondary Uterine Pathology

  Cesarean delivery
  Uterine curettage
  Manual removal of the placenta
  Cavity-entering myomectomy
  Hysteroscopic surgery (endometrial resection)
  In vitro fertilization procedures
  Uterine artery embolization
  Chemotherapy and radiotherapy

Epidemiology

- With the rapid increase in the incidence of cesarean delivery (CD) over the past several decades, this procedure has become associated with most cases of PA, whereas other factors are now responsible for a relatively small proportion of PA (Box 21.1).

ULTRASOUND IMAGING

- Ultrasound has become the primary screening tool for women at risk of PA. Grayscale ultrasound features suggestive of PA include the loss of the myometrial interface or retroplacental clear space, reduced myometrial thickness, and chaotic intraplacental blood flow and intraplacental lacunae (Figs. 21.2 to 21.5).
- The most common sonographic finding associated with PA is the loss of myometrial interface with enlargement of the underlying uterine vasculature.

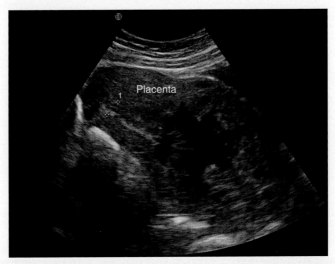

Fig. 21.2 Transabdominal grayscale ultrasound longitudinal view of the lower uterine segment at 10 weeks' gestation in a patient with placenta previa major covering the cervix. The basal plate is missing, over an area of 3 cm in diameter, and the placental tissue above it is distorted by a large intervillous lake or lacuna.

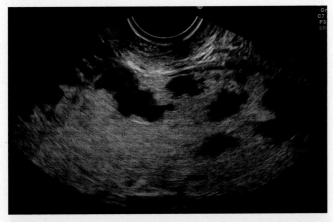

Fig. 21.3 Transvaginal grayscale ultrasound longitudinal view of the lower uterine segment at 22 weeks' gestation in a patient with placenta previa major covering the cervix. The basal plate is missing, and the placental anatomy is distorted by large intervillous lakes, or lacunae, which gives the placenta a "moth-eaten" appearance.

MAGNETIC RESONANCE IMAGING

- The degree of invasion to adjacent pelvic tissues and organs may be better ascertained with MRI than with ultrasound.

Management

- Delivery at approximately 34 weeks of gestation among women with a placenta previa and suspected PA, even without confirmation of fetal lung maturity, is the gestational age associated with optimal overall maternal and perinatal outcomes.

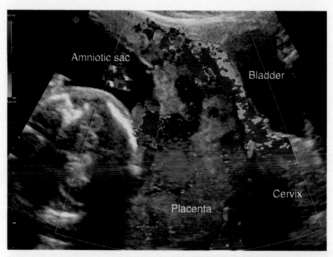

Fig. 21.4 Transabdominal color mapping ultrasound longitudinal view of the lower uterine segment at 20 weeks' gestation in a patient with anterior placenta previa covering the cervix after previous cesarean delivery and a delivery defect detected before pregnancy showing chaotic intraplacental blood flow, the presence of altered blood flow in the retroplacental space, and aberrant vessels crossing between placental surfaces.

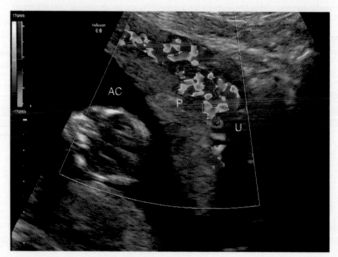

Fig. 21.5 Transabdominal color mapping ultrasound longitudinal view of the lower uterine segment at 38 weeks' gestation in a patient with anterior placenta previa after previous cesarean delivery showing the presence of altered blood flow in the retroplacental space and aberrant vessels crossing between placental surfaces. AC, amniotic cavity; P, placenta; U, uterus.

- Women with placenta accreta, increta, or percreta for whom no attempt is made to remove any part of their placenta have reduced levels of hemorrhage and a reduced need for blood transfusion.
- Women with PA managed by a multidisciplinary care team, compared with standard obstetric care, are less likely to require large-volume blood transfusion and reoperation within 7 days of delivery for bleeding complications.

SURGICAL MANAGEMENT

- Hysterectomy remains the most commonly performed procedure for the control of postpartum hemorrhage (PPH; see Chapter 20).
- Prior to skin incision, blood products should be made available (see Chapter 18).
- The role of interventional radiology at the time of primary CD and hysterectomy remains uncertain.
- The genitourinary tract is at substantial risk for injury during these procedures.
- Retrograde ureteral stents can be placed via cystoscopy to facilitate ureteral identification.

CONSERVATIVE MANAGEMENT

- The conservative surgical approach often involves the use of a fundal/classical incision to deliver the fetus without disturbing the placenta. The uterine incision is closed after delivery, and the placenta is left in situ.
- The utility of embolization and balloon occlusion catheters remains controversial, and it has not been demonstrated that the routine use of these interventions has benefits that outweigh the risks.

REPRODUCTIVE OUTCOMES FOLLOWING PLACENTA ACCRETA

- Women are at increased risk for adverse maternal outcomes that include recurrent PA, uterine rupture, PPH, and peripartum hysterectomy.

References for this chapter are available at **ExpertConsult.com.**

PART IV

Postpartum Care

CHAPTER 22

The Neonate

Paul J. Rozance ■ Adam A. Rosenberg

KEY POINTS

- Surfactant maintains lung expansion on expiration by lowering surface tension at the air-liquid interface in the alveolus.
- Antenatal corticosteroids accelerate fetal lung maturation and decrease neonatal mortality and RDS in preterm infants. In addition, corticosteroids are associated with a decrease in intracranial hemorrhage and necrotizing enterocolitis.
- Transition from intrauterine to extrauterine life requires removal of fluid from the lungs, switching from fetal to neonatal circulation
- The most important step in neonatal resuscitation is to achieve adequate expansion of the lungs.
- Meconium aspiration syndrome is likely the result of intrauterine asphyxia with mortality related to associated persistent pulmonary hypertension.
- The best predictor of neurologic sequelae of birth asphyxia is the presence of hypoxic-ischemic encephalopathy in the neonatal period. The neurologic sequelae of birth asphyxia is CP. However, the great majority of CP is of unknown origin or has some etiology other than perinatal asphyxia.
- The major neurologic complications seen in premature infants are periventricular hemorrhage/intraventricular hemorrhage and periventricular leukomalacia.
- Hypoglycemia is a predictable and preventable complication in the newborn.
- With improved methods of neonatal intensive care, survival has increased—in particular for infants weighing less than 1000 g—but it comes at the price of medical and neurodevelopmental sequelae.

Cardiopulmonary Transition

PULMONARY DEVELOPMENT

- Five stages of morphologic lung development have been identified in the human fetus.[1]
- Several million alveoli will form before birth, which emphasizes the importance of the last few weeks of pregnancy to pulmonary adaptation.
- Because of the development of high surface forces along the respiratory epithelium when breathing begins, the availability of surfactants in terminal airspaces is critical to postnatal lung function. As the radius of the alveolus decreases, surfactant serves to reduce surface tension, which prevents collapse of the alveolus.
- Surfactant deficiency is characterized by high opening pressure, low maximal lung volume, and lack of deflation stability at low pressures.

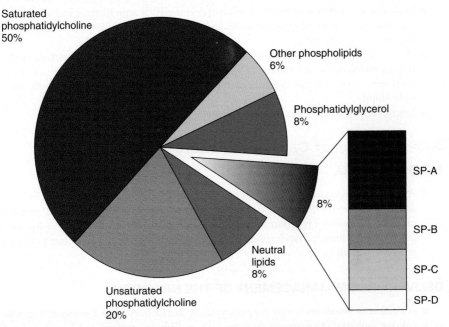

Fig. 22.1 Composition of pulmonary surfactant. SP, surfactant protein. (*Modified from Jobe AH. Lung development and maturation. In Fanaroff AA, Martin RJ [eds]:* Neonatal-Perinatal Medicine: Diseases of the Fetus and Infant, *7th ed. St Louis: Mosby; 2002:973.*)

- Natural surfactant contains mostly lipids, phospholipids specifically, and some protein (Fig. 22.1).
- A significant reduction of about 50% in the incidence of respiratory distress syndrome (RDS) is seen in infants born to mothers who received antenatal corticosteroids. The effects of antenatal corticosteroids and postnatal surfactant appear to be additive in terms of decreasing the severity of RDS and the mortality caused by it.[2]

FETAL BREATHING

- Respiratory activity is essential to the development of chest wall muscles, including the diaphragm, and serves as a regulator of lung fluid volume and thus lung growth.

MECHANICS OF THE FIRST BREATH

- With its first breaths, the neonate must overcome several forces that resist lung expansion: (1) viscosity of fetal lung fluid, (2) resistance provided by lung tissue itself, and (3) the forces of surface tension at the air-liquid interface.
- Normal expansion and aeration of the neonatal lung is dependent on removal of fetal lung liquid.[3] Once labor is initiated, a reversal of liquid flow occurs across the lung epithelium.

CIRCULATORY TRANSITION

- The diversion of right ventricular output away from the lungs through the ductus arteriosus is caused by the high pulmonary vascular resistance (PVR) in the fetus.

- With delivery, a variety of factors interact to decrease PVR acutely; these include mechanical ventilation, increased oxygen tension, and the production of endothelium-derived relaxing factor or nitric oxide.
- With occlusion of the umbilical cord, the low-resistance placental circulation is interrupted, which causes an increase in systemic pressure. This coupled with the decrease in PVR serves to reverse the shunt through the ductus arteriosus to a predominantly left-to-right shunt.
- Ductal closure occurs in two phases: constriction and anatomic occlusion.

Abnormalities of Cardiopulmonary Transition

BIRTH ASPHYXIA

- A variety of circumstances can result in respiratory depression in the infant, including (1) acute interruption of umbilical blood flow, as occurs during cord compression; (2) premature placental separation; (3) maternal hypotension or hypoxia; (4) any of the above-mentioned problems superimposed on chronic uteroplacental insufficiency; and (5) failure to execute a proper resuscitation.

DELIVERY ROOM MANAGEMENT OF THE NEWBORN

- A number of situations during pregnancy, labor, and delivery place the infant at increased risk for asphyxia: (1) maternal diseases, such as diabetes mellitus and hypertension; (2) fetal conditions, such as prematurity, growth restriction, fetal anomalies; and (3) conditions related to labor and delivery, including fetal distress, breech presentation, and administration of anesthetics and analgesics.
- The steps in the resuscitation process are described by the American Heart Association and American Academy of Pediatrics.[4]
- Most neonates can be effectively resuscitated with a bag and face mask.
- Normal healthy term infants require approximately 10 to 15 minutes to achieve oxygen saturations above 90%. Overall, 2% to 9% of children born through meconium-stained fluid are diagnosed with meconium aspiration.

SEQUELAE OF BIRTH ASPHYXIA

- The incidence of birth asphyxia is about 0.1% in term infants. Hypothermia (whole-body or selective head cooling) improves outcomes at 6 to 7 years of age.
- Low Apgar scores at 1 and 5 minutes are not predictive, but infants with low scores that persist at 15 and 20 minutes after birth have a 50% chance of manifesting cerebral palsy (CP) if they survive. Cord pH is predictive of adverse outcome only if the pH is less than 7. The best predictor of outcome is the severity of the neonatal neurologic syndrome.[5]
- To attribute CP to peripartum asphyxia, there must be an absence of other demonstrable causes, substantial or prolonged intrapartum asphyxia (fetal heart rate abnormalities, fetal acidosis), and clinical evidence during the first days of life of neurologic dysfunction in the infant (Box 22.1).

Birth Injuries

- Factors that predispose to birth injury include macrosomia, cephalopelvic disproportion, shoulder dystocia, prolonged or difficult labor, precipitous delivery, abnormal presentations (including breech), and use of operative vaginal delivery.

BOX 22.1 ■ Relationship of Intrapartum Events and Cerebral Palsy

Neonatal Signs Consistent With an Acute Peripartum or Intrapartum Event
- Evidence of a metabolic acidemia in fetal umbilical cord arterial blood obtained at delivery (pH <7.00 and base deficit ≥12 mmol/L)
- Apgar score of <5 at 5 and 10 minutes
- Neuroimaging evidence of acute brain injury seen on brain magnetic resonance imaging or magnetic resonance spectroscopy consistent with hypoxia-ischemia
- Presence of multisystem organ failure consistent with hypoxic-ischemic encephalopathy

Type and Timing of Contributing Factors Consistent With an Acute Peripartum or Intrapartum Event
- Sentinel hypoxic or ischemic event occurring immediately before or during labor and delivery such as a severe placental abruption
- Fetal heart rate monitor patterns consistent with an acute peripartum or intrapartum event
- Timing and type of brain injury patterns based on imaging studies consistent with an etiology of an acute peripartum or intrapartum event
- No evidence of other proximal or distal factors that could be contributing factors
- Developmental outcome is spastic quadriplegia or dyskinetic cerebral palsy

Modified from American College of Obstetricians and Gynecologists (ACOG), American Academy of Pediatrics (AAP). *Neonatal Encephalopathy and Neurologic Outcome.* Washington DC: ACOG; 2014.

- Primary subarachnoid hemorrhage is the most common variety of neonatal intracranial hemorrhage.
- Brachial plexus injuries are caused by stretching of the cervical roots during delivery, usually when shoulder dystocia is present. Upper arm palsy (Erb-Duchenne paralysis), the most common brachial plexus injury, is caused by injury to the fifth and sixth cervical nerves; lower arm paralysis (Klumpke paralysis) results from damage to the eighth cervical and first thoracic nerves.

Neonatal Thermal Regulation

- The range of environmental temperatures over which the neonate can survive is narrower than that of an adult. This range narrows with decreasing gestational age.
- Nonshivering thermogenesis is the most important means of increased heat production in the cold-stressed newborn.
- Heat transfer from the surface to the environment involves four routes: radiation, convection, conduction, and evaporation.

Clinical Applications

DELIVERY ROOM

- Room temperature can be elevated as an added precaution for the low-birthweight (LBW) infant.

NURSERY

- Adequate thermal protection of the LBW infant is essential.
- The most economical means of thermal support for the LBW infant is skin-to-skin contact with a parent.

Infant Feeding

- Breast milk remains the standard on which formulas are based. Breast milk's immuno-chemical and cellular components provide protection against infection.

NEONATAL HYPOGLYCEMIA

- Glucose falls over the first 1 to 2 hours after birth. *Low glucose* concentrations can be defined as less than 45 mg/dL. Infants at risk for low blood glucose concentrations and in whom glucose should be monitored include preterm infants, small for gestational age (SGA) infants, hyperinsulinemic infants (infant of a diabetic mother), large for gestational age (LGA) infants, and infants with perinatal stress or asphyxia. Because of the risk of subsequent brain injury, hypoglycemia should be aggressively treated.

NECROTIZING ENTEROCOLITIS

- This is the most common acquired gastrointestinal emergency in the NICU.
- Antenatal betamethasone may decrease the incidence.

NEONATAL JAUNDICE

- The most common problem encountered in a term nursery population is jaundice.
- Pathologic jaundice during the early neonatal period is indirect hyperbilirubinemia.
- Recent descriptions of bilirubin encephalopathy in breastfed infants, and in late preterm infants in particular, with dehydration and hyperbilirubinemia in whom an adequate supply of breast milk has not been established mandates close follow-up of all breastfeeding mothers.

Neonatal Hematology

ANEMIA

- Normal hemoglobin levels at term range from 13.7 to 20.1 g/dL.

POLYCYTHEMIA

- Although 50% of polycythemic infants are average for gestational age, the proportion of polycythemic infants is greater in the SGA and LGA populations.

THROMBOCYTOPENIA

- Neonatal thrombocytopenia can be isolated or it can occur associated with deficiency of clotting factors.
- Vitamin K_1 oxide (1 mg) should be given intramuscularly to all newborns to prevent hemorrhagic disease caused by a deficiency in vitamin K–dependent clotting factors (II, VII, IX, X).

Perinatal Infection

EARLY-ONSET BACTERIAL INFECTION

- Maternal colonization with group B *Streptococcus*, rupture of membranes for more than 12 to 18 hours, and chorioamnionitis increase the risk of infection.[6]

Respiratory Distress

- The presentation of respiratory distress is among the most common symptom complexes seen in the newborn and may be secondary to both noncardiopulmonary and cardiopulmonary etiologies (Table 22.1).
- The two presentations of serious structural heart disease in the first week of life are cyanosis and congestive heart failure. It is now recommended that all newborns have pulse oximetry screening at 24 hours to identify critical heart disease.
- The lungs represent the most common primary site of infection in the neonate.
- Hyaline membrane disease remains the most common etiology for respiratory distress in the neonatal period. The major long-term consequences are chronic lung disease that requires prolonged ventilator and oxygen therapy and includes bronchopulmonary dysplasia and significant neurologic impairment.

TABLE 22.1 ■ **Respiratory Distress in the Newborn**

Noncardiopulmonary	Cardiovascular	Pulmonary
Hypothermia or hyperthermia	Left-sided outflow obstruction	Upper airway obstruction
Hypoglycemia	Hypoplastic left heart	Choanal atresia
Metabolic acidosis	Aortic stenosis	Vocal cord paralysis
Drug intoxications, withdrawal	Coarctation of the aorta	Meconium aspiration
Polycythemia	Cyanotic lesions	Clear fluid aspiration
Central nervous system insult	Transposition of the great vessels	Transient tachypnea
Asphyxia	Total anomalous pulmonary venous return	Pneumonia
Hemorrhage	Tricuspid atresia	Pulmonary hypoplasia
Neuromuscular disease	Right-sided outflow obstruction	Primary
Werdnig-Hoffman disease		Secondary
Myopathies		Hyaline membrane disease
Phrenic nerve injury		Pneumothorax
Skeletal abnormalities		Pleural effusions
Asphyxiating thoracic dystrophy		Mass lesions
		Lobar emphysema
		Cystic adenomatoid malformation

INTRAVENTRICULAR HEMORRHAGE AND PERIVENTRICULAR LEUKOMALACIA

- Periventricular/intraventricular hemorrhage and periventricular leukomalacia are the most common neurologic complications of prematurity.
- The other important clinical correlate with periventricular leukomalacia is maternal chorioamnionitis and neonatal infection.
- Antenatal corticosteroids decrease the frequency of these complications and likely represent the most important antenatal strategy to prevent intracranial hemorrhage.[7]

Nursery Care

- *Level I nurseries* care for infants presumed healthy, with an emphasis on screening and surveillance.
- *Level II nurseries* can care for infants at more than 32 weeks' gestation who weigh at least 1500 g but who require special attention but will probably not need subspecialty services.
- *Level III nurseries* care for all newborn infants who are critically ill regardless of the level of support required.

CARE OF THE PARENTS

- Klaus and Kennell have outlined the steps in maternal-infant attachment. The 60- to 90-minute period after delivery is a very important time. Mothers with high-risk pregnancies are at increased risk for subsequent parenting problems.

KANGAROO CARE

- In the LBW population (<2500 g), kangaroo care improves rates of mortality, nosocomial infection/sepsis, and length of hospital stay.

Outcome of Neonatal Intensive Care and Threshold of Viability

- Predictions of survival can be significantly improved by consideration of clinical data in addition to birthweight and gestational age. Data from the National Institute of Child Health and Human Development can be referenced as well.
- The rate of severe neurologic disability is fairly constant at 10% of all very-LBW survivors from 1000 to 1500 g.
- If the end point of survival without major disability is considered, this occurs in 0% at 22 weeks, less than 10% at 23 weeks, approximately 20% to 25% at 24 weeks, and approximately 45% to 50% at 25 weeks.[8]

Late Preterm Infant

- Compared with term infants, late preterm infants have a higher mortality and prevalence of acute neonatal problems that include respiratory distress, temperature instability, hypoglycemia, apnea, jaundice, and feeding difficulties.

References for this chapter are available at ExpertConsult.com.

CHAPTER 23

Postpartum Care and Long-Term Health Considerations

Michelle M. Isley ■ Vern L. Katz

KEY POINTS

- By 6 weeks postpartum, only 28% of women have returned to their prepregnant weight.
- About 50% of parturients experience diminished sexual desire during the 3 months that follow delivery.
- Postpartum uterine bleeding of sufficient quantity to require medical attention occurs in 1% to 2% of parturients. Of patients who require curettage, 40% will be found to have retained placental tissue.
- Long-acting reversible contraceptive methods are the most effective contraceptive available and are safe methods for postpartum women, including those who are breastfeeding.
- In nonbreastfeeding postpartum women, combined hormonal contraceptive methods (pill, patch, ring) should not be used prior to 21 days because of the risk of venous thromboembolism; in postpartum women with additional risk factors, combined hormonal contraceptives should not be used until after 42 days.
- Breastfeeding results in 98% contraceptive protection when the woman is exclusively breastfeeding on demand both day and night, is amenorrheic, and the infant is less than 6 months old.
- Progestin-only contraceptives do not diminish lactation performance.
- Postpartum major depression occurs in 8% to 20% of parturients; if possible, risk factors should be considered to identify patients for increased screening and surveillance.
- Puerperal hypothyroidism often presents with symptoms that include mild dysphoria; consequently, thyroid function studies are suggested in the evaluation of patients with suspected postpartum depression that occurs 2 to 3 months after delivery.

Physiologic Changes

UTERUS

- The specific time course of uterine involution has not been fully elucidated, but within 2 weeks after birth the uterus has usually returned to the pelvis; by 6 weeks, it is usually normal size as estimated by palpation.
- Hemostasis immediately after birth is accomplished by arterial smooth muscle contraction and compression of vessels by the involuting uterine muscle.
- Frequently, a sudden but transient increase is observed in uterine bleeding between 7 and 14 days postpartum. Although it can be profuse, this bleeding episode is usually self-limited and requires nothing more than reassurance of the patient.

- In cases of abnormal postpartum bleeding, ultrasound examination may be a useful adjunct in detecting patients who have retained tissue or clot and who will therefore benefit from uterine evacuation and curettage.

OVARIAN FUNCTION

- Ovulation occurs as early as 27 days after delivery, with the mean time being about 70 to 75 days in nonlactating women. Among women who are breastfeeding their infants, the mean time to ovulation is about 6 months.
- In a woman exclusively breastfeeding, the likelihood of ovulation within the first 6 months postpartum is 1% to 5%.

WEIGHT LOSS

- For most women, weight loss postpartum does not tend to compensate for weight gain during gestation. By 6 weeks postpartum, only 28% of women will have returned to their prepregnant weight.

THYROID FUNCTION

- Postpartum thyroiditis (PPT) is an autoimmune disease that may present with hyperthyroid or hypothyroid symptoms, and it occurs in 2% to 17% of women with a mean incidence of about 10%. PPT occurs in up to 25% of women with type 1 diabetes.
- From 5% to 30% of women with PPT eventually develop hypothyroidism.

CARDIOVASCULAR SYSTEM, IMMUNITY, AND COAGULATION

- Even 1 year after delivery, a significantly higher cardiac output was observed in both nulliparous and multiparous women compared with prepregnancy values.
- A large multicenter study[1] over a 4.5-year period in California found that in 1,688,000 primiparous deliveries, the incidence of thrombotic events was higher in the first 6 weeks after delivery compared with the same period 1 year later (odds ratio, 10.8; 95% confidence interval, 7.8 to 15.1).
- Autoimmune thyroiditis, multiple sclerosis, and lupus erythematosus are examples of some of the diseases that may show an increase in disease activity in the first few months postpartum.

URINARY TRACT AND RENAL FUNCTION

- Because of the variable changes in renal clearance, mothers who take medications whose dosages have been changed because of the physiologic adaptations of pregnancy will need to have medication levels rechecked. This should be done at 4 to 6 weeks postpartum.

Management of the Puerperium

- Home nursing visits can be helpful in providing support, education, and advice to mothers in selected situations.
- Before discharge, women should be offered any vaccines that may be necessary to protect immunity.

- As recommended in 2012 by the Centers for Disease Control and Prevention, Tdap should be administered during pregnancy to all pregnant women, regardless of the interval since the last Tdap.[2] If Tdap was not given during pregnancy, it should be given immediately after delivery. The varicella vaccine should be initiated postpartum in those with a negative varicella titer.
- Physical activity such as walking up and down stairs, lifting moderately heavy objects, riding in or driving a car, and performing muscle-toning exercises can be resumed without delay if the delivery has been uncomplicated.
- Sexual activity may be resumed when the perineum is comfortable and when bleeding has diminished.
- Cesarean delivery is associated with a decreased incidence of dyspareunia compared with vaginal birth only for the first 6 months, after which the rates become similar.
- Similar to the return to exercise and sexual activity, the return to work should be individualized.

Health Maintenance

- The postpartum visit is scheduled at the time of discharge and routinely occurs 4 to 6 weeks after delivery. Some women may benefit from a visit sooner, such as women at risk for depression, those with a more complicated labor and delivery, and women who underwent a cesarean section for delivery.
- At the routine postpartum visit, questions regarding depression, energy, sexuality, contraception, and future pregnancies should be addressed.
- Women with chronic medical diseases such as collagen vascular disease, autoimmune disorders, and neurologic conditions should be considered for visits at closer intervals because many patients with these disorders experience flare-ups of their symptoms after delivery.

PERINEAL AND PELVIC CARE

- Urinary and anal incontinence is a significant problem in women after delivery.
- If symptoms of either urinary or flatal incontinence persist for more than 6 months, evaluation should be undertaken to define the specific neuromuscular or anatomic abnormality so that the appropriate treatment can be initiated.

DELAYED POSTPARTUM HEMORRHAGE AND POSTPARTUM ANEMIA

- Delayed postpartum uterine bleeding of sufficient volume to require medical attention occurs in 1% to 2% of patients. One of the most common causes of postpartum hemorrhage seen 2 to 5 days after delivery is von Willebrand disease.
- In the management of patients with heavy delayed bleeding, ultrasound examination can be used to help determine whether a significant amount of retained material is present, although it is sometimes difficult to distinguish between blood clot and retained placental fragments (Fig. 23.1).

POSTPARTUM INFECTION

- The most common cause of postpartum fever is endometritis, which occurs after vaginal delivery in about 2% of patients and after cesarean delivery in about 10% to 15%.

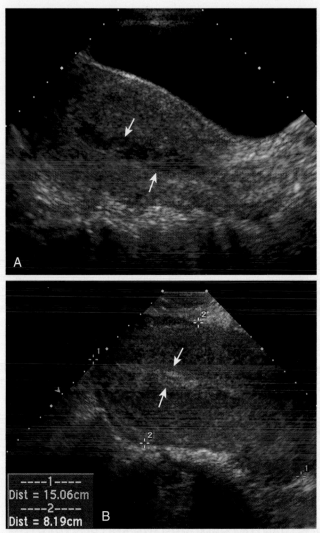

Fig. 23.1 **A,** Sonogram of a normal postpartum uterus. **B,** Postpartum uterus with retained tissue. (*From Poder L. Ultrasound evaluation of the Uterus. In Callen PW:* Ultrasonography in Obstetrics and Gynecology, *5th ed. Philadelphia: Saunders; 2000:939, 940.*)

MATERNAL-INFANT ATTACHMENT

■ It is now recognized that constant opportunities should be provided for parents to be with their newborns, particularly from the first few moments after birth and as frequently as possible during the first days thereafter. Immediate skin-to-skin contact is recommended.

■ Delaying the first bath, eliminating well-baby nurseries, putting the baby onto the mother's chest in skin-to-skin contact (even during cesarean delivery), and keeping the baby in the room with the mother during the first pediatric evaluation are all steps to support and promote that interaction.

Pregnancy Prevention

- A recent meta-analysis found that birth intervals shorter than 18 months are significantly associated with small size for gestational age, preterm birth, and infant death in the first year of life.[3]
- If a woman is exclusively breastfeeding on demand both day and night, is amenorrheic, and the infant is less than 6 months old, the contraceptive efficacy of lactational amenorrhea is 98%.

LONG-ACTING REVERSIBLE CONTRACEPTION

- Long-acting reversible contraception methods, which include intrauterine devices and contraceptive implants, are the most effective reversible methods available to women, with failure rates of less than 1%.
- The use of a single-rod implant in postpartum women does not result in changes in milk volume, milk constituents, or infant growth rates.

INJECTABLE CONTRACEPTION

- Use of depot medroxyprogesterone acetate immediately after delivery does not result in higher rates of postpartum depression.

ORAL HORMONAL CONTRACEPTION

- In nonbreastfeeding postpartum women, combined hormonal contraceptive methods (pill, patch, ring) should not be used prior to 21 days because of the risk of venous thromboembolism; in postpartum women with additional risk factors, combined hormonal contraceptives should not be used until after 42 days.
- Progestin-only contraceptives do not diminish lactation performance.

STERILIZATION

- Male and female sterilization are the most frequently used methods of contraception in the United States, used by 37% of all contraceptive users.
- Obstetricians must remember that vasectomy is often a more advisable and desirable alternative for a couple considering sterilization.
- Most women who choose sterilization do not regret their decision.

BARRIER METHODS

- Because of the physical changes of pregnancy and delivery, a diaphragm should not be fitted until 6 weeks postpartum.

NATURAL FAMILY PLANNING METHODS

- Typical use failure rates for natural family planning methods range from 12% to 25%.

Postpartum Psychological Reactions

- The psychological reactions experienced following childbirth include the common, relatively mild physiologic and transient "maternity blues" (occurring in 50% to 70% of women), true depression (occurring in 8% to 20% of women), and frank puerperal psychosis (occurring in 0.14% to 0.26% of women).

- When a patient and her family experience a loss associated with a pregnancy, special attention must be given to the grieving patient and her family.

POSTPARTUM POSTTRAUMATIC STRESS DISORDER

- Posttraumatic stress disorder may occur after any physical or psychological trauma. The disorder commonly occurs after a labor and delivery experience in which a woman is confronted with circumstances (pain, loss, trauma) that her defenses or sense of well-being cannot overcome.
- Whenever an emergency procedure is indicated, debriefing afterward—both early and a few weeks later—may help to decrease the incidence of this problem.

References for this chapter are available at ExpertConsult.com.

CHAPTER 24

Lactation and Breastfeeding

Edward R. Newton

KEY POINTS

- The WHO, the U.S. Surgeon General, the American Academy of Pediatrics, the American Academy of Family Practice, ACOG, and the Academy of Breastfeeding Medicine endorse breastfeeding as the gold standard for infant feeding.[1,2]
- Breastfeeding accrues many health benefits for the infant, including protection against infection, fewer allergies, better growth, better neurologic development, and lower rates of chronic diseases, such as type 1 diabetes and childhood cancer.
- Breastfeeding accrues more health benefits for the mother, including faster postpartum involution, improved postpartum weight loss, less premenopausal breast cancer, lower rates of cardiovascular disease, less type 2 diabetes mellitus, and better mother-infant bonding. Breastfeeding also decreases the economic burden.
- Formula lacks key components of breast milk, including defenses against infection, hormones and enzymes to aid digestion, polyunsaturated fatty acids necessary for optimal brain growth, and adequate composition for efficient digestion.
- Prolactin is the major promoter of milk synthesis, and oxytocin is the major initiator of milk ejection. The release of prolactin and oxytocin results from the stimulation of the sensory nerves that supply the areola and nipple.
- Oxytocin released from the posterior pituitary can be operantly conditioned and is influenced negatively by pain, stress, or loss of self-esteem.
- Contact with the breast within 30 minutes of birth increases the duration of breastfeeding. A frequency of nursing greater than eight feedings per 24 hours, night nursing, and a duration of nursing longer than 15 minutes are needed to maintain adequate prolactin levels and milk supply.
- Poor lactation is the major cause of nipple injury and poor milk transfer. Perceived or real lack of milk transfer is the major reason for the discontinuation of nursing.
- Milk production is reduced by an autocrine pathway through a protein that inhibits milk production by the alveolar cells and by distention and pressure against the alveolar cells.
- Breastfeeding and breast milk are the global standard for infant feeding in undeveloped and developed countries. Exclusive breastfeeding is recommended for the first 6 months and continued breastfeeding at least through 12 months with subsequent weaning as a mutual decision by the mother and infant dyad in the subsequent months and years.
- Women of lower socioeconomic status, those with less education, and teenagers initiate breastfeeding at about half to two-thirds the rate of mature high school graduates of middle and upper socioeconomic statuses.

Breast Anatomy and Development

- The adequacy of glandular tissue for breastfeeding is ascertained by inquiring whether a woman's breasts have enlarged during pregnancy.
- The tip of the nipple contains the openings (0.4 to 0.7 mm diameter) of 15 to 20 milk ducts (2 to 4 mm diameter).
- The alveoli are the critical units in the production and ejection of milk. The alveolar cells are stimulated by prolactin to produce milk.
- The most common site for accessory breast tissue is the axilla.

Physiology of Lactation

- The physiology of lactation has three major components: (1) the stages of lactogenesis, (2) endocrinology of lactogenesis, and (3) nursing behavior/milk transfer.

STAGES OF LACTOGENESIS

- Colostrum has more protein, especially secretory immunoglobulins, and more lactose; it also has a lower fat content than mature milk.
- The secretion of milk is copious, 500 to 700 mL/day when the milk "comes in."

ENDOCRINOLOGY OF LACTOGENESIS

- The alveolar cell is the principal site for the production of milk. Glucose is the major substrate for milk production.
- Given that milk is produced during the nursing episode, variation in content during a feed is expected.
- If a woman limits feedings to less than 4 minutes but nurses more frequently, the calorie density of the milk is lower and the infant's hunger may not be satiated.
- Moderate dieting and weight loss postpartum (4.5 lb/month) are not associated with changes in milk volume, nor does aerobic exercise have any adverse effect.[3]
- By 14 days, the breast-fed infant should have returned to its birthweight.
- The prolactin and oxytocin travel to their target cells: prolactin goes to the alveolar epithelium in the breast, and oxytocin goes to the myoepithelial cells that shroud the alveolar epithelium.
- If nursing frequency is maintained the prolactin levels will suppress the luteinizing hormone surges and ovarian function. Oxytocin levels also rise with nipple stimulation.
- Uterine involution is enhanced with breastfeeding.

MILK TRANSFER

- The milk is extracted not by negative pressure but by a peristaltic wave from the tip to the base of the tongue. Audible swallowing of milk is a good sign of milk transfer.
- From 80% to 90% of the milk is obtained in the first 5 minutes the infant nurses on each breast, but the fat-rich and calorie-dense hind milk is obtained in the remainder of the time sucking at each breast, usually less than 20 minutes total.
- The football hold and side-lying positions are more comfortable when the mother has an abdominal incision.
- Breast milk has the nutritional content to satisfy the growth needs of the infant for at least 6 months postpartum.

- One of the errors in Western child care is the early, forced introduction of solids.
- Inhibition of the let-down reflex and failure to empty the breasts completely leads to ductal distention and parenchymal swelling from extravascular fluid. This is termed *engorgement*.

Breast Milk: The Gold Standard

- One of the most common misconceptions by physicians and the lay public, and marketed by the formula industry, is that "formulas" are equivalent to breast milk.

OVERVIEW

- Artificial breast milk manufacturers add constituents (e.g., palm- or coconut-based oils) to make artificial breast milk appear rich and creamy.
- Current formulas have major differences in the total quantities and qualities of proteins, carbohydrates, minerals, vitamins, and fats compared with human milk.
- Breast-fed infants have faster linear and head growth, whereas formula-fed infants tend to have greater weight gain and fat deposition.
- Regardless of the cause, formula has important adverse effects on the metabolic competence of the child, adolescent, and future adult (Table 24.1).
- Breastfeeding enhances cognitive development.[4]
- Breastfeeding enhances infant responses to infection and reduces allergic disease. The major mechanisms for the protective properties of breast milk include active leukocytes, antibodies, antibacterial products, competitive inhibition, enhancement of nonpathogenic commensal organisms, and suppression of proinflammatory immune responses.
- The neonate must rely on an innate host defense system to provide an immediate but controlled response during the first critical 7 days of breastfeeding.
- One of the most important breast milk constituents in the innate host defense system are human-specific oligosaccharides.
- Iron and vitamin B_{12} are two essential nutriments for pathogenic bacteria. The free-iron form of lactoferrin competes with siderophilic bacteria for ferric iron and thus disrupts the proliferation of these organisms.
- Hormonal changes of lactation favor a reduction in maternal reproductive cancers.

TABLE 24.1 ■ Effects of Infant Feeding on Somatic Growth and Cardiovascular Pathophysiology in Developed Countries

	Benefit of Breastfeeding Adjusted OR (95% CI)	Risk of "Formula" Adjusted OR (95% CI)
Childhood obesity	0.81 (0.77-0.84)	1.23 (1.14-1.3)
Child type 2 diabetes	0.61 (0.44-0.85)	1.64 (1.18-2.27)
Maternal cardiovascular disease	0.72 (0.53-0.97)	1.39 (1.03-1.89)
Maternal hypertension	0.87 (0.82-0.92)	1.15 (1.09-1.22)
Maternal vascular calcifications	0.19 (0.05-0.68)	5.26 (1.47-20.0)
Maternal myocardial infarction	0.77 (0.62-0.94)	1.3 (1.06-1.61)
Maternal type 2 diabetes	0.84 (0.78-0.91)	1.19 (1.10-1.28)

In general, odds ratio (OR) was adjusted for age, parity, race, and socioeconomic status.
CI, confidence interval.

- *Breastfeeding enhances mother–infant bonding and reduces poor social adaptation.*
- Infants were more likely to be breastfed if they have early skin-to-skin contact.
- Early skin-to-skin contact was a better predictor of duration of exclusive breastfeeding than the timing of the first sucking episode.[5]
- The adjusted odds ratio for maternal maltreatment cases among children fed exclusively formula was increased versus any breastfeeding.[6] Exclusive feeding with formula is associated with a dramatic increase in perceived childhood anxiety.
- Breastfeeding is cost effective for the family and society.[8] Increase in acute medical diseases will manifest as increased costs of medical care.[7–11] Data demonstrate fewer days for sick leave in women who work.

Role of the Obstetrician and Gynecologist

- Interventions that included individual-level professional support and lay counselors had the most impact.
- The 36-week visit is a good time to address medications and breastfeeding.
- In 1989, the essential 10 steps (Box 24.1) in protecting, promoting, and supporting breastfeeding were published in a joint statement by the WHO and the United Nations Children's Fund (UNICEF).[12] The WHO Ten Steps have become institutionalized in the Baby-Friendly Hospital Initiative accreditation process.
- When the obstetrician remains a verbal participant in the mother's breastfeeding experience at the 4- to 6-week postpartum visit, the likelihood that the mother will continue to breastfeed at 16 weeks is almost doubled.[13]

Focused Issues in the Successful Management of Breastfeeding

- Several issues are in the domain of the obstetric care provider: anatomic abnormalities of the breast, the impact of breast surgeries, labor and delivery management, breast milk expression, breast and nipple pain, maternal nutrition and exercise during lactation, mastitis and breast abscess and masses, milk transfer and infant growth, galactogogues, maternal disease, back-to-work issues, contraception, and weaning.

BOX 24.1 ■ 10 Steps to Successful Breastfeeding

1. Have a written policy to support breastfeeding.
2. Train all health care providers in Baby-Friendly Hospital Initiative protocols.
3. Inform all pregnant women about the benefits of breastfeeding.
4. Initiate breastfeeding within 1 hour after birth.
5. Show mothers how to express breast milk and maintain lactation even if they are separated from their infants.
6. Give newborn infants no food or drink other than breast milk unless medically indicated.
7. Allow mothers and infants to remain together 24 hours a day (i.e., rooming in).
8. Encourage breastfeeding on demand.
9. Give no artificial teats or pacifiers.
10. Foster the establishment of breastfeeding support groups and refer mothers to them on discharge from the hospital or clinic.

Modified from WHO/UNICEF. Protecting, promoting, and supporting breastfeeding: the special role of maternity services, a joint WHO/UNICEF statement. Geneva: World Health Organization; 1989.

Anatomic Abnormalities of the Breast

- Excluding inverted nipples, congenital abnormalities of the breasts are rare and occur in fewer than 1 in 1000 women. The most significant defect is glandular hypoplasia.

PREVIOUS BREAST SURGERIES

- Women who have had breast biopsy or breast or chest surgery, including augmentation, have a threefold higher incidence of unsuccessful breastfeeding.
- A circumareolar incision was the dominant predictor of insufficient lactation.
- Silicone implants have not shown excess adverse events.

Labor and Delivery Management

- Epidural anesthesia with local anesthetic agents seems to be better for breastfeeding than parenteral narcotics.
- The five basic principles of lactation physiology are (1) early imprinting, (2) frequent nursing, (3) good latch-on, (4) a confident and comfortable mother, and (5) no supplementation unless medically indicated.
- Nursing technique should be evaluated in three areas: (1) presentation and latching on, (2) maternal-infant positioning, and (3) breaking of the suction.

BREAST MILK EXPRESSION

- The mechanical, preferably electric breast pump is a critically important adaptation when breastfeeding is expected to be difficult or impossible.

Maternal Nutrition During Lactation

- The mother must consume an extra 794 kcal/day unless stored energy is used.
- The appropriate intake of vitamins can be ensured by continuing prenatal vitamins with 1 mg of folic acid throughout lactation.
- Calcium and vitamin D are of special importance in women whose infants are breastfeeding exclusively.

Breast and Nipple Pain

- Breast pain, nipple injury, and/or breast infection were the cited reasons in the majority of women who stopped breastfeeding early.
- Engorgement causes a dull, generalized discomfort in the whole breast that gets worse just before a feeding and is then relieved by it.
- The use of soaps, alcohol, and other drying agents on the nipples tends to increase nipple trauma and pain. The nipples should be air dried for a few minutes after each feeding; clean water is sufficient to cleanse the breast, if necessary.

Mastitis and Breast Abscess

- The management of mastitis includes (1) breast support, (2) intake of fluids, (3) nursing technique assessment, (4) nursing first on the uninfected side to establish let-down, (5) the infected side emptied by nursing with each feeding (a breast pump helps ensure complete drainage), and (6) dicloxacillin 250 mg every 6 hours for 14 days. Erythromycin may be used in patients allergic to penicillin.

■ The management of a breast abscess is similar to that for mastitis except that drainage of the abscess is indicated.

Milk Transfer and Infant Growth

■ A healthy and successfully breastfeeding mother can supply enough nutrition through breast milk alone for 6 months.

Jaundice in the Newborn

■ See Chapter 22.
■ It has been clearly demonstrated that feeding frequency greater than eight feedings per 24 hours is associated with lower bilirubin levels.

Galactogogues: Drugs to Improve Milk Production

■ Metoclopramide (Reglan) is used to prolactin levels. Domperidone increases prolactin levels and milk supply twofold to threefold. Sulpiride is a selective dopamine antagonist. Intranasal oxytocin has been studied in preterm deliveries.

Maternal Disease

■ The four acute infections in which breastfeeding is contraindicated are (1) herpes simplex lesions of the breast; (2) acute maternal varicella in the first 3 days of the neonate's life; (3) untreated active tuberculosis; and (4) human immunodeficiency virus disease when it occurs in developed countries.

Breast Masses During Lactation

■ The prognosis for breast cancer diagnosed during pregnancy or lactation is poorer than for breast cancer diagnosed at other times. The delay in diagnosis and the greater size at diagnosis in lactating women is a failure of the obstetric care provider and/or the lactating woman to aggressively pursue the evaluation of a breast mass.

Back-to-Work Issues

■ In March 2011, federal law amended Section 7 of the Fair Labor Standards Act to require employers to provide "reasonable break time for an employee to express breast milk for her nursing child for 1 year after the child's birth each time such employee has need to express the milk."

Contraception

■ Women not using long-acting reversible contraception were 22 times more likely to have an unintended pregnancy than women using long-acting reversible contraception.

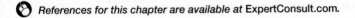 *References for this chapter are available at ExpertConsult.com.*

PART V

Complicated Pregnancy

CHAPTER 25

Surgery During Pregnancy

Nadav Schwartz ■ Jack Ludmir

KEY POINTS

- Care of the pregnant surgical patient requires a multidisciplinary approach with an understanding of the physiologic changes that accompany normal pregnancy.
- Expansion of maternal blood volume during pregnancy may mask signs of maternal hemorrhage, and clinically significant blood loss can occur before hemodynamic changes are evident.
- Delay in surgical intervention can result in increased maternal and fetal morbidity and mortality, which significantly increases the risk for preterm labor and fetal loss.
- Diagnostic doses of radiation (<5 cGy) from radiographs and CT scans are unlikely to pose any significant harm to the developing fetus. MRI and ultrasound can be safely used when appropriate to further minimize radiation exposure.
- No significant increased risk is apparent for congenital malformations in women who require nonobstetric surgery during pregnancy. Although the risk for preterm birth, low birthweight, and neonatal death may be increased, this may be due to the underlying illness rather than the surgical procedure.
- Although laparoscopy as a first approach to abdominal surgery in pregnancy seems reasonable, its safety continues to be studied. Abdominal insufflation pressures should be kept below 15 mm Hg whenever possible, and the Society of American Gastrointestinal and Endoscopic Surgeons guidelines should be followed. The use of a laparoscopic approach in the latter stages of pregnancy should be individualized based on indications and experience of the surgeon.
- Adnexal masses are commonly encountered in pregnancy, although most ovarian masses are benign. Pregnant women diagnosed with an adnexal mass should be counseled about the signs and symptoms of ovarian torsion. Surgical resection can generally be reserved for symptomatic women or for masses suspicious for malignancy.
- Data are lacking to recommend routine continuous fetal heart rate monitoring during surgery in pregnant women. In most cases, preoperative and postoperative fetal heart rate monitoring is appropriate.
- Preoperative corticosteroid administration to promote fetal lung maturity should be based on gestational age and the nature and risks of the planned surgery.
- Thromboembolic prophylaxis with pneumatic compression devices should be considered for all gravid surgical patients.
- Obesity presents unique management considerations during the perioperative period, most notably related to anesthesia risk, intraoperative risk, antibiotic prophylaxis, and thromboembolic prophylaxis. Early ambulation should be encouraged. If early ambulation is not possible, subcutaneous heparin prophylaxis should be considered.
- Bariatric surgery with subsequent weight loss may reduce the risk for medical complications in pregnancy. However, it may increase the risk for preterm delivery and intrauterine growth restriction. Women who have undergone bariatric surgery should be evaluated for nutritional deficiencies.

KEY POINTS—cont'd

- The gravid patient with a history of bariatric surgery who presents with vague abdominal complaints should be critically evaluated because delay in diagnosis of internal hernias, bowel obstruction, or anastomosis leaks can often lead to catastrophic events.
- Approximately 1 in 500 women will require nonobstetric surgery during pregnancy. The care of the pregnant surgical patient requires a multidisciplinary approach that involves the obstetrician, surgeon, anesthesiologist, and pediatrician.

Maternal Physiology

- Pregnancy-induced changes in maternal physiology and anatomy can confuse the clinical picture when evaluating the gravid patient who presents with abdominal symptoms.
- However, despite the altered location, the most consistent and reliable symptom in pregnant women with appendicitis remains right lower quadrant pain.[1,2]
- The gravid uterus may also limit diagnostic imaging of abdominal organs. After the first trimester, the maternal adnexa are displaced cephalad and may be difficult to image with ultrasound.

Diagnostic Imaging

IONIZING RADIATION

- The overwhelming concern related to diagnostic imaging is exposure of the developing fetus to ionizing radiation. The critical factors that determine the risk to the fetus are the dose of radiation to which the fetus is exposed and the gestational age at the time of the exposure.
- When evaluating a pregnant woman who presents with significant symptoms, the patient should be reassured that the radiation exposure to the fetus from diagnostic imaging does not confer a significant risk for fetal harm.[3,4]
- The "as low as reasonably achievable" principle applies to both mother and baby.
- Although patients should be counseled that no single diagnostic test should be considered harmful to the fetus, justification of the need for imaging should be confirmed with respect to maternal benefit.
- Exposure to less than 50 mGy (5 rads) has not been associated with an increase in fetal anomalies or pregnancy loss.

ULTRASOUND

- Overall, the safety and versatility of ultrasonography makes it the first-line diagnostic tool during pregnancy whenever appropriate to address the clinical question at hand.

MAGNETIC RESONANCE IMAGING

- There are numerous advantages to MRI use during pregnancy. Like ultrasound, MRI does not use ionizing radiation, and no harmful effects to the mother or fetus have been reported.

CONTRAST IN PREGNANCY

- Low-osmolarity iodinated contrast media does cross the placenta. However, the small quantities and transient exposure is not believed to be teratogenic.

ANESTHESIA AND TERATOGENICITY

- Most studies have been reassuring and have concluded that a significant risk for congenital malformations is unlikely when surgery is performed during the first trimester.[5]
- It may be preferable to defer most surgical interventions until the second trimester, when the theoretic risk of teratogenicity—as well as the established risk of spontaneous miscarriage—is further decreased.

ANESTHESIA AND PREGNANCY PHYSIOLOGY

- Therefore strategies to decrease the risk for aspiration are essential, such as preoperative fasting, antacid prophylaxis (e.g., 30 mL of sodium citrate), and airway protection.
- The Mallampati airway examination is often used to assess the airway and predict the degree of difficulty of intubation, with progression from low-risk airways (class I) to high-risk airways (class IV) A 34% increase in the frequency of class IV Mallampati airways is seen at term compared with the first trimester. These changes are more pronounced in the third trimester, in obese women, and in women with preeclampsia.

Nonobstetric Surgery and Pregnancy Outcome

- The rate of adverse perinatal outcome is relatively low for women undergoing surgery during pregnancy. In addition, although the risk for low birthweight, preterm birth, and neonatal demise exists, these risks may be associated with complications related to the underlying indication for surgery.
- The early second trimester is considered the optimal time for elective surgery that cannot be safely deferred until after the pregnancy.

Fetal Monitoring

- ACOG recommends that at a minimum, fetal monitoring should be conducted before and after the procedure in cases with a viable fetus. However, in select cases, intraoperative monitoring may be performed after consultation with an obstetrician who can properly counsel the pregnant woman facing surgery and individualize the decision based on factors such as gestational age, type of surgery, and facilities available.

Laparoscopy in Pregnancy

- The intraabdominal pressure required to obtain adequate laparoscopic visualization during surgery can have significant physiologic effects for both the pregnant woman and the fetus.
- Similar studies have shown significant changes in both maternal and fetal physiology at pressures greater than 15 mm Hg.

LAPAROSCOPY AND PREGNANCY OUTCOME

- In summary, no definitive data support a significantly increased risk for adverse pregnancy outcome using the laparoscopic approach for appendectomy during pregnancy.

Adnexal Masses in Pregnancy

- Fortunately, most adnexal masses encountered in pregnancy are benign and spontaneously resolve during the course of pregnancy. In fact, rates of spontaneous resolution have been reported to be as high as 72% to 96%.

- Although most adnexal masses encountered in pregnancy are benign, the rare possibility of malignancy should not be discounted. Between 1% and 3% of masses removed in pregnancy are found to be malignant.[6,7]
- Several sonographic features have been associated with an increased risk for malignancy, such as size greater than 7 cm, heterogeneity with solid and cystic components, papillary excrescences or mural nodules, thick internal septations, irregular borders, increased vascularity, and low-resistance blood flow.
- Another potential complication of an adnexal mass is ovarian torsion, which is estimated to occur in up to 7% of adnexal masses in pregnancy; 60% of torsions occur in the first trimester.
- Women with persistent adnexal masses in pregnancy should be counseled about the signs and symptoms of ovarian torsion, with surgical resection reserved for symptomatic patients and those in whom there is a suspicion of malignancy.
- Although pregnancy data are more limited, several reports are available of successful management of ovarian torsion in pregnancy with preservation of the ovary.
- Ultimately, the decision to untwist and preserve the torsed ovary should be individualized based on intraoperative findings and risk factors for recurrence.

Obesity, Bariatric Surgery, and Pregnancy

- Bariatric surgery is an increasingly common and effective treatment for obesity and has been associated with a significant improvement in overall health and a reduction in adverse pregnancy outcomes.
- Regional anesthesia should be considered if possible to avoid some of these risks, although the type of surgery and difficulty accomplishing regional anesthesia may not allow for this approach in some cases.
- Obesity is also an independent risk factor for venous thromboembolism in the postoperative period; therefore early ambulation should be encouraged. Prophylaxis with pneumatic compression devices should be undertaken until full ambulation is achieved. Subcutaneous heparin should also be considered. In addition, given the increased risk for wound infection and dehiscence in obese patients, adequate antibiotic prophylaxis is recommended.[8]
- The reduced absorptive capacity of the stomach and proximal small bowel often leads to deficiencies in several essential nutrients, including iron, vitamins B_{12} and D, folate, and calcium. Unfortunately, long-term compliance with vitamin supplementation is poor among bariatric surgery patients. Obtaining a baseline evaluation of these nutrients before conception or early in pregnancy is recommended. In addition, consultation with a nutritionist should be considered.[9]
- Complications associated with bariatric surgery including anastomotic leaks, obstruction, and hernias first manifest with symptoms commonly experienced during normal pregnancy—such as nausea, vomiting, and abdominal discomfort—so the potential exists for accurate diagnosis of these complications to be delayed in a pregnant patient, and maternal deaths have been reported.
- With the increasing prevalence of surgical treatment of obesity among young women, clinicians should familiarize themselves with some of the unique concerns that arise when managing these patients during pregnancy, and they should educate and monitor such patients for potential preterm delivery and intrauterine growth restriction.

References for this chapter are available at ExpertConsult.com.

CHAPTER 26

Trauma and Related Surgery in Pregnancy

Haywood L. Brown

KEY POINTS

- Maternal trauma is the most frequent cause of nonobstetric maternal death.
- In cases of significant trauma, such as motor vehicle accidents, maternal stabilization and evaluation in the emergency department should occur prior to transfer to labor and delivery.
- Fetal monitoring should occur as soon as possible while maternal evaluation takes place.
- Abruptio placentae complicates 1% to 2% of cases of minor blunt abdominal trauma and up to 40% of cases of severe abdominal trauma.
- Following cases of blunt trauma, fetal monitoring is recommended for a period of 4 to 24 hours depending on the findings.
- Placental abruption is the most frequent cause of fetal death after trauma.
- Most abruptions occur within 24 hours of an accident, but delayed abruption can occur.
- RhoGAM should be administered to Rh-negative women who experience trauma.
- Kleihauer-Betke testing is recommended for Rh-negative women who experience trauma beyond 20 weeks of gestation.
- Concerns about fetal effects of ionizing radiation should not delay imaging necessary to care for pregnant trauma victims.
- Seatbelt use may reduce adverse fetal outcome resulting from trauma by as much as 84%.
- All pregnant women should be screened for domestic violence during each trimester.

Incidence of Trauma in Pregnancy

- Traumatic injury has been reported to complicate 6% to 8% of all pregnancies and is the leading cause of nonobstetric maternal death.[1-3]
- In addition to risk for maternal morbidity and mortality, traumatic injuries can have significant fetal effects that include an increased risk for fetal death and other adverse outcomes. The incidence of spontaneous abortion, preterm birth, preterm premature rupture of membranes, uterine rupture, cesarean delivery (CD), placental abruption, and stillbirth are all increased.

Anatomic and Physiologic Changes of Pregnancy

- The importance of maternal physiologic changes during pregnancy and an understanding of fetal physiology are critical to effective resuscitation of the injured pregnant woman. This is especially important relative to the maternal response to stress and hypovolemia in the setting of trauma.

TRAUMA CONSIDERATIONS DURING PREGNANCY

- The leading cause of blunt abdominal trauma in pregnancy is motor vehicle accidents.
- Maternal mortality risk with penetrating trauma is more favorable than with blunt trauma because nonreproductive viscera are provided some protection by the gravid uterus, which absorbs the projectile objects.

MATERNAL ANATOMIC AND PHYSIOLOGIC CHANGES

- The dramatic increase in uterine blood flow, up to 600 mL/min, may result in rapid exsanguination in the event of an avulsion or injury to the uterine vasculature or rupture of the uterus. Retroperitoneal hemorrhage from remarkably hypertrophied pelvic vasculature is a common complication of pelvic fracture.

Blunt Trauma

- Blunt trauma to the maternal abdomen is an important cause of abruptio placentae. This is because blunt trauma exposes the gravid uterus to acceleration-deceleration forces that have a differential effect on the uterus and the attached placenta.
- As such, seemly minor or nonseverely injured pregnant women are at increased risk for placental abruption. Abruption may occur immediately after the abdominal impact or may be delayed for several hours after the trauma episode.

MOTOR VEHICLE CRASHES

- Motor vehicle crashes (MVCs) are the most common cause of trauma-associated fetal loss in the United States. The likelihood that an MVC will result in fetal loss is directly related to crash severity and to the severity of the maternal injury. Only about 1% of minor MVCs will result in abruptio placentae, whereas clinically evident abruption occurs in as many as 40% to 50% of cases of severe blunt maternal trauma.

FALLS

- 25% of pregnant women experience a fall at some time during pregnancy. Like MVCs, falls expose the placenta to the shearing forces associated with blunt trauma. However, compared with MVCs, the likelihood that a fall may result in placental abruption and fetal death is low.

DOMESTIC VIOLENCE AND INTIMATE PARTNER VIOLENCE

- The period prevalence of intimate partner violence during pregnancy has been reported to range from 6% to 22%, and up to 45% of pregnant women report a history of domestic abuse at some time during their lifetime.
- This analysis of pregnancy-associated homicides found that intimate partner homicides were most likely to occur during the first 3 months of pregnancy. In a United States study, 5% of female homicide victims were pregnant.

Specific Injuries

FRACTURES

- Fractures are the most common type of maternal injury to require hospitalization during pregnancy, and the lower extremities are the most common site of fractures that complicate pregnancy. Although pelvic fractures are less frequent than fractures of the extremities, pelvic fractures are most likely to result in adverse outcomes of pregnancy, including placental abruption and perinatal and infant mortality

- Pelvic fractures may also be associated with bladder and urethral trauma. Pelvic fractures are not a contraindication to vaginal delivery unless the fracture results in obstruction of the birth canal or if the pelvic fracture is unstable; more than 80% of women who have sustained pelvic fractures can deliver vaginally.

PENETRATING TRAUMA

- Gunshot and stab wounds are the most frequent types of penetrating trauma during pregnancy.[4,5] Penetrating trauma in a pregnant woman is less likely to result in death than penetrating trauma in a nonpregnant individual owing to the protective effect of the gravid uterus when penetrating wounds occur in the upper abdomen.
- However, penetrating trauma poses major risk for complex maternal bowel injury because of the compartmentalization of the bowel in the upper abdomen by the enlarged uterus.
- Gunshot wounds to the abdomen require exploratory surgery to determine the degree of abdominal viscera injury and debridement of damaged tissues.
- A stab wound in a pregnant woman should be managed the same as in a nonpregnant woman.

THERMAL INJURIES (BURNS)

- Maternal and fetal prognosis after thermal injury is a reflection of the percentage of body surface involved.
- Significant burns of 50% or more of the body surface have been associated with high maternal and fetal mortality.

DIRECT FETAL INJURIES

- Direct fetal injuries are uncommon because of the protection by the uterus and amniotic fluid. Fetal injury complicates fewer than 1% of pregnancies with blunt trauma but are most likely to occur with both direct and severe abdominal or pelvic impact and also in later pregnancy, when the fetal head is engaged in the maternal pelvis.

PREDICTORS OF FETAL MORTALITY

- Abruptio placentae is by far the leading cause of fetal death in published series and accounts for between 50% and 70% of all fetal losses due to trauma. Placental abruption complicates about 1% to 2% of cases of maternal trauma with low injury severity scores and up to 40% of severe maternal abdominal trauma. If a placental abruption occurs, the risk of fetal mortality has been reported to be as high as 50% to 80%.[4]
- MVCs (82%) are the most frequent mechanism of injury leading to fetal death, followed by gunshot wounds (6%) and falls (3%).[4] In particular, lack of seatbelt use is a substantial risk factor for poor fetal outcome, morbidity, and mortality.
- Because minor injuries are much more common than severe injuries, they are responsible for 60% to 70% of fetal losses attributable to trauma, even though a severe injury is much more likely to result in fetal loss than a nonsevere injury.

Management Considerations

INITIAL APPROACH

- The Centers for Disease Control and Prevention (CDC) has provided published guidelines for first responders and emergency medical personnel who provide care in the field to injured pregnant women. *Guidelines for emergency medical personnel include displacing the uterus from the inferior vena cava by positioning the mother in the lateral decubitus position. The CDC panel recommended that, if possible, women with a pregnancy of at least 20 weeks' gestation be transported to a trauma center with access to obstetric care.*
- All pregnant women who sustain or who are suspected to have sustained serious injuries should be first evaluated in the emergency department (ED) with the principle that maternal well-being is prioritized over fetal concerns.
- Stabilization of the mother with identification of the maternal injury is the initial priority. Fetal evaluation and interventions can be conducted in the ED as needed.

EVALUATION ON LABOR AND DELIVERY

- After clearance for severe maternal injury has been completed in the ED, the obstetrics team should provide a more thorough physical and obstetric assessment.
- Depending on the labor and delivery gestational age criteria for assumption of care at the facility, the stable patient with trauma at or beyond 23 weeks' gestation (the threshold of fetal viability) should be admitted to labor and delivery for further observation and monitoring for signs and symptoms of placental abruption and preterm labor.

FETAL MONITORING

- Fetal and uterine contraction monitoring is the most sensitive method for detecting abruptio placentae following trauma. In pregnant women who are beyond 23 to 24 weeks' gestation, frequent uterine contractions are nearly always present in women who develop placental abruption following trauma.
- Uterine contraction monitoring is unquestionably more sensitive than ultrasound in detecting placental abruption, and ultrasound detects only about 40% of abruptio placentae in the setting of trauma.
- The fetal heart rate tracing has been called the "fifth vital sign" because it may provide the earliest evidence of maternal hypovolemia or hypotension.
- The time within which a pregnant woman with trauma should receive fetal monitoring is variable. The rationale for a prolonged period of monitoring is the concern for delayed abruption, which has been reported up to 6 days after a traumatic event.[6] If uterine contractions occur less frequently than every 15 minutes over 4 hours of observation, placental abruption is unlikely to occur.[7-9]
- Therefore if the fetus is at or beyond 24 weeks' gestation, the recommended minimal time for monitoring is at least 4 hours from the occurrence of the trauma. Monitoring should be continued if uterine tenderness, contractions, or irritability; abnormal fetal heart activity; or vaginal bleeding are evident.
- If frequent contractions are noted (every 15 minutes or more often) even though no other signs and symptoms for abruption are present, 24 hours of monitoring is recommended because delayed abruptio placentae has been reported up to 48 hours or longer after maternal trauma.

LABORATORY TESTING

- Laboratory tests that may be helpful in the evaluation of trauma include a complete blood count with platelets, type, and Rhesus factor (Rh) testing; evaluation of coagulation function if abruptio placentae is a concern; and a Kleihauer-Betke (KB) test in the Rh-negative woman.
- The KB test may be used to determine whether additional vials of Rh immune globulin are required to prevent sensitization in Rh-negative women who experience trauma. For approximately 90% of pregnant women who experience trauma, fetal-maternal hemorrhage will be less than 30 mL, and 1 vial of Rh immune globulin will be sufficient to prevent sensitization.

Diagnostic Imaging

- Suggested guidelines for radiologic evaluation of trauma are provided in Fig. 26.1.

Exploratory Surgery for Traumatic Injuries During Pregnancy

- When nonobstetric surgery is necessary in a pregnant woman, attention to adequate maternal oxygenation, blood volume, and uterine perfusion is important in providing an environment to prevent fetal hypoxia. Penetrating trauma is the most common indication for nonobstetric surgery for traumatic injuries during pregnancy.
- Indications for surgical exploration include penetrating trauma to the upper abdomen, gunshot wounds to the abdomen, clinical evidence of active intraabdominal hemorrhage, or suspicion for bowel injury.
- In the event that fetal death has occurred prior to surgical exploration, vaginal delivery after induction of labor may be a preferable approach, although some recommend surgical uterine evacuation while the mother is under a current anesthetic if there is abruption and potential for coagulopathy.
- If the pregnancy is at or beyond 24 weeks, fetal monitoring should be carried out intermittently during the surgical procedure. If nonreassuring fetal status is detected during the procedure, in most instances it can be alleviated by attention to and correction of maternal hypovolemia or hypoxemia. If these supportive measures are not effective, CD may be necessary.

UTERINE RUPTURE

- Both blunt and penetrating injuries can result in uterine rupture, which occurs in approximately 0.6% to 1% of instances of maternal trauma.
- Uterine rupture most often results from direct abdominal impact and may occur at any gestational age, although the risk increases as the uterus becomes an abdominal organ later in pregnancy.[1,10]

IMPLICATIONS OF CARDIAC ARREST AND PERIMORTEM CESAREAN SECTION

- The chance of maternal survival after cardiac arrest despite aggressive attempts at resuscitation is significantly diminished compared with the nonpregnant state.

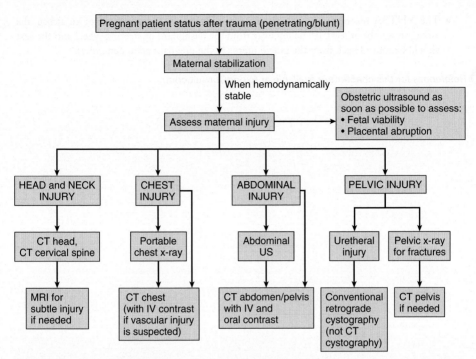

Fig. 26.1 Algorithm with suggested plan for diagnostic imaging studies for pregnant women who experience trauma. CT, computed tomography; IV, intravenous; MRI, magnetic resonance imaging; US, ultrasound. (*Modified from Patel SJ, Reede DL, Katz DS, et al. Imaging the pregnant patient for nonobstetric conditions: algorithms and radiation dose considerations. Radiographics. 2007;27:1719.*)

■ Long-term outcomes for children born after maternal cardiac arrest are more likely to be favorable if the child is delivered within 5 minutes of cessation of maternal circulation.

■ Perimortem cesarean section should be considered early in the resuscitation process in the trauma victim. If the pregnancy has extended beyond an acceptable gestation of viability, the decision to perform a perimortem cesarean section should be immediate and decisive.

■ If the pregnancy is at or beyond fetal viability (23 to 24 weeks' gestation), perimortem CD should commence within 4 minutes after maternal cardiac arrest if resuscitation has not restored maternal circulation.[11]

PREVENTION OF TRAUMA

■ Education and reinforcement of seatbelt use during pregnancy should be undertaken as a routine part of prenatal education and care.

■ The National Highway Traffic Safety Administration (NHTSA) recommends that pregnant women wear their seatbelts with the shoulder harness portion positioned over the collarbone between the breasts and the lap belt portion under the pregnant abdomen as low as possible on the hips and across the upper thighs and not above or over the abdomen.

■ The NHTSA recommends that when a pregnant woman rides in front of an airbag, the airbag should be at least 10 inches away from the dashboard or steering wheel and the seat should be moved back from the gravid uterus as the pregnant abdomen grows.

References for this chapter are available at ExpertConsult.com.

CHAPTER 27

Early Pregnancy Loss and Stillbirth

Joe Leigh Simpson ■ Eric R.M. Jauniaux

KEY POINTS

- About 50% to 70% of conceptions are lost, most in the first trimester. Losses in preimplantation embryos are especially high: 25% to 50% of morphologically normal and 50% to 75% of morphologically abnormal embryos.
- Sporadic pregnancy loss is age dependent, and 40-year-old women have twice the loss rate of 20-year-old women. Most of these pregnancies are lost before 8 weeks' gestation.
- At least 50% of clinically recognized pregnancy losses show a chromosomal abnormality, and those in miscarriages differ from those found in liveborn infants, although autosomal trisomies still account for 50% of abnormalities.
- A balanced translocation is present in 5% of couples with REPL. Many nongenetic causes of REPL have been proposed, but very few are proven. Efficacy of treatment in these cases often remains uncertain.
- Uterine anomalies are accepted causes of second-trimester losses, but their role in first-trimester losses is less clear. Couples who experience a second-trimester loss may benefit from metroplasty or hysteroscopic resection of a uterine septum.
- Drugs, toxins, and physical agents are uncommon causes of early pregnancy loss, especially repetitive loss. It should not be assumed that exposures to toxicants explain repetitive losses. Passive and active smoking and illicit drug use are associated with higher rates of both early pregnancy loss and stillbirth.
- Antiphospholipid syndrome (antibodies to lupus anticoagulant, antiphospholipid, and anti–β_2-glycoprotein) is an accepted cause of second-trimester losses but its role in first-trimester losses is arguable. Strict ACOG criteria exist for applying the diagnosis of antiphospholipid syndrome to a woman who had had repeated first-trimester REPL.
- In REPL, the overall prognosis is good even without therapy. The live birth rate is 60% to 70% even with up to four losses and no prior liveborn infants. Women who have had more than four losses are less likely to have a cytogenetic explanation and may have a different prognosis.
- An efficacious therapeutic regimen for REPL should show success rates greater than these expected background rates.
- The frequency of chromosomal abnormalities and nonchromosomal genetic factors (e.g., syndromes) in stillbirths (losses after 20 weeks' gestation or weighing at least 350 g) is underevaluated. Cultures initiated from postdelivery products (placenta or fetal skin) often lead to unsuccessful culture and thus tissue for cytogenetic studies should be obtained by amniocentesis or chorionic villus sampling when possible.

Introduction

- About 50% to 70% of spontaneous conceptions are lost before completion of the first trimester, most before implantation or during the first month after the last menstrual period. These very early losses are often not recognized as conceptions. Of clinically recognized pregnancies, 10% to 15% are lost.

Frequency and Timing of Pregnancy Loss

- Fewer than half of preimplantation embryos persist, as witnessed by assisted reproductive technology success rates rarely exceeding 30% to 40% of cycles initiated. Even immediately after implantation, judged preclinical or chemical by the presence of β-human chorionic gonadotropin (β-hCG) in maternal serum, about 30% of pregnancies are lost.[1] After clinical recognition, 10% to 12% are lost. Most clinical early pregnancy loss (EPL) occurs before 8 weeks.
- After the first trimester, pregnancy losses occur at a slower rate. Loss rates are only 1% in women confirmed by ultrasound to have viable pregnancies at 16 weeks.
- Maternal age is positively correlated with pregnancy loss rates at any gestational age. Prior pregnancy loss also increases loss rates, but far less than once believed.
- The clinical consequence of the above epidemiology facts is that in order to be judged efficacious in preventing recurrent early pregnancy loss (REPL), therapeutic regimens must show success rates substantially greater than 70%. Essentially no therapeutic regimen can make this claim.

Placental Anatomic Characteristics of Successful and Unsuccessful Pregnancies

- As judged by adult tissue criteria, the human fetus develops in a low-oxygen environment.
- Toward the end of the first trimester, the intrauterine environment undergoes radical transformation in association with onset of the maternal arterial circulation and the switch to hemotrophic nutrition (see Chapter 1).
- In about two-thirds of EPL, anatomic evidence of defective placentation is apparent.
- In about 80% of missed miscarriages, the onset of the maternal placental circulation is both precocious and generalized throughout the placenta.

Numerical Chromosomal Abnormalities: Most Frequent Cause of Early Pregnancy Loss

- Chromosomal abnormalities are the main cause of both preimplantation and clinically recognized pregnancy loss. At least 50% of *clinically recognized pregnancy losses* result from a chromosomal abnormality.[2]

TYPES OF NUMERICAL CHROMOSOMAL ABNORMALITIES
Autosomal Trisomy

- Autosomal trisomies represent the largest single class (about 50%) of chromosomal complements in cytogenetically abnormal early pregnancy failure.
- Aneuploidy usually results from errors at maternal meiosis I, and these are associated with advanced maternal age.[3,4]
- Errors in *paternal* meiosis account for 10% of acrocentric (13, 14, 15, 21, and 22) trisomies.[3]

Polyploidy

- Nonmosaic triploidy (3n = 69) and tetraploidy (4n = 92) are common in EPL. Tetraploidy is uncommon, rarely progressing beyond 2 to 3 weeks of embryonic life.
- An association exists between diandric (paternally inherited) triploidy and partial hydatidiform mole. This chromosomal abnormality can also be associated with persistent trophoblastic disease and thus needs to be identified in order to offer hCG follow-up.

Sex Chromosome Polysomy (X or Y)

- The complements 47,XXY and 47,XYY each occur in about 1 per 800 live-born male births; 47,XXX occurs in 1 per 800 female births but is increased in pregnancies conceived by intracytoplasmic sperm injection.

Monosomy X

- Monosomy X is the single most common chromosomal abnormality among early pregnancy failure, accounting for 15% to 20% of abnormal specimens (Table 27.1).

RELATIONSHIP BETWEEN RECURRENT LOSSES AND NUMERICAL CHROMOSOMAL ABNORMALITIES

- In a given family, successive EPL is likely to be either recurrently normal or recurrently abnormal.

GENETIC COUNSELING AND MANAGEMENT FOR RECURRENT ANEUPLOIDY

- Couples predisposed to recurrent aneuploidy are at increased risk not only for aneuploid EPL but also for aneuploid liveborn neonates.
- If the complement of the first miscarriage is abnormal, recurrence usually involves aneuploidy, although not necessarily of the same chromosome.
- Selective transfer of euploid embryos following preimplantation genetic diagnosis decreases the rate of clinical miscarriages in couples with REPL and live-born trisomies.

Chromosomal Rearrangements
TRANSLOCATIONS

- Translocations are the most common structural rearrangement and are found in about 5% of couples who experience REPL.
- Individuals with balanced translocations are phenotypically normal, but their offspring may show chromosomal duplications or deficiencies as result of normal meiotic segregation.
- Women are about twice as likely as men to carry a balanced translocation.[5]

TABLE 27.1 ■ Chromosomal Completion in Spontaneous Abortions Recognized Clinically in the First Trimester

Chromosomal Complement	Frequency	Percent
Normal 46,XX or 46,XY		54.1
Triploidy:		7.7
69,XXX	2.7	
69,XYX	0.2	
69,XXY	4.0	
Other	0.8	
Tetraploidy:		2.6
92,XXX	1.5	
92,XXYY	0.55	
Not stated	0.55	
Monosomy X		18.6
Structural abnormalities		1.5
Sex chromosome polysomy:		0.2
47,XXX	0.05	
47,XXY	0.15	
Autosomal monosomy (G)		0.1
Autosomal trisomy for chromosomes:		22.3
1	0	
2	1.11	
3	0.25	
4	0.64	
5	0.04	
6	0.14	
7	0.89	
8	0.79	
9	0.72	
10	0.36	
11	0.04	
12	0.18	
13	1.07	
14	0.82	
15	1.68	
16	7.27	
17	0.18	
18	1.15	
19	0.01	
20	0.61	
21	2.11	
22	2.26	
Double trisomy		0.7
Mosaic trisomy		1.3
Other abnormalities or not specified		0.9
		100.0

Data from Simpson JL, Bombard AT. Chromosomal abnormalities in spontaneous abortion: frequency, pathology and genetic counseling. In: Edmonds K (ed). *Spontaneous Abortion*. London: Blackwell; 1987.

- Reciprocal translocations involve not centromeric fusion but rather interchanges between two or more chromosomes. Overall, the risk is 12% for offspring of either female heterozygotes or male heterozygotes.[6,7]
- Detecting a chromosomal rearrangement thus profoundly affects subsequent pregnancy management. Antenatal cytogenetic studies should be offered.
- Preimplantation genetic diagnosis of embryos from couples who have a balanced translocation reveals that most embryos are unbalanced: 58% in robertsonian translocations and 76% in reciprocal translocations.[8]

INVERSIONS

- Inversions are uncommon parental chromosomal rearrangements where the order of the genes is reversed but are responsible for REPL at a rate similar to translocations.
- Women with a *pericentric* inversion have a 7% risk for abnormal liveborn infants, whereas men carry a 5% risk.[9]

MOSAICS

- Mosaicism may be restricted to the placenta, the fetus per se being normal. This phenomenon is termed *confined placental mosaicism.*

Nonchromosomal Causes of Early Pregnancy Loss

LUTEAL PHASE DEFECTS

- Once almost universally accepted as a common cause of EPL, luteal phase defects are now generally considered an uncommon explanation.
- The current consensus is that luteal phase defects are either an arguable entity or not proved to be treated successfully with progesterone or progestational therapy.

THYROID ABNORMALITIES

- Decreased conception rates and increased fetal losses are associated with overt hypothyroidism or hyperthyroidism (see Chapter 42).

DIABETES MELLITUS

- Women whose diabetes mellitus is poorly controlled are at increased risk for fetal loss during the entire pregnancy.

INTRAUTERINE ADHESIONS (SYNECHIAE)

- Intrauterine adhesions can interfere with implantation or early embryonic development.
- If adhesions are detected in a woman experiencing REPL, lysis under direct hyperoscopic visualization should be performed.

MÜLLERIAN FUSION DEFECTS

- Müllerian fusion defects are an accepted cause of *second-trimester* losses and pregnancy complications. REPL may be related to müllerian fusion defects, but other explanations are more likely even when such a defect is found.

- Losses are more likely to be associated with a uterine septum than a bicornuate uterus.[10]
- Women experiencing second-trimester abortions may benefit from uterine reconstruction, but reconstructive surgery is not necessarily advisable for REPL.

LEIOMYOMAS

- Location of leiomyomas is probably more important than size.
- More often, however, leiomyomas have no etiologic relationship to pregnancy loss.
- Surgical procedures to reduce leiomyomas may occasionally be warranted in women experiencing repetitive second-trimester pregnancy losses for women whose fetuses were both phenotypically and karyotypically normal and in whom viability until at least 9 to 10 weeks was documented.

CERVICAL INSUFFICIENCY

- Characterized by painless dilation and effacement of the cervix between 16 and 28 weeks of gestation, cervical insufficiency usually occurs during the middle second or early third trimester and usually follows traumatic events, although the etiology may be genetic. Indications for surgery and techniques to correct cervical insufficiency are discussed in Chapter 28.

INFECTIONS

- Infections are a known cause of late fetal losses and a rare cause of early fetal losses, but infection as a cause of REPL is unlikely.

THROMBOPHILIAS
Acquired

- An association between *second-trimester* pregnancy loss and certain autoimmune diseases is well accepted[11] (see Chapter 46). For first-trimester losses, consensus holds that a less significant relationship exists.
- Antiphospholipid syndrome includes lupus anticoagulant antibodies, anticardiolipin antibody, *or* anti-β_2–glycoprotein.
- In the most recent ACOG bulletin on the topic,[12] three or more losses before the tenth week of pregnancy are considered to fulfill diagnostic criteria for antiphospholipid syndrome in the sense of justifying prophylactic heparin therapy.

Inherited

- Inherited maternal hypercoagulable states are unequivocally associated with increased fetal losses in the second trimester but less convincingly in the first trimester (see Chapter 45).
- There is an association between recurrent (two or more) fetal losses earlier than 13 weeks for thrombophilias related to factor V Leiden (G1691A), activated protein-C resistance, prothrombin (*20210A0* gene), and protein-S deficiency but none for *MTHFR*, protein C, and antithrombin deficiencies.

Exogenous Agents

- Various exogenous agents have been implicated in fetal losses, although studies fail to stratify these by sporadic and recurrent losses (see Chapter 8).
- Physicians should be cautious about attributing pregnancy loss to exogenous agents.

RADIATION AND CHEMOTHERAPEUTIC AGENTS

■ Irradiation and antineoplastic agents in high doses are acknowledged abortifacients. It is therefore prudent for pregnant hospital workers to avoid handling chemotherapeutic agents and to minimize radiation exposures during diagnostic imaging.

ALCOHOL

■ Alcohol consumption should be avoided during pregnancy for reasons independent of pregnancy; thus women should not attribute a pregnancy loss to social alcohol exposure during early gestation.

CAFFEINE

■ In general, reassurance can be given concerning moderate caffeine exposure and pregnancy loss.

CONTRACEPTIVE AGENTS

■ Oral contraceptive use before or during pregnancy is not associated with fetal loss.

CHEMICALS

■ Various chemical agents have been claimed to be associated with fetal losses, but only a few are accepted as potentially causative.[13]

CIGARETTE SMOKING

■ Active and passive maternal smoking has a damaging effect in every trimester of human pregnancy. Cigarette smoke contains scores of toxins that exert a direct effect on the placental and fetal cell proliferation and differentiation and can explain the increased risk for miscarriage, fetal growth restriction, stillbirth, preterm birth, and placental abruption.
■ Secondhand (passive) smoke exposure during pregnancy increases the risk of miscarriage by 11%.

TRAUMA

■ The temptation to attribute a loss to minor traumatic events should be avoided.

PSYCHOLOGICAL FACTORS

■ Some studies have reported a beneficial effect of psychological well-being on REPL.

COMMON MEDICATIONS

■ Nonsteroidal antiinflammatory drugs are widely used during pregnancy but are not associated with an increased risk of early pregnancy loss.

Management of Recurrent Early Pregnancy Loss

■ Two main concepts have dominated the literature on this topic in the past 2 decades: (1) that REPL is mainly caused by aneuploid conceptions and other genetic errors and that the recurrence rate can be explained by the combination of chance and increased risk; and (2) that maternal thrombophilic, endocrine, or immune system abnormalities play a main role in causing loss of euploid conceptions.

WHEN IS FORMAL EVALUATION NECESSARY?

- A couple who experiences even one loss should be counseled and provided with recurrence risk rates. However, not every couple needs formal assessment and a battery of tests.
- Although a firm scientific basis for waiting until three losses is lacking, this is the benchmark for the Royal College of Obstetricians and Gynecologists and the European Society of Human Reproduction and Embryology.[14] The ACOG defines *recurrent loss* as either two or three consecutive losses.
- Any couple who has a stillborn or anomalous liveborn infant should undergo cytogenetic studies unless the stillborn was known to have a normal chromosomal complement.

RECOMMENDED EVALUATION

- Couples experiencing only one first-trimester loss should receive relevant information, but not necessarily be evaluated formally.
- Investigation may or may not be necessary after two spontaneous miscarriages, depending on the patient's age and personal desires. After three spontaneous EPLs, evaluation is usually indicated.
- Detection of a trisomic conceptus suggests recurrent aneuploidy, justifying prenatal cytogenetic studies in future pregnancies.
- Women with either acquired or inherited thrombophilias have an increased risk for late first-trimester REPL and should be tested accordingly.

Late Pregnancy Loss (Stillbirth)

- *Stillbirth* is the term used to describe pregnancy loss at 20 weeks' gestation or greater.
- Stillbirth occurs more often in primiparous women of a given age than in multiparous women of comparable age.
- Risks for stillbirth are highest (twofold) in women delivered of a growth-restricted infant earlier than 32 weeks' gestation.[15,16]

GENETIC FACTORS

- Chromosomal abnormalities or significant copy number variants (microdeletions, microduplications) are detected in 8% to 13% of stillbirths.[17-19] Thus special effort should be made to determine chromosomal status of a stillborn.
- Successful culture for chromosomal analysis occurs in 80% when amniocentesis is used to obtain cells.
- The major yield of autopsy for a stillborn fetus is detection of an unrecognized mendelian explanation.

POLYGENIC/MULTIFACTORIAL DISORDERS

- The multiple malformation syndrome could indicate mendelian etiology.

BOX 27.1 ■ **Maternal Laboratory Tests Recommended by the American College of Obstetricians and Gynecologists After Stillbirth**

All Mothers of Stillborn Infants
- Complete blood count
- Kleihauer-Betke or other test for fetal cells in the maternal circulation
- Human parvovirus-B19 immunoglobulin G; immunoglobulin M antibody
- Syphilis
- Lupus anticoagulant
- Anticardiolipin antibody
- Thyroid-stimulating hormone

Selected Mothers of Stillborn Infants
- Thrombophilia:
  - Factor V Leiden
  - Prothrombin gene mutation
  - Antithrombin III
  - Homocysteine (fasting)
- Protein-S and protein-C activity
- Parental karyotypes
- Indirect Coombs test
- Glucose screening (oral glucose tolerance test, hemoglobin A1c)
- Toxicology screen

Data from the American college of obstetricians and gynecologists (ACOG). Practice bulletin: management of stillbirth. *No. 102:1. Washington, DC: ACOG; 2009.*

MATERNAL EVALUATION

■ Certain maternal laboratory tests are recommended by ACOG (Box 27.1).

MANAGEMENT IN SUBSEQUENT PREGNANCIES

■ High-quality ultrasound and vigilant fetal surveillance are universally recommended. Induction is recommended at 38 weeks.

Obstetric Outcome After Early Pregnancy Complications

■ Recent meta-analyses and reviews have indicated an increased risk for adverse outcome in ongoing pregnancies after an early pregnancy event.
■ In particular, the risk for premature labor and delivery is increased after most first-trimester complications.

⊗ *References for this chapter are available at ExpertConsult.com.*

CHAPTER 28

Cervical Insufficiency

Jack Ludmir ■ John Owen ■ Vincenzo Berghella

KEY POINTS

- Cervical insufficiency is primarily a clinical diagnosis characterized by recurrent painless dilatation and spontaneous midtrimester loss.
- Cervical insufficiency is rarely a distinct and well-defined clinical entity, but only one component of the larger and more complex spontaneous preterm birth syndrome.
- Current evidence suggests that cervical competence functions along a continuum, influenced by both endogenous and exogenous factors, such as uterine contractions and decidual/membrane activation.
- The traditional nomenclature of cerclage type as prophylactic, therapeutic, and emergent should be replaced by history-indicated, ultrasound-indicated, and physical examination–indicated cerclage.
- There is no objective preconceptional diagnostic test for cervical insufficiency.
- History-indicated cerclage for patients with a clinical history of cervical insufficiency remains a reasonable approach.
- Cervical ultrasound for cervical insufficiency has been proven to be a clinically useful screening and diagnostic tool in selected high-risk populations such as those with a prior sPTB who may have a treatable *component* of cervical insufficiency.
- In the vast majority of women with prior sPTBs, and even those with nonclassic clinical histories of cervical insufficiency, serial sonographic evaluations of the cervix may be an acceptable alternative approach to history-indicated cerclage.
- Physical examination–indicated cerclage may be beneficial in reducing PTB in a subgroup of patients without markers of infection.
- Abdominal cerclage may be considered for those rare patients with a history of failed vaginal cerclage.
- Ultrasound-indicated cerclage in twin gestation should not be performed because of the possible increase risk for preterm delivery with this intervention.
- There is a need for randomized studies to evaluate alternative treatments for cervical insufficiency such as pharmacologic therapy and vaginal pessary.

Overview

■ The incidence of cervical insufficiency in the general obstetric population is reported to vary between approximately 1/100 and 1/2000.[1] If women with a singleton gestation, a prior spontaneous preterm birth (sPTB), and a current transvaginal ultrasound (TVU) cervical length (CL) less than 25 mm are labeled as having cervical insufficiency, the incidence is about 3% to 4%.[2]

- *Cervical insufficiency,* as classically defined, is recurrent painless cervical dilation that leads to three or more midtrimester births.[3]
- In a proposed model of cervical competence as a continuum, a poor obstetric history attributed to cervical insufficiency likely results from a process of premature cervical ripening induced by myriad underlying processes that include infection, inflammation, local or systemic hormonal effects, or even genetic predisposition.

Short Cervix

- A new description defines cervical insufficiency by the presence of both (1) TVU cervical length less than 25 mm and/or cervical changes detected on physical examination before 24 weeks of gestation and (2) prior sPTB at less than 37 weeks.
- TVU CL screening should be done using the technique described by the Cervical Length Education and Review program[4] and the Society for Maternal-Fetal Medicine through its Perinatal Quality Foundation.
- The sensitivity of a short CL is much higher, about 70%, in a singleton pregnancy with a prior sPTB.[5]

Risk Factors for Cervical Insufficiency

- Risk factors include prior cervical destructive surgery (e.g., trachelectomy, loop electrosurgical excision procedure, large loop excision of the transformation zone, laser conization, or cold-knife cone biopsy), in utero diethylstilbestrol exposure, prior induced or spontaneous first- and second-trimester abortions, uterine anomalies, multiple gestations, or even prior sPTBs that did not meet typical clinical criteria for cervical insufficiency.

Tests for Cervical Insufficiency

- Because no universally applicable standard exists for the diagnosis of cervical insufficiency, and because the results of such tests were never evaluated and linked to a proven effective treatment, their clinical utility was at best theoretic. Because no test for cervical insufficiency in the nonpregnant patient has been validated, none of these tests are in common use today.

Clinical Diagnosis of Cervical Insufficiency
PATIENT HISTORY

- Cervical insufficiency has primarily been a clinical diagnosis characterized by a history of recurrent painless dilation and spontaneous midtrimester (16 to 24 weeks) birth of a nonanomalous living fetus that usually suffers neonatal death or serious long-term morbidities from extreme prematurity.
- The physician managing a patient who experiences a spontaneous midtrimester birth is in the optimal position to assess and document whether the clinical criteria for cervical insufficiency were met (e.g., hourglassing membranes without painful regular uterine contractions) and to rule out other causes of midtrimester birth (e.g., placental abruption, antecedent fetal death, or fetal anomaly).

Sonographic Diagnosis of Cervical Insufficiency

- The relative risk of sPTB increases steadily as the measured CL shortened.

- Cervical sonography has a lower sensitivity (about 30% to 40%) as a screening test in low-risk women (i.e., singleton gestations without prior sPTB),[6] but it appears to have significant utility for identifying clinically significant cervical pathology in women with a prior early sPTB.[5,7]

Diagnosis of Cervical Insufficiency on Physical Examination

- Uncommonly, a patient in the midtrimester will present with vague pelvic symptoms such as increased pressure and vaginal discharge with increased urinary frequency but without other symptoms of urinary tract infection.
- Fetal parts or the umbilical cord might be seen behind the membranes or even contained in the prolapsing sac.
- This is termed *acute cervical insufficiency.* Presumably, these findings were antecedent events in most if not all cases of midtrimester birth later attributed to cervical insufficiency based on historic criteria. However, this presentation provides a unique clinical opportunity to witness the natural history of cervical insufficiency, explore possible etiologies, and consider the effectiveness of different interventions (Box 28.1).

Treatment

CERCLAGE TECHNIQUE
History-Indicated Cerclage

- Owing to its simplicity and effectiveness, a McDonald technique is recommended as the first-line procedure.
- Currently, no evidence suggests that placing two sutures results in better outcomes than placing one.
- It appears that for a history-indicated cerclage, the rate of subclinical intraamniotic infection is very low, and amniocentesis does not seem justifiable.
- The suture is usually removed electively at 36 to 37 weeks.
- In patients with a prior failed vaginal cerclage, an abdominal cerclage has been recommended.[8]
- Cesarean delivery is necessary, and the suture is left in place if future fertility is desired.
- In the past few years, a laparoscopic abdominal approach to the cervix has been described using the same principles as an abdominal cerclage.[9]

Physical Examination–Indicated Cerclage

- Although some clinicians offer this therapeutic modality up to 28 weeks, we do not advocate the use of cerclage beyond 24 weeks' gestation because of concerns about fetal viability should the procedure contribute to a preterm delivery.[10]
- Although clinicians have been reluctant to offer cerclage in patients with protruding membranes, some reports have suggested a salvage rate in excess of 70% despite advanced cervical dilation, with only 40% delivering before 35 weeks.[11]

BOX 28.1 ■ Criteria for the Diagnosis of Cervical Insufficiency on Physical Examination

- Midtrimester cervical dilation and membranes visible at or beyond the external os in the absence of clinically defined antecedent labor or overt intrauterine infection
- Significant (serial) asymptomatic cervical dilation detected by palpation at midtrimester

Cerclage in the Presence of Premature Rupture of Membranes or Preterm Labor

- Decisions to remove the suture at the time of ruptured membranes should be individualized until more information becomes available.

Effectiveness Based on Evidence

History-Indicated Cerclage

- Because of its unproven efficacy in randomized clinical trials and the attendant surgical risks, the recommendation for history-indicated cerclage should be limited to women with multiple midtrimester sPTBs when a careful history and physical examination suggest a dominant cervical component. Unless the physical examination confirms a significant cervical anatomic defect consistent with disruption of its circumferential integrity, the clinician should assess the history for other components of the PTB syndrome. Cervical insufficiency remains a diagnosis of exclusion.

Ultrasound-Indicated Cerclage

- A patient-level analysis confirmed significant benefit of ultrasound-indicated cerclage for CLs less than 25 mm observed before 24 weeks' gestation in women with prior sPTB. Cerclage reduced PTB at cutoffs of less than 37, 35, 32, 28, and 24 weeks, and composite neonatal mortality and morbidity were also significantly lower (relative risk, 0.64; 95% confidence interval, 0.45 to 0.91).
- Collective results have established the utility of cervical length screening and ultrasound-indicated cerclage for a short cervix less than 25 mm in women with a prior sPTB (Box 28.2).

Physical Examination–Indicated Cerclage

- Although not currently standard practice, the evaluation of amniotic fluid for markers of infection and/or inflammation appears to have important prognostic value, but it is still unclear whether and to what extent the results should direct patient management.
- Although physical examination–indicated cerclage may benefit some, patient selection remains largely empiric. The earlier the gestational age at presentation, the more advanced the cervical dilation, and the presence of prolapsed membranes and intraamniotic infection imparts greater risk of poor neonatal outcome.

ACTIVITY RESTRICTION

- The validity of bed rest for treatment has not been scientifically proven, and some data suggest *worse* outcomes in patients placed on bed rest.[12]

BOX 28.2 ■ Patient at Risk for Cervical Insufficiency: History-Indicated Versus Ultrasound-Indicated Cerclage

- Preterm births will occur regardless of strategy chosen.
- Both strategies have similar rates of preterm birth.
- Fewer cerclages are performed with the ultrasound-indicated cerclage strategy.
- It seems reasonable to follow at-risk patients with sonography and to perform a cerclage based on sonographic findings.

PESSARY

- We must await the results of ongoing trials and assess the need for further prospective, randomized trials that compare pessary, cerclage, and progesterone before conclusions regarding the efficacy of any of these interventions can be established.

PROGESTERONE

- Further research is necessary to evaluate the possible cumulative effects of other interventions for short TVU CL, including not only cerclage and progesterone but also perhaps nonsteroidal antiinflammatory agents, other tocolytics, and other pharmacologic agents.

References for this chapter are available at ExpertConsult.com.

CHAPTER 29

Preterm Labor and Birth

Hyagriv N. Simhan ■ Jay D. Iams ■ Roberto Romero

KEY POINTS

- More than 70% of fetal, neonatal, and infant morbidity and mortality occurs in infants born preterm.
- The rate of PTB peaked in 2006 as the result of the increased use of assisted reproductive technology, ultrasound dating, and indicated preterm births. It has since declined largely because of the adoption of fertility practices to reduce the multifetal gestations associated with infertility treatment.
- Major risk factors for PTB are a history of previous preterm delivery, multifetal gestation, and bleeding after the first trimester of pregnancy; however, most women who deliver preterm have no apparent risk factors; therefore every pregnancy is potentially at risk.
- Four interventions have been shown to reduce perinatal morbidity and mortality: (1) transfer of the mother and fetus to an appropriate hospital before PTB; (2) administration of maternal antibiotics to prevent neonatal GBS infection; (3) administration of maternal corticosteroids to reduce neonatal RDS, IVH, and neonatal mortality; and (4) administration of maternal magnesium sulfate at the preterm delivery at less than 32 weeks to reduce the incidence of CP.
- The risk of recurrent PTB may be reduced in women with a prior PTB with 17-α-hydroxyprogesterone caproate and in women with a short cervix (<20 mm) by administration of prophylactic supplemental progesterone. Cervical cerclage should be indicated for women with a prior PTB and a short cervix.

Overview

■ Complications related to preterm birth (PTB) account for more newborn and infant deaths than any other cause.[1] Although advances in neonatal care have led to increased survival and reduced short- and long-term morbidity for infants born preterm, surviving infants have increased risks of visual and hearing impairment, chronic lung disease, cerebral palsy (CP), and delayed development in childhood.

■ The causes of PTB are diverse but can be usefully considered according to whether the parturition process—which includes cervical remodeling, decidual membrane activation, and myometrial contractions—had begun before birth occurred. Preterm births that do not follow spontaneous initiation of parturition most often are iatrogenic, when the health of the mother or fetus is at risk (e.g., with major hemorrhage, hypertension, or poor fetal growth).

Definitions

■ A *preterm birth* is commonly defined as one that occurs after 20 weeks' gestation and before the completion of 37 menstrual weeks of gestation regardless of birthweight.

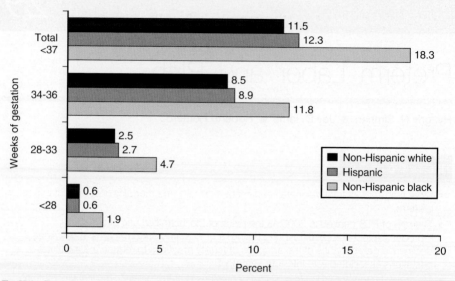

Fig. 29.1   Percentage of live preterm births by racial group. (Data from Martin JA, Hamilton BE, Sutton PD, et al. Births: final data for 2008.*Natl Vital Stat Rep.* 2010;59[1]:1, 3-71.)

- Recognition that some infants born after 37 weeks are not fully mature and that many births before 20 weeks arise from the same causes that lead to preterm births has led to reevaluation of these definitions and boundaries.[2]

Frequency of Preterm and Low-Birthweight Delivery

- About 9.6% of all births in 2005 were preterm—almost 13 million worldwide.
- Blacks have rates of PTB that are almost twofold higher than those of other racial/ethnic groups (Fig. 29.1).

INFANT MORTALITY

- Infant and childhood mortality and morbidity in surviving preterm infants rise as gestational age at birth declines.

PERINATAL MORBIDITY

- Common complications in premature infants include respiratory distress syndrome (RDS), intraventricular hemorrhage (IVH), bronchopulmonary dysplasia, patent ductus arteriosus, necrotizing enterocolitis (NEC), sepsis, apnea, and retinopathy of prematurity.

LONG-TERM OUTCOMES

- Major neonatal morbidities related to PTB that carry lifetime consequences include chronic lung disease, grades 3 and 4 intraventricular hemorrhage (associated with CP), NEC, and vision and hearing impairment. Follow-up studies of infants born preterm and of low birthweight (LBW) infants reveal increased rates of CP, neurosensory impairment, reduced cognition and motor performance, academic difficulties, and attention-deficit disorders.

BOX 29.1 ■ Diagnosis of Preterm Labor and Initial Assessment

- What is the gestational age, and what is the level of confidence about the accuracy of the gestational age?
- In the absence of advanced labor (cervical effacement >80% with dilation >2 cm) and a clear cause of preterm labor, what is the accuracy of the diagnosis of preterm labor?
- Are confirmatory diagnostic tests such as cervical sonography, fetal fibronectin, or amniocentesis for infection necessary?
- What is the anticipated neonatal morbidity and mortality at this gestational age in this clinical setting?
- Should labor be stopped?
- Is transfer to a more appropriate hospital required?
- Should fetal lung maturity be tested?
- What interventions can be applied that will reduce the risks of perinatal morbidity and mortality?
- Should drugs to arrest labor (tocolytics), glucocorticoids, or antibiotics be given?

Clinical Care for Women in Preterm Labor

- Clinical evaluation of preterm parturition begins with assessment of potential causes of labor, looking first for conditions that threaten the health of the mother and fetus.
- Conditions that suggest specific therapy, such as preterm ruptured membranes or cervical insufficiency, should then be sought and treated accordingly.
- The next concerns are the accuracy of preterm labor diagnosis and the balance of risks and benefits that accompany active attempts to inhibit labor versus allowing delivery (Box 29.1).

Diagnosis of Preterm Labor

- Preterm labor must be considered whenever a pregnant woman reports recurrent abdominal or pelvic symptoms that persist for several hours in the second half of pregnancy.
- For decades, the clinical diagnosis of preterm labor has been based on the presence of regular, painful uterine contractions accompanied by cervical dilation and/or effacement.
- The inability to accurately distinguish women with an episode of preterm labor who will deliver preterm from those who deliver at term has greatly hampered the assessment of therapeutic interventions because as many as 50% of untreated (or placebo-treated) subjects do not actually deliver preterm. Optimal criteria for initiation of treatment are unclear.
- The practice of initiating tocolytic drugs for contraction frequency without additional diagnostic criteria results in unnecessary treatment of women who are not at increased risk of imminent sPTB.[3]

DIAGNOSTIC TESTS FOR PRETERM LABOR

- Diagnostic accuracy may be improved in these patients by testing other features of parturition such as cervical ripening; measurement of cervical length (CL) by transvaginal ultrasound; and decidual activation, tested by an assay for fetal fibronectin in cervicovaginal fluid.[4,5]

Treatment for Women in Preterm Labor

- Four interventions that have been shown to reduce neonatal morbidity and mortality.

MATERNAL TRANSFER

- Many states have adopted systems of regionalized perinatal care in recognition of the advantages of concentrating care for preterm infants, especially those born before 32 weeks.

ANTIBIOTICS

- Women with preterm labor should be treated with antibiotics to prevent neonatal group B *Streptococcus* (GBS) infection if colonized with GBS (see Chapters 53 and 54).
- Antibiotic therapy in women with preterm labor and intact membranes is not effective in prolonging pregnancy or preventing preterm delivery.
- Antimicrobial therapy for women in preterm labor should be limited to GBS prophylaxis, women with preterm premature rupture of membranes, or treatment of a specific pathogen (e.g., urinary tract infection).

ANTENATAL CORTICOSTEROIDS

- Glucocorticoids act generally in the developing fetus to promote maturation over growth. In the lung, corticosteroids promote surfactant synthesis, increase lung compliance, reduce vascular permeability, and generate an enhanced response to postnatal surfactant treatment.
- A single rescue course of antenatal corticosteroids may be considered if the antecedent treatment was given more than 2 weeks prior, the gestational age is less than $32^{6/7}$ weeks, and the woman is judged by the clinician to be likely to give birth within the coming week. However, regularly scheduled repeat courses or multiple courses (i.e., more than two) are not recommended.[6]
- A course of treatment consists of two doses of 12 mg of betamethasone; the combination of 6 mg each of betamethasone acetate and betamethasone phosphate, administered intramuscularly twice, 24 hours apart; or four doses of 6 mg of dexamethasone given intramuscularly every 12 hours.

Fetal Effects

- Infants born to treated women were significantly less likely to experience RDS (odds ratio [OR], 0.53), IVH (OR, 0.38), or neonatal death (OR, 0.60). The beneficial effects on IVH are independent of the effects on respiratory function. Other morbidities of PTB are also reduced by antenatal glucocorticoids, including NEC, patent ductus arteriosus, and bronchopulmonary dysplasia. Although both are considered effective, betamethasone may be superior to dexamethasone with respect to reduction of morbidity and mortality in the preterm newborn.

Other Fetal Effects of Glucocorticoids

- Transient reduction in fetal breathing and body movements sufficient to affect the interpretation of the biophysical profile have been described with both drugs but are more common after administration of betamethasone, typically lasting 48 to 72 hours after the second dose.

Maternal Effects

- Antenatal glucocorticoids produce a transient rise in maternal platelet and white blood cell counts that lasts 72 hours; a count in excess of 20,000 is rarely due to steroids.

Duration of Benefit

- Neonatal benefit has been most easily observed when the interval between the first dose and delivery exceeds 48 hours, but some benefit is evident after an incomplete course.

Risks of Antenatal Corticosteroid Treatment

■ The safety and benefit of one course of steroids has never been questioned. Long-term follow-up studies of infants in the original cohorts of infants treated with a single course of antenatal steroids have displayed no differences in physical characteristics or mental function when compared with gestational age–matched controls.

SEQUELAE OF ANTENATAL TREATMENTS TO REDUCE FETAL/ NEONATAL MORBIDITY
Respiratory Distress

■ Neonatal treatment with surfactant is an effective adjunctive therapy that adds independently and synergistically to the benefit of corticosteroids in reducing RDS-related morbidity.

Neurologic Morbidity

■ A randomized placebo-controlled trial of antenatal magnesium conducted in 1062 women who delivered before 30 weeks' gestation found significantly lower rates of gross motor dysfunction and nonsignificant trends of reduced mortality and CP in surviving infants in the treated group at 2 years of age.
■ However, the available evidence suggests that magnesium sulfate given before anticipated early PTB reduces the risk of CP in surviving infants.[7]
■ The largest reduction in risk was for moderate to severe CP.
■ A 4-g bolus of magnesium sulfate with a 1-g/h maintenance dose is a regimen anticipated to have a more favorable side effect and safety profile than a higher-dose regimen.
■ Administration of magnesium sulfate is appropriate for women with preterm premature rupture of the membranes or preterm labor who have a high likelihood of imminent delivery (e.g., within 24 hours) or before an indicated preterm delivery. If emergency delivery is necessary given maternal or fetal status, it should not be delayed to administer magnesium sulfate.

TOCOLYSIS IN PRETERM LABOR

■ Although no medications have been approved for the indication of tocolysis by the U.S. Food and Drug Administration (FDA), a number of classes of drugs are used for this purpose.

Efficacy

■ No studies have consistently shown that any tocolytic can reduce the rate of PTB and improve neonatal outcomes.
■ Recent Cochrane meta-analyses of tocolytic agents indicate that calcium channel blockers and oxytocin antagonists can delay delivery by 2 to 7 days with the most favorable ratio of benefit to risk, that β-mimetic drugs delay delivery by 48 hours but carry greater side effects, that evidence is insufficient regarding cyclooxygenase (COX) inhibitors, and that magnesium sulfate is ineffective.
■ Meta-analyses of studies of individual tocolytic drugs typically report limited prolongation of pregnancy but no decrease in PTB, and they rarely offer information about whether prolongation of pregnancy was accompanied by improved infant outcomes. Delayed delivery for 48 hours to allow antenatal transport and corticosteroids to reduce neonatal morbidity and mortality are thus the main rationale for use of these drugs.

Choosing a Tocolytic Agent

Pharmacology

- The activity of tocolytic agents can be explained by their effect on the factors that regulate the activity of this enzyme, notably calcium and cyclic adenosine monophosphate.

Contraindications to Tocolysis

- Common maternal contraindications to tocolysis include preeclampsia or gestational hypertension with severe features, hemorrhage, and significant maternal cardiac disease.
- Fetal contraindications to tocolysis include gestational age of greater than 37 weeks, fetal demise or lethal anomaly, chorioamnionitis, and evidence of acute or chronic fetal compromise.
- Tocolytic drugs may be safely used when standard protocols are followed. The choice of tocolytic requires consideration of the efficacy, risks, and side effects for each patient.

Calcium Channel Blockers

- The Cochrane Collaboration meta-analyses support calcium channel blockers as short-term tocolytics, compared with other available agents, because of relatively greater suppression of contractions and fewer side effects than other agents in 12 reported trials.

Maternal Effects

- Concomitant or sequential use of calcium channel blockers with β-mimetics is not recommended, nor is concurrent administration of magnesium, owing to reports of skeletal muscle blockade when nifedipine was given with magnesium sulfate.

Magnesium Sulfate

- A meta-analysis that compared magnesium to controls observed no difference in the risk of birth within 48 hours of treatment for women given magnesium (relative risk [RR], 0.85; 95% confidence interval [CI], 0.58 to 1.25; 11 trials, 881 women). Magnesium appeared to confer no benefit on the risk of preterm birth (<37 weeks' gestation) or very preterm birth (<34 weeks' gestation).
- An agent such as indomethacin may be a reasonable choice for tocolysis in the woman receiving magnesium sulfate for neuroprotection of the fetus.

Cyclooxygenase Inhibitors

- Prostaglandin synthesis is increased when the COX-2 form of this enzyme is induced by cytokines, bacterial products such as phospholipases and endotoxins, and corticosteroids; it is reduced by the inhibition of COX with nonsteroidal antiinflammatory drugs.
- Unlike aspirin, indomethacin binds reversibly to COX, so that inhibition lasts only until the drug is cleared metabolically.

β-Mimetic Tocolytics

- The most commonly used β-mimetic in the United States is terbutaline, marketed as a drug for asthma.
- The Cochrane Database reported an analysis of 1332 women enrolled into 11 randomized placebo-controlled trials of β-mimetic drugs and found that treated subjects were less likely to deliver within 48 hours (RR, 0.63; 95% CI, 0.53 to 0.75) but not within 7 days.

Atosiban and Other Tocolytic Agents

- The Food and Drug Administration declined to approve the use of atosiban for tocolysis because of concerns about the drug's safety when used in fetuses at less than 28 weeks' gestation.[8]

Care After Acute Treatment for Preterm Labor

Maintenance Tocolytic Treatment

- The duration of hospitalization for an episode of preterm labor varies according to several factors, including the examination of the cervix, ease of tocolysis, gestational age, obstetric history, distance from the hospital, and the availability of home and family support.

Conduct of Labor and Delivery for the Preterm Infant

- Intrapartum care for women in labor before term is often complicated by conditions that increase the chance of intrapartum fetal compromise such as malpresentation, hypertension, amnionitis, abruption, oligohydramnios, or fetal growth restriction.

INTRAPARTUM ASSESSMENT OF THE PRETERM FETUS

- Ominous heart rate tracings in preterm fetuses have the same associations with fetal acidosis as they do later in gestation.

LABOR AND DELIVERY

- The duration of labor in preterm gestation may be shorter than that of term pregnancy. The active phase of the first stage and the second stage may be particularly brief. Care should be taken to ensure that the fetus does not have a precipitous delivery without control of the fetal head.
- The neonatal care team should be alerted to the circumstances of a PTB well in advance of the delivery so that appropriate personnel and equipment can be made available.

CESAREAN DELIVERY

- Routine cesarean delivery for all preterm or very LBW (VLBW) infants is not justified.

DELAYED CORD CLAMPING

- Early cord clamping and delayed cord clamping are quite varied in the literature. General consensus and review of numerous articles suggest that early cord clamping occurs within 30 seconds of delivery; late cord clamping occurs when the delay is greater than 30 seconds and up to 5 minutes, although most of the benefit occurs within the first 60 to 120 seconds.[9]
- In the VLBW population, delayed cord clamping reduces the need for any delivery room resuscitation intervention, supplemental oxygen, or bag-mask ventilation.[10]

Prevention of Preterm Birth

- Care of PTB may be described according to the public health model as *tertiary* (treatment initiated *after* the parturition process has begun to limit perinatal morbidity and mortality), *secondary* (identification and treatment for individuals with increased risk), or *primary* (prevention and reduction of risk in the population).

SECONDARY PREVENTION OF PRETERM BIRTH

Before Pregnancy

- Prepregnancy medical risk factors occur in as many as 40% of PTBs, but preconception medical interventions to reduce PTB in these women have been disappointing.

TABLE 29.1 ■ Selected Studies of Progestogens to Reduce Preterm Birth

Study	Year	Population	Effect on PTB Rate
Keirse[24]*	1990	Meta-analysis	↓40%
da Fonseca[17]†	2003	History of PTB	↓40%
Meis[18]*	2003	History of PTB	↓35%
Fonseca[14]†	2007	Short cervix <15 mm	↓44%
O'Brien[15]†	2007	History of PTB without short cervix‡	No ↓
DeFranco[13]†	2007	History of PTB with short cervix§	↓
Hassan[16]†	2011	Short cervix 10 to 20 mm	↓45%

*17-α-hydroxyprogesterone caproate.
†Vaginal progesterone in various formulations.
‡Women likely to receive cerclage not enrolled. Mean cervical length at entry was 37 mm.
§Secondary analysis of O'Brien study subjects who later had a short cervix (<28 mm).
PTB, preterm birth variably defined.

During Pregnancy

Modification of Maternal Activity
- Grobman and coworkers[11] reported no relation between reduced activity and frequency of PTB in nulliparous women with CL less than 30 mm before 24 weeks.

Nutritional Supplements
- Trials of supplemental vitamins C and E and calcium have not demonstrated a reduction in PTB risk.[12]

Progestogens
- Randomized trials have demonstrated an approximately 40% decrease in the rate of PTB in women with a prior PTB and/or a short cervix (<15 to 20 mm before 24 weeks' gestation) who were treated with either intramuscular 17-α-hydroxyprogesterone caproate 250 mg weekly or with vaginal progesterone suppositories or cream daily between 16 and 36 weeks' gestation (Table 29.1).[13–18]
- Several randomized placebo-controlled trials have found that progestogen supplementation does not affect the rate of PTB in women with multifetal gestations, indicating that the mechanism of progesterone's action to reduce risk of PTB in singletons is not related to uterine stretch.[19–22]
- Taken together, these studies indicate that a *short cervix*, rather than *prior PTB*, is the most appropriate criterion for institution of vaginal progesterone therapy. However, a history of PTB will continue to be an indication for 17-α-hydroxyprogesterone caproate treatment until additional studies demonstrate that such treatment is unnecessary in women with a prior PTB who maintain a normal CL beyond 24 weeks' gestation.
- The optimal strategy to identify candidates for progesterone therapy has not been determined.

Cervical Cerclage
- The relationship between a short cervix and the risk of PTB was initially interpreted as evidence of diminished cervical strength or competence, but subsequent clinical experience and interventional studies do not support that conclusion. Cerclage is an effective treatment for women with a history of PTB and a short cervix (see Chapter 28).

CLINICAL USE OF PROGESTERONE AND CERCLAGE TO PREVENT PRETERM BIRTH

■ The body of evidence that shows progesterone is effective in reducing the risk of PTB in women with a short cervix with or without a history of PTB has influenced the clinical care of women who would previously have been considered to be candidates for prophylactic history-indicated cervical cerclage.

PRIMARY PREVENTION OF PRETERM BIRTH

■ Primary prevention strategies for PTB will require consistent efforts through education and public policy because the public and government currently underestimate the magnitude of the societal burden.

Public Educational Interventions

Public and Professional Policies

■ Risk of PTB was increased among women who worked more than 42 hours per week (OR, 1.33; CI, 1.1 to 1.6) and who were required to stand for more than 6 hours per day (OR, 1.26; CI, 1.1 to 1.5).

Social Determinants of Health

■ The social determinants of health are (1) promotion of school attendance and completion, (2) food security, (3) neighborhood nutritional programs, (4) job fairs, and (5) an increasing role for hospital and health providers as local leaders.[23]

References for this chapter are available at ExpertConsult.com.

CHAPTER 30

Premature Rupture of the Membranes

Brian M. Mercer

KEY POINTS

- PROM complicates about 8% to 10% of pregnancies and is a significant cause of gestational age–dependent and infectious perinatal morbidity and mortality.
- Latency from membrane rupture to delivery is typically brief and decreases with increasing gestational age at membrane rupture.
- Chorioamnionitis is common after PPROM and increases in frequency with decreasing gestational age at membrane rupture.
- Women with a prior preterm birth due to PROM have a 3.3-fold higher risk for subsequent preterm birth due to PROM and a 13.5-fold higher risk for PPROM before 28 weeks' gestation.
- Some potentially preventable causes of PPROM include urogenital tract infections, poor maternal nutrition with a low body mass index (<19.8 kg/m^2), and cigarette smoking.
- Vaginally collected amniotic fluid can reliably predict the presence of fetal pulmonary maturity after PPROM.
- Conservative management after PPROM with documented fetal pulmonary maturity near term (32 to 36 weeks) prolongs latency only briefly but increases the risk for perinatal infection and does not improve neonatal outcomes.
- Antenatal corticosteroid administration and limited-duration broad-spectrum antibiotic administration have been shown to reduce newborn complications when given in the setting of PROM remote from term.
- Cervical cerclage retention after PPROM has not been shown to improve neonatal outcomes.
- Lethal pulmonary hypoplasia is common after PROM that occurs before 20 weeks and can be predicted with serial ultrasound assessment of lung and chest growth.

Overview

- Membrane rupture that occurs spontaneously before the onset of labor is described as premature rupture of the membranes (PROM) regardless of the gestational age at which it occurs.
- PROM at any gestational age is associated with brief latency from membrane rupture to delivery and also increased risks for perinatal infection and umbilical cord compression due to oligohydramnios.
- Regardless of the gestational age, the patient should be well informed regarding the potential maternal, fetal, and neonatal complications of PROM and preterm birth.

TABLE 30.1 ■ **Risk for Preterm Birth Due to Premature Rupture of the Membranes Among Multiparas**

	N	<37 Weeks (%)	<35 Weeks (%)
All multiparas	1711	5.0	2.3
No risk factors present	1351	3.2	0.8
Prior preterm birth due to PROM only	124	10.5	4.8
Prior preterm birth due to PROM and positive fFN*	13	15.4	15.4
Prior preterm birth due to PROM and short cervix†	26	23.1	15.4
All three risk factors present	8	25.0	25.0

fFN, fetal fibronectin; *PROM*, premature rupture of the membranes.
*Positive fFN, cervicovaginal fFN screen positive (>50 ng/mL) at 22 to 24 weeks' gestation.
†Short cervix, cervix length <25 mm on transvaginal ultrasound at 22 to 24 weeks' gestation.
Modified from Mercer BM, Goldenberg RL, Meis PJ, et al, for the NICHD-MFMU Network. The preterm prediction study: prediction of preterm premature rupture of the membranes using clinical findings and ancillary testing. Am J Obstet Gynecol. 2000;183:738.

Fetal Membrane Anatomy and Physiology

- Preterm PROM likely results from a variety of factors that ultimately lead to accelerated membrane weakening through an increase in local cytokines and an imbalance in the interaction between matrix metalloproteinases and tissue inhibitors of metalloproteinase, increased collagenase and protease activity, or other factors that cause increased intrauterine pressure (e.g., polyhydramnios).[1-5]

Etiology of Premature Rupture of the Membranes

- Preterm PROM has also been linked to infections that involve the urogenital tract.
- Group B *Streptococcus* bacteriuria is associated with preterm PROM and low-birthweight infants.[6,7] Ascending bacterial colonization and infection are integral to the pathogenesis of preterm PROM in many cases.
- Prior preterm birth (PTB) and especially prior preterm PROM (PPROM) have been associated with PPROM in a subsequent pregnancy.[8] The risk of recurrence increases with decreasing gestational age of the index PTB.
- Among women with prior deliveries, prior PTB due to preterm labor or PROM and a positive cervicovaginal fetal fibronectin (fFN) screen were statistically significant clinical markers for subsequent PPROM after controlling for other factors.
- Among multiparas, women with a prior PTB due to PROM, a short cervix on ultrasound, and positive cervicovaginal fFN screen had a 31-fold higher risk for PROM with delivery before 35 weeks' gestation (25% vs. 2.3%) than those without risk factors (Table 30.1).
- Current evidence supports 17-α-hydroxyprogesterone caproate treatment for women with a prior PTB due to PROM or preterm labor and also supports treatment with vaginal progesterone for asymptomatic women with a short cervical length.[9-11]
- Vitamin C supplementation to prevent PPROM is not currently recommended.

Clinical Course After Premature Rupture of the Membranes

MATERNAL RISKS

■ Hallmarks of PROM include a brief latency from membrane rupture to delivery. On average, latency increases with decreasing gestational age at membrane rupture. At term, half of expectantly managed gravidas deliver within 5 hours and 95% deliver within 28 hours of membrane rupture.[12] Of all women with PROM before 34 weeks, 93% deliver in less than 1 week.

Risks of Premature Rupture of the Membranes

MATERNAL RISKS

■ Chorioamnionitis is the most common maternal complication after PPROM.
■ Abruptio placentae can cause PROM or can occur subsequent to membrane rupture, and it affects 4% to 12% of these pregnancies.[13] Uncommon but serious complications of PROM managed conservatively near the limit of viability include retained placenta and hemorrhage, requiring dilation and curettage (12%); maternal sepsis (0.8%); and maternal death (0.14%).[14]

FETAL AND NEONATAL RISKS

■ Fetal complications after membrane rupture include infection and fetal distress due to umbilical cord compression or placental abruption.
■ Fetal death complicates 1% to 2% of cases of conservatively managed PROM.[15]
■ The frequency and severity of neonatal complications after PROM vary inversely with gestational age at membrane rupture and at delivery.
■ PPROM increases the risk of neonatal sepsis twofold over that seen after PTB due to preterm labor with intact membranes.[16]
■ Although no data suggest that immediate delivery on admission with PROM will avert these sequelae, these findings highlight the importance of restricting conservative management after PROM to circumstances in which there is the potential to reduce neonatal morbidity through either antenatal corticosteroid administration or extended pregnancy prolongation for fetal maturation.
■ Pulmonary hypoplasia is a severe complication of oligohydramnios in the second trimester that results from a lack of terminal bronchiole and alveolar development during the canalicular phase of pulmonary development.[17]

Management of Premature Rupture of the Membranes

GENERAL CONSIDERATIONS

■ Management of PROM is based primarily on an individual assessment of the estimated risk for fetal and neonatal complications should conservative management or delivery be pursued. The risks for maternal morbidity should also be considered, particularly when PROM occurs before the limit of potential viability.
■ In general, digital cervical examinations should be avoided until it is determined that delivery is inevitable because such examination has been associated with a shortening of latency from membrane rupture to delivery.[18]

■ If conservative management of PPROM is to be pursued, the patient should be admitted to a facility capable of providing emergent delivery for placental abruption, fetal malpresentation in labor, and fetal distress due to umbilical cord compression or in utero infection. The facility should also be capable of providing 24-hour neonatal resuscitation and intensive care because conservative management should generally be performed only when significant risk for neonatal morbidity and mortality is present.

MANAGEMENT OF PREMATURE RUPTURE OF THE MEMBRANES AT TERM

■ Women with PROM at term should be offered early delivery, generally with a continuous oxytocin infusion, to reduce the risk for maternal and neonatal complications.

MANAGEMENT OF PROM NEAR TERM (32 TO 36 WEEKS)

■ Conservative management after PROM at 34 to 36 weeks' gestation only briefly prolongs pregnancy while increasing the likelihood of chorioamnionitis.
■ As such, conservative management of PROM that occurs at 34 to 37 weeks might be an option if the risk of intrauterine infection is considered to be low.
■ Management of the woman with PROM at 32 to 33 weeks' gestation is more controversial because pulmonary and other gestational age–dependent complications can occur, but the likelihood of survival at this gestation is high and long-term complications are uncommon.
■ At 32 to 33 weeks' gestation, it can be helpful to assess fetal pulmonary maturity and to treat with antenatal corticosteroids those pregnancies without documented fetal maturity.
■ Vaginal pool specimen collection is preferable if an adequate specimen can be obtained.
■ Delivery should be initiated before complications ensue if there is documented fetal pulmonary maturity after PROM at 32 to 33 weeks.

MANAGEMENT OF PROM REMOTE FROM TERM (23 TO 31 WEEKS)

■ Infants born at 23 to 31 weeks' gestation are at increased risk for perinatal death, and survivors commonly suffer acute and long-term complications. Pregnancy prolongation can reduce these risks, and because of this, inpatient conservative management is generally attempted unless intrauterine infection, significant vaginal bleeding, placental abruption, or advanced labor is evident or fetal testing becomes nonreassuring.
■ During conservative management, initial care generally consists of prolonged continuous fetal heart rate and maternal contraction monitoring for evidence of umbilical cord compression and occult contractions and to establish fetal well-being.
■ Although a low initial amniotic fluid index is associated with shorter latency and an increased risk for chorioamnionitis, it does not accurately predict who will ultimately develop these complications and should not be used in isolation to make management decisions.
■ The clinical diagnosis is made when maternal fever (temperature ≥38°C [100.4°F]) with uterine tenderness and maternal or fetal tachycardia are identified in the absence of another evident source of infection. The maternal white blood cell count can be helpful if clinical findings are equivocal.
■ Once chorioamnionitis is diagnosed, broad-spectrum antibiotics should be initiated and delivery should be pursued.

CORTICOSTEROID ADMINISTRATION

- Meta-analysis regarding antenatal corticosteroid administration after PPROM has confirmed steroid therapy to significantly reduce the risks for respiratory distress syndrome (20% vs. 35.4%), intraventricular hemorrhage (7.5% vs. 15.9%), and necrotizing enterocolitis (0.8% vs. 4.6%) without increasing the risks for maternal (9.2% vs. 5.1%) or neonatal (7.0% vs. 6.6%) infection.[19]

ANTIBIOTIC ADMINISTRATION

- Antibiotic treatment significantly prolongs latency after membrane rupture and reduces chorioamnionitis, and treatment also reduces the frequencies of newborn complications that include neonatal infection, the need for oxygen or surfactant therapy, and intraventricular hemorrhage.
- There is a role for a 7-day course of parenteral and oral antibiotic therapy with erythromycin and amoxicillin-ampicillin during conservative management of PROM remote from term, to prolong latency and to reduce infectious and gestational age–dependent neonatal complications. Extended-spectrum ampicillin–clavulanic acid treatment is not recommended because it may be harmful.

MAGNESIUM SULFATE FOR NEUROPROTECTION

- Administration of magnesium sulfate before early PTB will improve long-term infant outcomes and is recommended for anticipated deliveries before 32 weeks' gestation after PPROM.

TOCOLYSIS

- Tocolysis and progesterone therapy are not recommended during conservative management of PPROM.

CERVICAL CERCLAGE

- No well-controlled study has found cerclage retention to improve newborn outcomes after PROM; early cerclage removal is recommended when PROM occurs.

MANAGEMENT OF PREVIABLE PREMATURE RUPTURE OF THE MEMBRANES

- The cause of PROM before the limit of viability has implications for the anticipated pregnancy outcome and can be helpful in guiding counseling and management.
- Maternal risks during conservative management of PROM at 24 weeks or less include chorioamnionitis (35%), abruptio placentae (19%), retained placenta (11%), and endometritis (14%).[20] Maternal sepsis (0.8%) and death (1 in 619 pregnancies overall) are rare but serious complications.
- Consensus has not yet been reached regarding the advantages of inpatient versus outpatient management for the patient who elects conservative management after previable PROM.
- Typically, women with previable PROM who have been managed as outpatients are readmitted to the hospital once the pregnancy reaches the limit of viability.
- During conservative management, serial ultrasound studies performed every 1 to 2 weeks can evaluate for reaccumulation of amniotic fluid and interval pulmonary growth.

References for this chapter are available at ExpertConsult.com.

CHAPTER 31

Preeclampsia and Hypertensive Disorders

Baha M. Sibai

KEY POINTS

- Hypertension is the most common medical complication during pregnancy.
- Preeclampsia is a leading cause of maternal mortality and morbidity worldwide.
- The pathophysiologic abnormalities of preeclampsia are numerous, but the etiology is unknown.
- At present, there is no proven method to prevent preeclampsia. However, low-dose aspirin may have a role in certain women.
- HELLP syndrome may develop in the absence of maternal hypertension and proteinuria.
- Expectant management improves perinatal outcome in a select group of women with severe preeclampsia before 32 weeks' gestation.
- Magnesium sulfate is the preferred agent to prevent or treat eclamptic convulsions.
- Rare cases of eclampsia can develop before 20 weeks' gestation and beyond 48 hours postpartum.
- Antihypertensive agents do not improve pregnancy outcome in women with mild uncomplicated chronic hypertension.
- Labetalol is the drug of choice for the treatment of chronic hypertension during pregnancy; angiotensin-converting enzyme inhibitors should not be used.

Definitions

- *Gestational hypertension* is defined as a systolic blood pressure (BP) greater than 140 mm Hg but less than 160 mm Hg or a diastolic BP greater than 90 mm Hg but less than 110 mm Hg. The pressures must be observed at least 4 hours apart but no more than 7 days apart.
- *Severe hypertension* refers to sustained systolic BP to at least 110 mm Hg and/or diastolic BP of at least 110 mm Hg for at least 4 hours or once the patient is receiving oral antihypertensive medication or received IV antihypertensive therapy prior to the 4-hour period.

PREECLAMPSIA AND ECLAMPSIA

- *Preeclampsia* is gestational hypertension (GH) plus proteinuria (Table 31.1).
- It is recognized that some women with GH may have undiagnosed chronic hypertension, whereas others will subsequently progress to develop the clinical syndrome of preeclampsia.

TABLE 31.1 ■ Hypertensive Disorders of Pregnancy

Clinical Findings	Chronic Hypertension	Gestational Hypertension*	Preeclampsia
Time of onset of hypertension	<20wk	>20wk	Usually in third trimester
Degree of hypertension	Mild or severe	Mild	Mild or severe
Proteinuria*	Absent	Absent	Usually present
Cerebral symptoms	May be present	Absent	Present in 30%
Hemoconcentration	Absent	Absent	Severe disease
Thrombocytopenia	Absent	Absent	Severe disease
Hepatic dysfunction	Absent	Absent	Severe disease

*Defined as 1+ or more (or protein/creatinine ratio >0.30) by dipstick testing on two occasions or 300mg or more in a 24-hour urine collection or protein.

Criteria for Preeclampsia or Gestational Hypertension With Severe Features

■ Systolic BP greater than 160 mm Hg or diastolic BP greater than 110 mm Hg on two occasions at least 4 hours apart. Note that prompt treatment is recommended for severe hypertension sustained for longer than 30 minutes.
■ New-onset cerebral symptoms (headaches) or visual disturbances
■ Impaired liver function or persistent right upper quadrant or epigastric pain unresponsive to medications not accounted for by an alternative diagnosis
■ Pulmonary edema
■ Thrombocytopenia (<100,000/μL)
■ Progressive renal insufficiency (serum creatinine >1.1 mg/dL)
■ *Eclampsia* is defined as the occurrence of seizures after the second half of pregnancy not attributable to other causes.
■ Chronic hypertension is defined as hypertension present prior to 20 weeks gestation or hypertension that persists for more than 3 months postpartum. Women with chronic hypertension may develop superimposed preeclampsia.

Preeclampsia

■ Preeclampsia is a form of hypertension that is unique to human pregnancy. The clinical findings of preeclampsia can manifest as either a maternal syndrome (Fig. 31.1) or a fetal syndrome (Fig. 31.2).[1]
■ The incidence of preeclampsia ranges between 2% and 7% in healthy nulliparous women. In these women preeclampsia is generally mild, with the onset near term or during labor (75% of cases), and the condition conveys only a minimally increased risk for adverse fetal outcome.

CAPILLARY LEAK SYNDROME: FACIAL EDEMA, ASCITES AND PULMONARY EDEMA, AND GESTATIONAL PROTEINURIA

■ Hypertension is considered to be the hallmark for the diagnosis of preeclampsia. However, in some patients with preeclampsia, the disease may manifest as either a capillary leak (proteinuria, facial and vulvar edema, ascites, pulmonary edema); excessive weight gain, particularly during the second and early third trimester; or a spectrum of abnormal hemostasis with multiple-organ dysfunction.

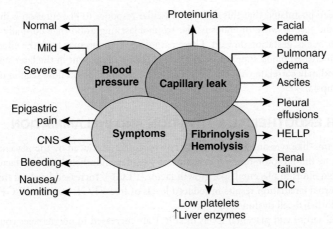

Fig. 31.1 Maternal manifestations in preeclampsia. CNS, central nervous system; DIC, disseminated intravascular coagulation; HELLP, hemolysis, elevated liver enzymes, and low platelets.

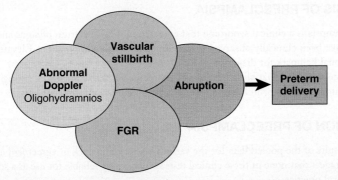

Fig. 31.2 Fetal manifestations of preeclampsia. FGR, fetal growth restriction.

Gestational Proteinuria (Urine Protein Excretion of >300 mg/24 Hours)

■ In the absence of other pathology, the patient should be treated as having potential preeclampsia and requires evaluation for the presence of symptoms; evaluation should include blood tests and frequent monitoring of BP (at least twice per week or, alternatively, ambulatory home BP measurements), and the patient should be educated about the signs and symptoms of preeclampsia.

RISK FACTORS FOR PREECLAMPSIA

■ Generally, preeclampsia is considered a disease of primigravid women. Other risk factors include advanced maternal age, multiple gestation, diabetes, and obesity.

PATHOPHYSIOLOGY

■ The human placenta receives its blood supply from numerous uteroplacental arteries that are developed by the action of migratory interstitial and endovascular trophoblasts into the walls *of the spiral arterioles.* This transforms the uteroplacental arterial bed into a low-resistance, low-pressure, high-flow system.

- It has been postulated that this defective vascular response to placentation is due to inhibition of the second wave of endovascular trophoblast migration that normally occurs from about 16 weeks' gestation onward. These pathologic changes may have the effect of curtailing the increased blood supply required by the fetoplacental unit in the later stages of pregnancy and may correlate with the decreased uteroplacental blood flow seen in most cases of preeclampsia.

VASCULAR ENDOTHELIAL ACTIVATION AND INFLAMMATION

- Soluble fms-like tyrosine kinase 1 (sFlt-1) is a protein produced by the placenta. It acts by binding to the receptor-binding domains of vascular endothelial growth factor (VEGF), and it also binds to placental-like growth factor (PLGF). Increased levels of this protein in the maternal circulation results in reduced levels of free VEGF and free PLGF with resultant endothelial cell dysfunction.
- Maternal serum and placental levels of sFlt-1 are increased in pregnancies complicated by preeclampsia values above those seen during normal pregnancies.

DIAGNOSIS OF PREECLAMPSIA

- Preeclampsia is a clinical syndrome that embraces a wide spectrum of signs and symptoms that have been clinically observed to develop alone or in combination. Elevated BP is the traditional hallmark for diagnosis of the disease.
- It is recommended that all BP values be recorded with the woman in a sitting position for ambulatory patients or in a semireclining position for hospitalized patients.

PREDICTION OF PREECLAMPSIA

- The results of the pooled data for the various tests and the lack of agreement among serial tests suggest that none of these clinical tests is sufficiently reliable for use as a screening test in clinical practice.
- During the past decade, several prospective and nested case-control studies have found that certain maternal risk factors, biophysical clinical factors, and serum biomarkers obtained in the first trimester are associated with subsequent development of hypertensive disorders of pregnancy, GH, or preeclampsia. Based on the results of this study and other reports in recent years, it is clear that evaluation of maternal clinical factors and other biophysical and biomarkers measured in the first trimester is useful only for the prediction of those who will ultimately progress to preeclampsia that will require delivery prior to 34 weeks of gestation.
- Currently, no prospective studies or randomized trials have evaluated the benefits and risks of first-trimester screening for prediction of preeclampsia. Until then, the use of such tests for screening should remain investigational.
- Pregnancies complicated by abnormal uterine artery Doppler findings in the second trimester are associated with more than a sixfold increase in the rate of preeclampsia.
- Current data do not support Doppler studies for routine screening of pregnant women for preeclampsia, but uterine artery Doppler could be beneficial as a screening test in women at very high risk for preeclampsia if an effective preventive treatment should become available.
- The ACOG task force report on hypertension in pregnancy recommends only using risk factors for identifying women considered at increased risk for preeclampsia.

PREVENTION OF PREECLAMPSIA

- In short, randomized trials have evaluated protein or salt restriction; zinc, magnesium, fish oil, or vitamin C or E supplementation; the use of diuretics and other antihypertensive agents; and the use of heparin to prevent preeclampsia in women with various risk factors. These trials have had limited sample sizes, and results have revealed minimal to no benefit.

Antiplatelet Agents Including Low-Dose Aspirin

- The rationale for recommending low-dose aspirin (LDA) prophylaxis is the theory that the vasospasm and coagulation abnormalities in preeclampsia are caused partly by an imbalance in the thromboxane A_2/prostacyclin ratio.
- Antiplatelet agents, largely LDA, have small to moderate benefits when used for prevention of preeclampsia.
- LDA administered after 12 weeks' gestation reduced the risk of preeclampsia by an average of 24% (pooled relative risk [PRR], 0.76; 95% confidence interval [CI], 0.62 to 0.95), reduced the average risk of preterm birth by 14% (PRR, 0.86; 95% CI, 0.76 to 0.98), and reduced the risk of fetal growth restriction (FGR) by 20% (PRR, 0.80; 95% CI, 0.65 to 0.99).
- The U.S. Preventive Services Taskforce has recommended that women considered at increased risk for preeclampsia—that is, those with a history of preeclampsia, preexisting chronic hypertension or renal disease, pregestational diabetes, autoimmune disease, or multifetal gestation—should receive LDA (81 mg/day) starting at 12 to 28 weeks until delivery to reduce the likelihood of developing subsequent preeclampsia, preterm birth, or FGR.

LABORATORY ABNORMALITIES IN PREECLAMPSIA

Renal Function

- Despite the fact that uric acid levels are elevated in women with preeclampsia, this test is not sensitive or specific for the diagnosis of preeclampsia or for predicting adverse perinatal outcome.

Hepatic Function

- Liver function abnormalities are seen in only 10% of women with severe preeclampsia.

Hematologic Changes

- Plasma fibrinopeptide A, D-dimer levels, and circulating thrombin-antithrombin complexes are higher in women with preeclampsia than in normotensive gravidas. In contrast, plasma antithrombin III activity is decreased.
- Thrombocytopenia is the most common hematologic abnormality in women with severe preeclampsia. It is correlated with the severity of the disease process and the presence or absence of placental abruption.
- Fibrinogen levels, prothrombin time, and partial thromboplastin time should be obtained only in women with a platelet count of less than 100,000/mm^3.

Hemolysis, Elevated Liver Enzymes, and Low Platelets (HELLP) Syndrome

Laboratory Criteria for Diagnosis

- Various diagnostic criteria have been used for HELLP. Hemolysis, defined as the presence of microangiopathic hemolytic anemia, is the hallmark of the triad of HELLP syndrome.

- *Class 1* HELLP syndrome was defined as a platelet nadir below 50,000/mm³, *class 2* as a platelet nadir between 50,000 and 100,000/mm³, and *class 3* as a platelet nadir between 100,000 and 150,000/mm³.
- Most researchers do not regard HELLP syndrome to be a variant of disseminated intravascular coagulation (DIC) because coagulation parameters such as prothrombin time, partial thromboplastin time, and serum fibrinogen are normal.

Clinical Findings
- The syndrome appears to be more common in white women and is also more common in preeclamptic women who have been managed conservatively.

Differential Diagnosis
- The presenting symptoms, clinical findings, and many of the laboratory findings in women with HELLP syndrome overlap with a number of medical syndromes, surgical conditions, and obstetric complications
- Pregnant women with probable preeclampsia who present with atypical symptoms should have a complete blood count, a platelet count, and liver enzyme determinations irrespective of maternal BP findings.

Management of HELLP Syndrome
- There is also a consensus of opinion that prompt delivery is indicated if the syndrome develops beyond 34 weeks' gestation or earlier if obvious multiorgan dysfunction, DIC, liver infarction or hemorrhage, renal failure, suspected abruption, or nonreassuring fetal status are apparent.
- Considerable disagreement exists about the management of women with HELLP syndrome at or before 34 weeks of gestation when the maternal condition is stable, except for mild to moderate abnormalities in blood tests, and fetal condition is reassuring. In such patients, some authors recommend the administration of corticosteroids to accelerate fetal lung maturity followed by delivery after 24 hours, whereas others recommend prolonging pregnancy until the development of maternal or fetal indications for delivery or until achievement of fetal lung maturity.

Expectant Management of HELLP Syndrome
- Few large case series describe expectant management of women with true HELLP, partial HELLP, or severe preeclampsia with isolated liver enzyme elevation. In general, these reports suggest that transient improvement in laboratory values or pregnancy prolongation from a few days to a few weeks is possible in a select group of women with HELLP syndrome. It is important to note that most of the patients included in these studies were ultimately delivered within 1 week of expectant management.
- The ACOG Task Force recommended delivery of such patients after completion of a course of corticosteroids for fetal lung maturity or if the gestational age is less than 24 weeks.

Maternal and Perinatal Outcome
- The presence of HELLP syndrome is associated with an increased risk for maternal death (1%) and increased rates of maternal morbidities such as pulmonary edema (8%), acute renal failure (3%), DIC (15%), abruptio placentae (9%), liver hemorrhage or failure (1%), acute respiratory distress syndrome, sepsis, and stroke (<1%).
- It is generally agreed that perinatal mortality and morbidity are substantially increased in pregnancies complicated by the HELLP syndrome. The reported perinatal death rate in recent series ranged from 7.4% to 34%, and this high perinatal death rate is mainly experienced at a very early gestational age (<28 weeks) in association with severe FGR or placental abruption.

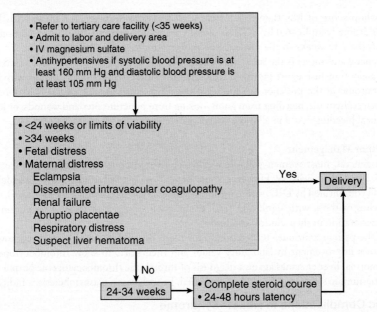

Fig. 31.3 An algorithm for the management of hemolysis, elevated liver enzymes, and low platelets (HELLP) syndrome. IV, intravenous.

- The HELLP syndrome may develop antepartum or postpartum.
- Laboratory assessment for potential HELLP syndrome should be considered during the first 48 hours postpartum in women with significant hypertension or symptoms of severe preeclampsia.

Recommended Management
- Patients with a suspected diagnosis of HELLP syndrome should be hospitalized immediately and observed in a labor and delivery unit (Fig. 31.3). Such patients should be managed as if they have preeclampsia with severe features and should initially receive IV magnesium sulfate as prophylaxis against convulsions and antihypertensive medications to maintain systolic BP below 160 mm Hg or diastolic BP below 105 mm Hg. A 5-mg bolus dose of hydralazine repeated as needed every 20 minutes for a maximal dose of 25 mg/h. BP is recorded every 20 minutes during therapy and every hour once the desired values are achieved.
- The recommended dose of labetalol is 20 to 40 mg given intravenously every 10 minutes for a maximum of 300 mg, and the dose of nifedipine is 10 to 20 mg orally every 20 minutes for a maximum dose of 50 mg within 1 hour. During the observation period, maternal and fetal conditions should be followed carefully.
- The recommended regimen of magnesium sulfate is a loading dose of 6 g given over 20 minutes, followed by a maintenance dose of 2 g/h as a continuous IV solution.

Intrapartum Management
- The presence of HELLP syndrome is not an indication for immediate cesarean delivery (CD), and such an approach might prove detrimental for both mother and fetus. The decision to perform a CD should be based on gestational age, fetal condition, the presence of labor, and the cervical Bishop score. Elective CD is recommended for all women with HELLP syndrome before 30 weeks' gestation who are not in labor and have a

Bishop score of less than 5. Elective CD is also undertaken for those with HELLP syndrome complicated by FGR or oligohydramnios, particularly if the gestational age is less than 32 weeks in the presence of an unfavorable cervical Bishop score.

- General anesthesia is the method of choice for CD in most thrombocytopenic women.
- Platelet transfusions are indicated either before or after delivery in all patients with HELLP syndrome in the presence of significant bleeding—such as subcapsular hematoma of the liver, ecchymosis, bleeding from gums, oozing from puncture sites and wounds, or intraperitoneal bleeding—and in all those with a platelet count less than 20,000/mm³.

Postpartum Management

- In general, most women will show evidence of resolution of the disease process within 48 hours after delivery. However, some patients—especially those with placental abruption complicated by DIC, severe thrombocytopenia (platelet count <20,000/mm³), or severe ascites or those with significant renal dysfunction—may show delayed resolution or even deterioration in their clinical condition.
- If the patient continues to deteriorate for more than 72 hours after delivery, however, or shows improvement in laboratory values and then starts to show thrombocytopenia and abnormal liver enzymes again, a diagnosis of thrombotic thrombocytopenic purpura/hemolytic-uremic syndrome should be considered. In such cases, plasmapheresis is indicated.

Hepatic Complications in HELLP Syndrome

- Marked elevations in serum aminotransferases (>1000 to 2000 IU/L) are not typical of uncomplicated HELLP syndrome; however, when they do occur, the possibility of hepatic infarction and subcapsular hematoma of the liver must be considered.

Antepartum Management of Gestational Hypertension–Preeclampsia

Gestational Hypertension

- Women with gestational hypertension–preeclampsia (GH-PE) are at risk for progression to severe hypertension, preeclampsia with severe features, HELLP syndrome, or eclampsia. The risks are increased with a lower gestational age at the time of diagnosis; therefore these patients require close observation of maternal and fetal conditions.
- The results of several randomized trials reveal that control of maternal BP with antihypertensive drugs does not improve pregnancy outcome in these women.
- In the absence of progression to severe disease, women with GH-PE can continue pregnancy until 37 weeks' gestation.

Hospitalization

- Women with mild hypertension and nonsevere preeclampsia suggest that most of these women can be safely managed at home or in a day care facility provided they undergo frequent maternal and fetal evaluation.

Bed Rest

- Complete or partial bed rest for the duration of pregnancy is often recommended for women with nonsevere hypertension-preeclampsia. No evidence to date suggests that this practice improves pregnancy outcome.

Blood Pressure Medications

- Several randomized trials have described the use of antihypertensive drugs compared with no treatment or a placebo in the management of women with nonsevere hypertension or preeclampsia remote from term. Overall, these trials revealed lower rates of progression to severe disease with no improvement in perinatal outcome.

- It is recommended that antihypertensive medications not be used routinely to control mild levels of hypertension.

Fetal and Maternal Surveillance

- It is universally agreed that fetal testing is indicated during expectant management of women with GH or preeclampsia.
- Maternal surveillance is indicated in all women with GH-PE. The goal of monitoring in women with GH is to observe progression of the condition to severe hypertension or to preeclampsia. In women with preeclampsia, the goal is early detection of progression to preeclampsia with severe features.
- The frequency of laboratory testing will depend on the initial findings, the severity of the maternal condition, and the ensuing clinical progression.

Recommended Management

- In general, women with disease that develops at 37 weeks' gestation or later should undergo induction of labor.
- Those who are managed as outpatients are also advised to come to the hospital or outpatient facility immediately if they develop abdominal pain, significant headache, uterine contractions, vaginal spotting, or decreased fetal movement.
- In women with preeclampsia at less than 37 weeks' gestation but at more than 32 weeks, outpatient management can be considered for reliable patients with a systolic BP of 155 mm Hg or less or diastolic BP of 105 mm Hg or less and no symptoms. Women who do not satisfy these criteria are hospitalized, particularly those with preeclampsia before 32 weeks.

EXPECTANT MANAGEMENT

- Because these pregnancies have been associated with increased rates of maternal morbidity and mortality and with significant risks for the fetus (growth restriction, hypoxemia, and death), it is generally agreed that all such patients should be delivered if the disease develops after 34 weeks' gestation.
- During expectant management, women should be aware that the decision to continue such management will be made on a daily basis and that the median time of pregnancy prolongation is 7 days with a range of 2 to 35 days.
- Expectant management is associated with reduced short-term neonatal morbidity in a select group of women with a gestational age between 24 and 32 weeks.
- The data support the use of steroids to reduce neonatal complications in women with severe preeclampsia at 34 weeks' gestation or less.

RECOMMENDED MANAGEMENT OF PREECLAMPSIA WITH SEVERE FEATURES

- The presence of severe disease mandates immediate hospitalization in labor and delivery. IV magnesium sulfate is begun to prevent convulsions, and antihypertensive medications are administered to lower severe levels of hypertension
- Patients with resistant severe hypertension despite maximal doses of IV labetalol (300 mg within an hour) plus maximum doses of hydralazine (25 mg) or oral rapid-acting nifedipine

(50 mg) or persistent cerebral symptoms while on magnesium sulfate are delivered irrespective of gestational age.

- For pregnancies at $24^{0/7}$ weeks or greater without any indication for prompt delivery, corticosteroids are administered to accelerate fetal lung maturity. With a gestational age between $33^{0/7}$ and $33^{6/7}$ weeks, severe FGR with absent or reversed umbilical artery diastolic flow, largest amniotic fluid vertical pocket less than 2 cm, preterm labor or premature rupture of the membranes, HELLP syndrome or partial HELLP syndrome, or persistent symptoms—such as headaches, visual changes, epigastric or right upper quadrant pain, nausea, or vomiting—the fetus should be delivered no later than 24 hours after the last dose of corticosteroids. These gravidas should remain on magnesium sulfate with continuous monitoring of uterine contractions and fetal heart rate (FHR) until delivery.
- Because of the potential for rapid deterioration in maternal and fetal conditions during expectant management, these women should generally be managed in a tertiary care hospital with adequate maternal and neonatal intensive care facilities. They should be cared for in consultation with a maternal-fetal medicine specialist, and the mother should receive counseling from a neonatologist.
- A suggested regimen consists of an initial dose of labetalol of 200 mg every 8 hours to be increased up to 800 mg every 8 hours (600 to 2400 mg/day) as needed. If the maximal dose is inadequate to achieve the desired BP goal, short-acting oral nifedipine is added with an initial dose of 10 mg every 6 hours and is subsequently increased up to 20 mg every 4 hours. If severe hypertension persists despite combined maximal doses of oral medications, delivery should be considered.
- Patients with resistant severe hypertension after maximal doses of IV hydralazine (25 mg) or labetalol (300 mg) should receive magnesium sulfate and be delivered.

Intrapartum Management

- Some women with GH-PE progress to severe disease as a result of changes in cardiac output and stress hormones during labor.
- Epidural analgesia is considered to be the preferred method of pain relief in women whose GH and preeclampsia are nonsevere.
- Evidence suggests that epidural anesthesia is safe in these women.
- In women with preeclampsia with severe features, general anesthesia carries the risk for aspiration and failed intubation owing to airway edema, and it is associated with marked increases in systemic and cerebral pressures during intubation and extubation. Women with airway or laryngeal edema may require awake intubation under fiberoptic observation with the availability of immediate tracheostomy.

Prevention of Eclamptic Seizures

- Magnesium sulfate is the drug of choice to prevent convulsions in women with preeclampsia. The results of recent randomized trials revealed that magnesium sulfate is superior to placebo or no treatment for prevention of convulsions in women with preeclampsia with severe features.
- Whether magnesium sulfate treatment benefits women with mild preeclampsia remains unclear.

Control of Severe Hypertension

- Antihypertensive medications are indicated with sustained elevations in systolic BP to levels of 160 mm Hg or greater and/or when diastolic BP is 105 mm Hg or higher for at least 60 minutes.[2]

- Hydralazine, labetalol, or nifedipine can be used to treat severe hypertension in preeclampsia. The provider should be familiar with the dosage to be used, the expected response, and potential side effects of each of these drugs.
- For the treatment of severe hypertension in pregnancy, the recommended dosage is IV hydralazine given as bolus injections of 5 to 10 mg every 20 minutes for a maximal dose of 25 mg in 60 minutes. The recommended dose of labetalol is 20 to 80 mg intravenously every 10 minutes for a maximal dose of 300 mg; and the dosage of nifedipine is 10 to 20 mg orally every 20 minutes for a maximal dose of 50 mg within 60 minutes.[2]

Mode of Delivery

- No randomized trials have compared the optimal method of delivery in women with GH-PE. A plan for vaginal delivery should be attempted in all women with disease without other indications for CD and in most women with severe disease, particularly those beyond 30 weeks' gestation.
- In general, the decision to perform a CD versus a trial of labor in such patients should be individualized and based on one or more of the following factors: fetal gestational age, fetal presentation, presence or absence of severe FGR, oligohydramnios, results of umbilical artery Doppler, ultrasound biophysical profile (BPP), FHR monitoring, presence of labor, and cervical Bishop score. On the basis of the available data, CD is recommended for all women with a gestation of less than 28 weeks and for those with severe FGR, severe oligohydramnios, BPP of 4 or less, or reverse umbilical artery Doppler flow at less than 32 weeks of gestation.

Postpartum Management

- Women with severe preeclampsia—particularly those with abnormal renal function, capillary leak, or early-onset disease—are at increased risk for pulmonary edema and exacerbation of severe hypertension postpartum. Careful evaluation of the volume of IV fluids, oral intake, blood products, and urine output are advised in addition to monitoring by pulse oximetry and chest auscultation.
- In general, most women with GH become normotensive during the first week postpartum. In contrast, in women with preeclampsia, hypertension often takes longer to resolve. In addition, in some women with preeclampsia, an initial decrease in BP is seen immediately postpartum, followed by development of hypertension again between days 3 and 6.
- Severe hypertension or preeclampsia with severe features may develop for the first time during the postpartum period. Hence, postpartum women should be educated about the signs and symptoms of severe hypertension or preeclampsia. These women are at increased risk for eclampsia, pulmonary edema, stroke, and thromboembolism. Therefore medical providers and personnel who respond to patient phone calls should be educated and instructed about symptoms of severe postpartum hypertension.

MATERNAL AND PERINATAL OUTCOMES WITH PREECLAMPSIA

- Maternal and perinatal outcomes in preeclampsia are usually dependent on one or more of the following four factors: (1) gestational age at onset of preeclampsia and at the time of delivery, (2) the severity of the disease process, (3) the presence of multifetal gestation, and (4) the presence of preexisting medical conditions such as pregestational diabetes, renal disease, or thrombophilias.

COUNSELING WOMEN WHO HAVE HAD PREECLAMPSIA IN PRIOR PREGNANCIES

- The incidence of chronic hypertension is significantly higher in women with a history of preeclampsia.
- Severe preeclampsia in the second trimester increases the risk for subsequent hypertension.
- For women with preeclampsia complicated by placental abruption, the risk for abruption in subsequent pregnancies ranges from 5% to 20%.
- Women with a history of HELLP syndrome are at increased risk for all forms of preeclampsia in subsequent pregnancies In general, the rate of preeclampsia in subsequent pregnancies is about 20%, with significantly higher rates if the onset of HELLP syndrome is during the second trimester.

Eclampsia

- Eclampsia is the occurrence of convulsions or coma unrelated to other cerebral conditions with signs and symptoms of preeclampsia.
- Eclampsia is defined as the development of convulsions or unexplained coma during pregnancy or postpartum in patients with signs and symptoms of preeclampsia.

DIAGNOSIS

- The diagnosis of eclampsia is secure in the presence of generalized edema, hypertension, proteinuria, and convulsions. However, women in whom eclampsia develops exhibit a wide spectrum of signs that range from severe hypertension, severe proteinuria, and generalized edema to absent or minimal hypertension, no proteinuria, and no edema.
- The diagnosis of eclampsia is usually associated with proteinuria (at least 1+ on a dipstick).[1]
- Several clinical symptoms are potentially helpful in establishing the diagnosis of eclampsia. These include persistent occipital or frontal headaches, blurred vision, photophobia, epigastric or right upper quadrant pain, and altered mental status.

TIME OF ONSET OF ECLAMPSIA

- Although most cases of postpartum eclampsia occur within the first 48 hours, some cases can develop beyond 48 hours postpartum and have been reported as late as 23 days postpartum. In the latter cases, an extensive neurologic evaluation may be required to rule out the presence of other cerebral pathology.
- Eclampsia that occurs before the 20th week of gestation is generally associated with molar or hydropic degeneration of the placenta with or without a coexistent fetus.
- *Late postpartum eclampsia* is defined as eclampsia that occurs more than 48 hours but less than 4 weeks after delivery.

CEREBRAL PATHOLOGY

- Autoregulation of the cerebral circulation is a mechanism for the maintenance of constant cerebral blood flow during changes in BP, and it may be altered in eclampsia.
- Although eclamptic patients may initially manifest a variety of neurologic abnormalities— including cortical blindness, focal motor deficits, and coma—fortunately, most have no permanent neurologic deficits.

- Cerebral imaging findings in eclampsia are similar to those found in patients with hypertensive encephalopathy.
- Cerebral imaging is not necessary for the diagnosis and management of most women with eclampsia; however, it is indicated for patients with focal neurologic deficits or prolonged coma.

MATERNAL AND PERINATAL OUTCOME

- Eclampsia is associated with a slightly increased risk for maternal death in developed countries (0% to 1.8%), but the maternal mortality rate may be as high as 14% in developing countries.
- The greatest risk for death was found among women with pregnancies at or before 28 weeks' gestation.
- Pregnancies complicated by eclampsia are also associated with increased rates of maternal morbidities such as placental abruption (7% to 10%), DIC (7% to 11%), pulmonary edema (3% to 5%), acute renal failure (5% to 9%), aspiration pneumonia (2% to 3%), and cardiopulmonary arrest (2% to 5%)

IS ECLAMPSIA PREVENTABLE?

- Some of the recommended preventive therapies have included close monitoring (in-hospital or outpatient), use of antihypertensive therapy to keep maternal BP below a certain level (less than severe range or to normal values), timely delivery, and prophylactic use of magnesium sulfate during labor and immediately postpartum in those considered to have preeclampsia.
- 20% to 40% of eclamptic women do not have any premonitory signs or symptoms before the onset of convulsions.
- Magnesium sulfate has been compared with diazepam, phenytoin, and a lytic cocktail. Overall, these trials revealed that magnesium sulfate was associated with a significantly lower rate of recurrent seizures (9.4% vs. 23.1%; RR, 0.41; 95% CI, 0.32 to 0.51) and a lower rate of maternal death (3% vs. 4.8%; RR, 0.62; 95% CI, 0.39 to 0.99) than that observed with other agents.

TREATMENT OF ECLAMPTIC CONVULSIONS

- Drugs such as diazepam should *not* be given in an attempt to stop or shorten the convulsion, especially if the patient does not have an IV line in place and someone skilled in intubation is not immediately available.

Prevention of Maternal Injury During the Convulsions

- The first priority in the management of eclampsia is to prevent maternal injury and to support cardiovascular function. During or immediately after the acute convulsive episode, supportive care should be given to prevent serious maternal injury and aspiration, assess and establish airway patency, and ensure maternal oxygenation.
- Transcutaneous pulse oximetry to monitor oxygenation is recommended.

Prevention of Recurrent Convulsions

- Magnesium sulfate is the drug of choice to treat and prevent subsequent convulsions in women with eclampsia. A loading dose of 6 g over 15 to 20 minutes is recommended, followed by a maintenance dose of 2 g/h as a continuous IV solution. Severe hypertension should be treated with parenteral antihypertensive therapy.

INTRAPARTUM MANAGEMENT OF ECLAMPSIA

- Maternal hypoxemia and hypercarbia cause FHR and uterine activity changes during and immediately after a convulsion. The FHR tracing may reveal bradycardia, transient late decelerations, decreased beat-to-beat variability, and compensatory tachycardia. Uterine contractions can increase in frequency and tone. These changes usually resolve spontaneously within 3 to 10 minutes after the termination of convulsions and correction of maternal hypoxemia.
- Fetal outcome is generally good after an eclamptic convulsion. The mechanism for the transitory fetal bradycardia may be a decrease in uterine blood flow caused by intense vasospasm and uterine hyperactivity.
- The presence of eclampsia is not an indication for CD. The decision to perform a CD should be based on gestational age, fetal condition, presence of labor, and cervical Bishop score.

POSTPARTUM MANAGEMENT OF ECLAMPSIA

- Parenteral magnesium sulfate should be continued for at least 24 hours after delivery or for at least 24 hours after the last convulsion. If oliguria is present (<100 mL/4 h), both the rate of fluid administration and the dose of magnesium sulfate should be reduced.

Chrionic Hypertension

DEFINITION AND DIAGNOSIS

- In women whose prepregnancy BP is unknown, the diagnosis is based on the presence of *sustained hypertension* before 20 weeks of gestation, defined as either systolic BP of at least 140 mm Hg or diastolic BP of at least 90 mm Hg on at least two occasions measured at least 4 hours apart.
- Women with chronic hypertension are at increased risk for superimposed preeclampsia. The development of superimposed preeclampsia is associated with high rates of adverse maternal and perinatal outcomes.

ETIOLOGY AND CLASSIFICATION

- The patient is considered to be at low risk when she has mild essential hypertension without any organ involvement. The BP criteria are based on measurements at the initial visit irrespective of treatment with antihypertensive medications.

MATERNAL AND PERINATAL RISKS

- Pregnancies complicated by chronic hypertension are at increased risk for the development of superimposed preeclampsia, placental abruption, and fetal growth restriction. The reported rates of preeclampsia in the literature in mild hypertension range from 14% to 28%.
- The overall rate of superimposed preeclampsia is approximately 25%.
- The reported rate of placental abruption in women with mild chronic hypertension has ranged from 0.7% to 2.7% The rate in those with severe or high-risk hypertension may be 5% to 10%.
- Fetal and neonatal complications are also increased in women with chronic hypertension. The risk for perinatal mortality is three to four times greater compared with that of the general obstetric population. The likelihood of premature delivery and a growth-restricted infant is also increased in women with chronic hypertension.

GOALS OF ANTIHYPERTENSIVE THERAPY IN PREGNANCY

- In nonpregnant individuals, long-term BP control can lead to significant reductions in the rates of stroke and cardiovascular morbidity and mortality. In contrast to hypertension in pregnancy, the duration of therapy is shorter, the benefits to the mother may not be obvious during the short time of treatment, and the exposure to medication will include both mother and fetus. In this respect, the clinician must balance the potential short-term maternal benefits against possible short-term and long-term benefits and risks to the fetus and infant.
- No available data suggest that short-term antihypertensive therapy is beneficial for the mother or the fetus in the setting of low-risk hypertension except for a reduction in the rate of exacerbation of hypertension. However, only three trials have had a sufficient sample size to evaluate the risks for superimposed preeclampsia and placental abruption.
- Antihypertensive therapy is necessary in women with severe hypertension to reduce the acute risks for stroke, congestive heart failure, and renal failure. In addition, control of severe hypertension can permit pregnancy prolongation and thereby improve perinatal outcome. However, no evidence suggests that control of severe hypertension reduces the rate of either superimposed preeclampsia or placental abruption.

SAFETY OF ANTIHYPERTENSIVE DRUGS IN PREGNANCY

- Limited data in the literature suggest potential adverse fetal effects, such as oligohydramnios and fetal-neonatal renal failure, when angiotensin-converting enzyme inhibitors are used in the second or third trimester.
- The use of atenolol during the first and second trimesters has been associated with significantly reduced fetal growth along with decreased placental growth and weight. On the other hand, no such effects on fetal or placental growth have been reported with other β-blockers—such as metoprolol, pindolol, and oxprenolol—but data on the use of these agents in early pregnancy are very limited.
- The available evidence suggests that the use of calcium channel blockers, particularly nifedipine, in the first trimester was not associated with increased rates of major birth defects.

RECOMMENDED MANAGEMENT OF CHRONIC HYPERTENSION IN PREGNANCY

Evaluation and Classification

- Women with chronic hypertension should ideally be counseled before pregnancy, when extensive evaluation for target organ damage can be undertaken. Assessment of the etiology and severity of the hypertension, as well as the coexistence of other medical illnesses should be undertaken.
- Evaluation should include urinalysis, urine culture and sensitivity, 24-hour urine evaluations for protein, electrolytes, complete blood cell count, and screening for diabetes.
- Women with long-standing hypertension for several years, particularly those with a history of poor compliance or poor BP control, should be evaluated for target-organ damage that includes left ventricular hypertrophy, retinopathy, and renal injury. These women should undergo an electrocardiogram examination and echocardiography if the electrocardiogram is abnormal, ophthalmologic evaluation, and creatinine clearance.

Low-Risk Hypertension

- Women with low-risk chronic hypertension without superimposed preeclampsia usually have a pregnancy outcome similar to that of the general obstetric population.

- Antihypertensive treatment with either nifedipine or labetalol is initiated if the patient develops severe hypertension before term. The development of severe hypertension, pre-eclampsia, or abnormal fetal growth requires immediate fetal testing with a nonstress test or biophysical profile. Women who develop severe hypertension require hospitalization.

High-Risk Hypertension

- Hospitalization of women with high-risk uncontrolled hypertension at the time of the first prenatal visit is recommended.
- Antihypertensive therapy is initiated in all women with systolic BP of 160 mm Hg or more or diastolic BP of 110 mm Hg or more. In women without target-organ damage, the aim of antihypertensive therapy is to keep systolic BP between 140 and 150 mm Hg and diastolic BP between 90 and 100 mm Hg.
- The recommended drug of choice for control of hypertension in pregnancy is labetalol, starting at 100 mg twice daily to be increased to a maximum of 2400 mg/day. If maternal BP is not controlled with maximal doses of labetalol, a second drug such as a thiazide diuretic or nifedipine may be added.
- The development of uncontrolled severe hypertension or preeclampsia requires maternal hospitalization for more frequent evaluation of maternal and fetal well-being. The development of FGR also requires intensive surveillance, and the development of these complications at or beyond 34 weeks' gestation should be considered an indication for delivery.

⊗ *References for this chapter are available at ExpertConsult.com.*

CHAPTER 32

Multiple Gestations

Roger B. Newman ■ Elizabeth Ramsey Unal

KEY POINTS

- Twinning is one of the most common high-risk conditions in all of obstetrics with a reported rate of 33.1 per 1000 births in 2012. Both maternal and perinatal morbidity and mortality are significantly higher in multifetal gestations than in singleton pregnancies.
- Chorionicity is a critical determinant of pregnancy outcome and management, and as such it should be ascertained by ultrasound as early in gestation as possible.
- Monochorionic pregnancies are at higher risk than dichorionic pregnancies and have increased rates of spontaneous abortion, congenital anomalies, IUGR, and IUFD in addition to a 10% to 15% risk for TTTS, a complication unique to monochorionic pregnancies.
- Multiple gestations benefit from specialized care, which includes attention to maternal nutrition and weight gain, serial assessment of fetal growth by ultrasound, and careful surveillance for signs of preterm labor.
- Routine bed rest, prophylactic tocolytics, prophylactic cerclage, prophylactic progesterone, and prophylactic pessary have not been shown to be effective in prolonging multiple gestations. However, none of these interventions has been adequately studied in the highest-risk women based on prior obstetric history or current short cervical lengths.
- The nadir of perinatal complications and an increase in stillbirth risk occurs earlier in twin gestations than in singletons. Uncomplicated dichorionic twins appear to have the best outcomes between 37 and 38 weeks, and uncomplicated monochorionic diamniotic twin outcomes are best when delivery occurs between 36 and 37 weeks. We recommend scheduled delivery at the later end of this range.
- Monoamniotic twin outcomes are best when managed with a combination of prophylactic antenatal corticosteroids, hospitalization for daily fetal assessment, and elective CD between 32 and 34 weeks.
- Mode of delivery should take into account gestational age, fetal presentations, estimated weights, and the experience and skill of the obstetrician; a trial of labor is appropriate when both twins are vertex.
- Mode of delivery should be individualized for vertex-nonvertex twins, and CD is optimal when the presenting twin is nonvertex.

Zygosity and Chorionicity

- Zygosity refers to the genetic makeup of the twin pregnancy.
- Chorionicity indicates the placental composition (Fig. 32.1) and is determined by the mechanism of twinning and, in monozygotic (MZ) twins, by the timing of embryo division (Table 32.1).

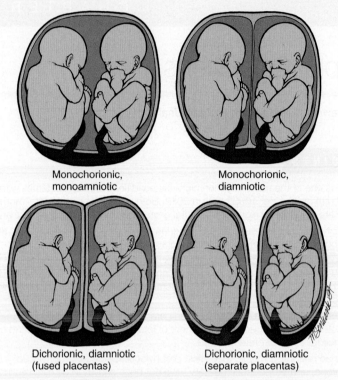

Monochorionic,
monoamniotic

Monochorionic,
diamniotic

Dichorionic, diamniotic
(fused placentas)

Dichorionic, diamniotic
(separate placentas)

Fig. 32.1   Placentation in twin pregnancies.

TABLE 32.1 ■ **Determination of Monozygotic Twin Placentation**

Timing of Cleavage of Fertilized Ovum	Resulting Placentation	Percentage of Monozygotic Twins
<72 hours	Diamniotic dichorionic	25-30
Days 4-7	Diamniotic monochorionic	70-75
Days 8-12	Monoamniotic monochorionic	1-2
≥Day 13	Conjoined	Very rare

- MZ twins are at higher risk for adverse outcomes than are dizygotic (DZ) twins. Not only do MZ twins have higher rates of anomalies than DZ twins, they also deliver earlier, have a lower birthweight, and have higher rates of intrauterine and neonatal death.
- Among natural conceptions, DZ twins arise in about 1% to 1.5% of pregnancies from multiple ovulation, and MZ twins occur in 0.4% of pregnancies. Rates of spontaneous DZ twinning are greatly affected by maternal age, family history, and race. The risk for DZ twinning increases with maternal age and peaks at 37 years of age.

Diagnosis of Multiple Gestations

- Using transvaginal ultrasound, separate gestational sacs with individual yolk sacs can be identified as early as 5 weeks from the first day of the last menstrual period, and embryos with cardiac activity can usually be seen by 6 weeks.

TABLE 32.2 ■ Determination of Chorionicity and Amnionicity in First-Trimester Pregnancies

Placentation	Gestational Sacs	Yolk Sacs	Amniotic Cavities
Dichorionic diamniotic	2	2	2 (thick dividing membrane)
Monochorionic diamniotic	1	2	2 (thin dividing membrane)
Monochorionic monoamniotic	1	1*	1

*Although this is nearly always true, there have been case reports of two yolk sacs in early pregnancy in twins later confirmed to be monoamniotic.

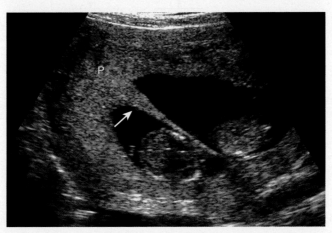

Fig. 32.2   Twin peak sign in a dichorionic twin pregnancy. P, fused dichorionic placentae.

DETERMINATION OF CHORIONICITY

- Knowledge of chorionicity is essential in counseling patients on obstetric and neonatal risks because chorionicity is a major determinant of pregnancy outcome. Chorionicity is also crucial in making a surveillance and management plan because monochorionic twin gestations require closer surveillance for complications unique to monochorionic placentation, such as twin-twin transfusion syndrome (TTTS).
- Determination of chorionicity is easiest and most reliable when assessed in the first trimester (Table 32.2).
- At 11 to 14 weeks' gestation, sonographic examination of the base of the intertwin membrane for the presence or absence of the lambda, or twin peak, sign provides reliable distinction between a fused dichorionic and a monochorionic pregnancy (Fig. 32.2).
- After the early second trimester, determination of chorionicity and amnionicity becomes less accurate, and different techniques are used to assess placentation (Fig. 32.3).
- Dichorionicity could be determined with 97.3% sensitivity and 91.7% specificity, and monochorionicity with 91.7% sensitivity and 97.3% specificity, in twin gestations first scanned at 22.6 ± 6.9 weeks.

Maternal and Fetal Risks of Multiple Gestation

- The degree of maternal physiologic adaptation to pregnancy (see Chapter 3) is exaggerated with a multiple gestation. By 25 weeks' gestation, the average twin gestation uterine size is equal to a term singleton pregnancy.

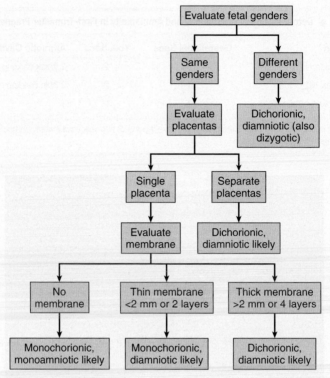

Fig. 32.3 Algorithm for determination of chorionicity and amnionicity in the second and third trimesters.

- Virtually every obstetric complication, with the exception of macrosomia and postterm gestation, is more common with multiple gestations, and in general the risk rises proportionally to increasing plurality and is more severe (Table 32.3).
- Atypical presentations of preeclampsia are also more common in multifetal gestations, especially triplets and higher-order multiples.
- Although fortunately still a very rare event, maternal death is also increased in multifetal gestations.

PERINATAL MORBIDITY AND MORTALITY

- Infants who are products of multiple gestations have higher rates of low birthweight (LBW), very low birthweight (VLBW), earlier gestational age at delivery, and higher rates of neonatal and infant death and cerebral palsy (Table 32.4).
- The overall evidence supports an approximately twofold increased risk for congenital anomalies in twins versus singletons, with most of this risk occurring in MZ twins.

Issues and Complications Unique to Multiple Gestations

"VANISHING TWIN"

- Loss of one fetus of a multiple gestation early in pregnancy.

TABLE 32.3 ■ Maternal Complications in Multiple Gestations

	Singleton (n = 71,851) (%)	Twin (n = 1694) (%)	RR	95% CI
Hyperemesis	1.7	5.1	3.0	2.1 to 4.1
Threatened spontaneous abortion	18.6	26.5	1.4	1.3 to 1.6
Anemia	16.2	27.5	1.7	1.5 to 1.9
Abruption	0.5	0.9	2.0	1.2 to 3.3
Gestational hypertension	17.8	23.8	1.3	1.2 to 1.5
Preeclampsia	3.4	12.5	3.7	3.3 to 4.3
Eclampsia	0.1	0.2	3.4	1.2 to 9.4
Antepartum thromboembolism	0.1	0.5	3.3	1.3 to 8.1
Manual placental extraction	2.5	6.7	2.7	2.2 to 3.2
Evacuation of retained products	0.6	2.0	3.1	2.0 to 4.8
Primary PPH (>1000 mL)	0.9	3.1	3.4	2.9 to 4.1
Secondary PPH	0.6	1.7	2.6	1.8 to 4.6
Postpartum thromboembolism	0.2	0.6	2.6	1.1 to 5.9

From Campbell DM, Templeton A. Maternal complications of twin pregnancy. Int J Gynecol Obstet. 2004;84:71-73.
CI, confidence interval; PPH, postpartum hemorrhage; RR, relative risk.

TABLE 32.4 ■ Birth Outcomes for Multiple Gestations

	Mean Birthweight (g)	Mean Gestational Age at Delivery (wk)	Delivery <32 wk Gestation (%)	LBW (%) (<2500 g)	VLBW (%) (<1500 g)
Singleton	3296	38.7	1.6	6.4	1.1
Twins	2336	35.3	11.4	56.6	9.9
Triplets	1660	31.9	36.8	95.1	35.0
Quadruplets	1291	29.5	64.5	98.6	68.1
Quintuplet and higher-order	1002	26.6	95	94.6	86.5

From Martin JA, Hamilton BE, Ventura SJ, etal. Births: Final data for 2009. National vital statistics reports; vol
60 no 1. Hyattsville, MD: National Center for Health Statistics, 2011.
LBW, low birthweight; VLBW, very low birthweight.

FIRST-TRIMESTER MULTIFETAL PREGNANCY REDUCTION

- Because the risk for pregnancy loss, preterm delivery, and long-term physical and neurodevelopmental morbidity for children who are products of multiple gestations is directly proportional to the number of fetuses being carried, first-trimester multifetal pregnancy reduction has been advocated as a method to reduce the risks associated with prematurity.
- Unless reduction of the entire monochorionic component is planned, the use of this technique is contraindicated in monochorionic pregnancies because of the vascular communications within the placenta.

- Although perinatal morbidity and mortality are clearly improved when pregnancies with quadruplets or greater are reduced to smaller numbers, the obstetric and perinatal advantages of reducing triplets to twins remain debatable.
- In monochorionic twins, selective termination is far more challenging. Ablation of the umbilical cord of the anomalous fetus is needed to avoid back-bleeding through communicating vessels, which may precipitate death or neurologic injury in the remaining normal co-twin.

INTRAUTERINE FETAL DEMISE OF ONE TWIN

- Intrauterine fetal demise (IUFD) of one fetus in a multiple gestation in the second or third trimester complicates about 2.4% to 6.8% of twin pregnancies, but it can have more severe sequelae for the surviving fetus including brain injury.
- The most widely accepted hypothesis as to the cause of neurologic injury in surviving co-twins in a monochorionic pregnancy is that significant hypotension occurs at the time of the demise.
- Clinical management depends on the gestational age, maternal status, or detection of in utero compromise of the surviving fetus or fetuses.
- In the authors' practices, a single IUFD in a monochorionic diamniotic pregnancy at or after 34 weeks would be an indication for delivery.

TWIN-TWIN TRANSFUSION SYNDROME

- TTTS is exclusively a complication of monochorionic multifetal pregnancies. It occurs in 10% to 15% of monochorionic diamniotic gestations and is thus the most common life-threatening complication specific to this type of twinning.
- TTTS results in underperfusion of the donor twin and overperfusion of the recipient. The donor twin develops oligohydramnios, and if it is chronic, intrauterine growth restriction (IUGR) ensues; the recipient twin experiences volume overload.
- TTTS can present at any gestational age, but earlier onset is associated with a poorer prognosis.

Diagnosis and Staging

- The antenatal diagnosis of TTTS is made by ultrasound. The two classic criteria are monochorionic diamniotic twin gestation and oligohydramnios (deepest vertical pocket [DVP] <2 cm) in one amniotic sac and polyhydramnios (DVP >8 cm) in the other sac.
- Although the Quintero staging is widely used and has proved enormously useful in our understanding of TTTS, many experts have noted its limitations (Table 32.5).

TABLE 32.5 ▪ Quintero Staging for Twin-Twin Transfusion Syndrome

Stage I	Oligohydramnios, polyhydramnios sequence. Donor twin bladder visible.
Stage II	Oligohydramnios, polyhydramnios sequence. Donor twin bladder not visible. Doppler scan normal.
Stage III	Oligohydramnios, polyhydramnios sequence. Donor twin bladder not visible, and Doppler scans abnormal (absent or reversed end-diastolic velocity in the umbilical artery, reversed flow in the ductus venosus, or pulsatile flow in the umbilical vein).
Stage IV	One or both fetuses have hydrops.
Stage V	One or both fetuses have died.

Management

- When TTTS is diagnosed, five management options are available: (1) expectant management, (2) septostomy, (3) serial amnioreduction, (4) selective termination/cord occlusion, and (5) fetoscopic laser photocoagulation.
- Management depends on the gestational age at diagnosis and on the severity of the clinical findings.

Septostomy

- Septostomy involves intentional perforation of the dividing membrane, usually performed with a 20- or 22-gauge needle under ultrasound guidance.

Serial Amnioreduction

- In serial reduction amniocentesis, a needle is placed into the polyhydramniotic sac under ultrasound guidance. Amniotic fluid is withdrawn until the fluid volume normalizes (i.e., DVP <8 cm).
- Based on observational data, amnioreduction appears to offer a twofold to threefold increase in overall survival compared with no intervention.

Laser Therapy

- Laser ablation of placental anastomoses is the favored treatment option for early-onset TTTS.
- Unlike both serial amnioreduction and septostomy, which are considered palliative procedures, laser ablation is the only therapeutic option that corrects the underlying pathophysiologic aberration that causes TTTS, and is the optimal therapy before 26 weeks' gestation.
- Compared with the amnioreduction group, the laser group had a higher likelihood of survival for at least one twin to 28 days of life (76% vs. 56%; $P = .009$) and 6 months of age.
- Short-term complications of laser ablation include placental abruption, preterm premature rupture of the membranes, IUFD, and labor.
- Even with optimal laser treatment of TTTS, it remains a serious disease with 20% to 50% overall perinatal mortality.

Selective Intrauterine Growth Restriction in Monochorionic Twin Pregnancies

- *Selective IUGR* (sIUGR) is defined as growth restriction, most commonly an estimated fetal weight (EFW) below the 10th percentile of one twin with appropriate growth in the co-twin but without full criteria for TTTS.
- Three management options are available for early-onset sIUGR in a monochorionic twin pregnancy including expectant, cord occlusion of the IUGR twin, and laser photocoagulation.

Twin Anemia-Polycythemia Sequence

- *Twin anemia-polycythemia sequence* (TAPS) refers to the occurrence of a chronic and severe hemoglobin discordance in a monochorionic diamniotic twin pair in the absence of other criteria for TTTS.
- Ideal management of TAPS is not yet clear, but intrauterine transfusions—both intraperitoneal and intravenous—and laser treatment have been reported with good success. Expectant management is also a reasonable option.

MONOAMNIOTIC TWINS

- Monoamniotic twinning is an uncommon form of MZ twinning (1%) in which both fetuses occupy a single amniotic sac.
- Historically, perinatal mortality rates for monoamniotic twins have been reported to approach 50%, attributed to premature delivery, growth restriction, and congenital anomalies (seen in up to 25% of monoamniotic twin pregnancies) but mostly to umbilical cord entanglement and cord accidents.
- Improved neonatal survival and decreased perinatal morbidity are achievable with monoamniotic twins admitted electively for daily fetal monitoring (two or three times per day for 1 to 2 hours) after viability. We recommend offering hospital admission to all women with monoamniotic twins.
- Most experts perform elective cesarean delivery (CD) following the administration of antenatal corticosteroid therapy between 32 and 34 weeks' gestation. Delivery at 32 to 34 weeks is associated with a low risk of serious neonatal morbidity counterbalanced against the unpredictable continuing IUFD risk.

TWIN REVERSED ARTERIAL PERFUSION SEQUENCE

- Patients with twin reversed arterial perfusion (TRAP) sequence have a monochorionic placenta with vascular anastomoses that sustain the life of the acardiac twin.
- This poorly oxygenated blood preferentially perfuses the acardiac twin's lower body, contributing to the bizarre anomalies seen in acardiac fetuses.
- Color Doppler is essential to confirm diagnosis.
- When faced with a monochorionic pregnancy complicated by TRAP sequence, three options are available: (1) expectant management, (2) delivery, or (3) interruption of the vascular communication between the twins.

CONJOINED TWINS

- Conjoined twins occur when a single embryo incompletely divides between 13 and 15 days after fertilization instead of splitting earlier.
- The mortality rate is high.
- Ultrasound can establish this diagnosis in utero as early as the first trimester based on visualization of monoamnionicity and a bifid fetal pole.
- If the patient desires expectant management, she should be counseled that the prognosis for survival and successful separation depends on the degree of organ and vascular sharing between the two fetuses, especially the heart. Of conjoined twins who are deemed appropriate for and survive to undergo elective separation, survival rates approach 80%.

Antepartum Management of Multifetal Pregnancy (Fig. 32.4)

MATERNAL NUTRITION AND WEIGHT GAIN

- The increased physiologic stress of a multifetal pregnancy demands a 10% higher maternal resting energy expenditure.
- The Institute of Medicine (IOM) issued new body mass index (BMI)-specific weight-gain recommendations for twin pregnancy in 2009 (Table 32.6). Normal-weight women who achieved the IOM weight gain recommendations had significantly larger infants and a greater likelihood of infants weighing more than 2500 g.

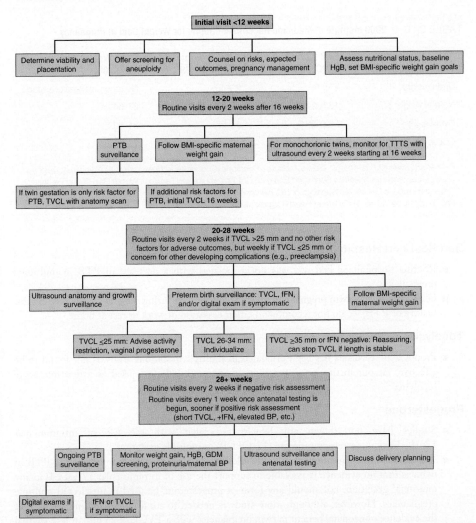

Fig. 32.4 Suggested algorithm for antepartum management of twin gestations. BMI, body mass index; BP, blood pressure; fFN, fetal fibronectin; GDM, gestational diabetes mellitus; HgB, hemoglobin; PTB, preterm birth; TVCL, transvaginal cervical length; TTTS, twin-twin transfusion syndrome.

SPONTANEOUS PRETERM BIRTH

- Patients with a multiple gestation are at significant risk for preterm labor and delivery.
- A 2010 meta-analysis of twins found that in asymptomatic women, a transvaginal cervical length (TVCL) of 20 mm or less between 20 and 24 weeks' gestation was the best predictor of preterm birth (PTB) before 32 and before 34 weeks.
- The degree of change in the cervical length over time may also be an important predictor of PTB in twins.
- In symptomatic mothers of twins, fetal fibronectin had good predictive value. The use of these tests can help guide management decisions, such as frequency of office visits or whether work or activity restriction is prudent.

TABLE 32.6 ■ 2009 Institute of Medicine Recommendations for Weight Gain in Pregnancy

Prepregnancy BMI	BMI (kg/m²) WHO Criteria	Total Weight Gain Singleton (lb)	Total Weight Gain Twins (lb)
Underweight	<18.5	28-40	No recommendations made
Normal weight	18.5-24.9	25-35	37-54
Overweight	25.0-29.9	15-25	31-50
Obese	≥30.0	11-20	25-42

From Rasmussen KM, Yaktine AL, editors. Institute of Medicine (Committee to Reexamine IOM Pregnancy Weight Guidelines, Food and Nutrition Board and Board on Children, Youth, and Families). Weight Gain During Pregnancy: Reexamining the Guidelines. Washington, DC: National Academies Press; 2009.
BMI, body mass index; WHO, World Health Organization.

Bed Rest and Hospitalization

- Routine hospitalized bed rest was not associated with a decrease in PTB in multifetal pregnancies.
- For asymptomatic twin pregnancies in women with a reassuring cervical length and no prior history of PTB, we do not recommend either cessation of work or rest at home.

Tocolysis

- Prophylactic tocolysis has been evaluated in multiple gestations and was not found to be effective. At our institution, intravenous magnesium sulfate is used as a first-line acute tocolytic.

Progesterone

- Studies have not shown any benefit associated with the use of intramuscular 17α-hydroxyprogesterone caproate (17-OH-P) in multiple gestation.
- The authors' interpretation of the available literature on progesterone to prevent PTB in twins is that no evidence is available to support the use of intramuscular 17-OH-P in any multifetal gestation, nor should any form of progesterone be used in unselected multiple pregnancies. However, although more study is needed to confirm this finding, because of the evidence of neonatal benefit in twin pregnancies with a TVCL of 25 mm or less, vaginal progesterone should be offered to these women. Evidence is insufficient to support a specific dose or to support gel versus a micronized progesterone suppository.

Cerclage

- Prophylactic cerclage has been studied and was found to be ineffective in both twins and triplets.
- Cerclage placement in multiple gestations should be restricted to women with either a strongly suggestive history of cervical insufficiency or objectively documented cervical insufficiency based on physical examination. Neither prophylactic nor ultrasound-indicated cerclage are of benefit in multifetal gestations.

Pessary

- No difference was seen in neonatal outcomes; gestational age at delivery; or delivery before 28 weeks, 32 weeks, or 37 weeks between women randomized to pessary and those randomized to expectant management.

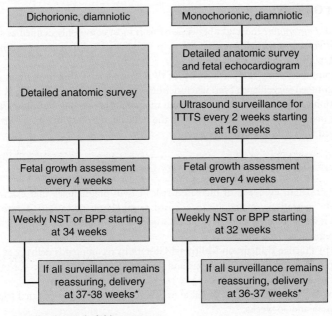

Fig. 32.5 Antenatal surveillance and delivery timing for uncomplicated diamniotic twins. This figure applies only to uncomplicated twins. If any fetal or maternal complications exist, more frequent ultrasounds and antenatal testing, as well as earlier delivery, may be indicated. BPP, biophysical profile; NST, nonstress test; TTTS, twin-twin transfusion syndrome.

- A subgroup analysis of women with TVCL below the 25th percentile suggests that pessary could be effective in women pregnant with twins who also have a short cervix.
- In the 2014 Practice Bulletin on Multifetal Gestation, ACOG cites the ProTWIN study and concludes that "based on available evidence, the use of prophylactic cervical pessary is not recommended in multifetal pregnancies."

ANTENATAL TESTING

- Multiple gestations are at increased risk for uteroplacental insufficiency, IUGR, and stillbirth; for this reason, antenatal surveillance in the form of nonstress tests or biophysical profiles is often performed (Fig. 32.5).
- A 2009 National Institute of Child Health and Human Development document lists initiation of antenatal testing at 28 weeks as a reasonable strategy for triplets.

FETAL GROWTH SURVEILLANCE

- Twins grow at the same rate as singletons until 30 to 32 weeks gestation, after which their growth velocity slows compared with singletons.
- It is recommended that all patients with twins undergo ultrasound evaluation of fetal growth at least every 4 weeks after 20 weeks and more frequently if IUGR or growth discordance is suspected. Additionally, ultrasounds should be performed every 2 weeks in monochorionic twins beginning at 16 weeks to screen for TTTS.

Discordant Growth

- *Significant discordance* in weight between twins is most commonly defined as a greater than 20% difference in actual or estimated twin weights (the difference between the weights divided by the weight of the larger twin).
- We recommend using the presence of EFW discordance of 20% or more as an indication for heightened surveillance even when neither fetus meets criteria for IUGR. This recommendation applies to both dichorionic and monochorionic twins, but more caution should be used in monochorionic gestations with the same degree of estimated growth discordance compared with a dichorionic pregnancy.

Timing of Delivery in Multiple Gestations

- Given consistent evidence of increased risk in twin pregnancies that extend past 38 to 39 weeks' gestation (analogous to a postdate singleton gestation), a rational delivery approach would be elective delivery at 38 weeks in well-dated, uncomplicated dichorionic twin pregnancies (see Fig. 32.5).
- The 2014 Practice Bulletin on Multifetal Gestations recommends delivery at 38 weeks for uncomplicated dichorionic gestations and between 34 and $37^{6/7}$ weeks for uncomplicated monochorionic diamniotic twins.
- Most experts agree that it is reasonable to offer delivery of uncomplicated triplets anytime between 35 and 36 weeks.

Mode of Delivery in Multiple Gestations

- A trial of labor and vaginal delivery is appropriate for all vertex-vertex twin gestations, regardless of gestational age or EFW.
- Twin pregnancies with a nonvertex presenting twin are nearly always managed by CD.
- Provided the obstetrician is sufficiently trained in breech extraction, breech extraction is the preferable option for achievement of vaginal delivery with a nonvertex second twin (see Chapter 17). Most experts recommend avoidance of breech extractions on second twins with EFWs of less than 1500 g.
- Elective CD of patients with three or more live fetuses of viable gestational age is in most cases the optimal management strategy.

Intrapartum Management of Twin Vaginal Delivery

- If a trial of labor is elected, both fetuses should be continuously monitored.
- We typically transfer the patient to the OR bed for delivery. Epidural anesthesia for labor and delivery is also advisable and is advocated by ACOG.
- Many reports have suggested that the interval between deliveries should ideally be 15 minutes or less and certainly not more than 30 minutes.
- Although some second twins may require rapid delivery, most can be safely followed with fetal heart rate surveillance and can remain undelivered for substantial periods of time if there are no signs of nonreassuring fetal status.

CHAPTER 33

Intrauterine Growth Restriction

Ahmet Alexander Baschat ■ Henry L. Galan

KEY POINTS

- Although the terms intrauterine growth restriction (IUGR), fetal growth restriction (FGR), and small for gestational age (SGA) are used interchangeably, IUGR and FGR identify pathologically small fetuses, whereas SGA indicates a fetus below a specific cutoff without designation of pathology.
- IUGR is a major cause of perinatal morbidity, perinatal mortality, and both short-term and life-long morbidities.
- Although IUGR is currently defined by fetal size alone, the four primary underlying etiologies—aneuploidy, viral infection, nonaneuploid syndromes, and placental insufficiency—produce quite different outcomes.
- Identification of growth restriction as a result of placental insufficiency requires a comprehensive diagnostic workup that includes measurement of the fetal abdominal circumference in combination with umbilical artery Doppler studies, exclusion of fetal anomalies, and possibly invasive testing to detect aneuploidy and viral infection.
- The combination of a small abdominal circumference, normal anatomy, low or normal amniotic fluid volume, and abnormal umbilical artery Doppler is strongly suggestive of placental insufficiency.
- Because mortality resulting from FGR can be reduced with appropriate antenatal surveillance, all pregnancies at risk for IUGR should be carefully monitored.
- Deterioration of fetal biophysical and cardiovascular parameters follows a relatively predictable pattern, progressing from early to late changes that can be used for the prediction of fetal acid-base imbalance and the risk for stillbirth.
- Antenatal surveillance in preterm IUGR requires the combination of several testing modalities to provide fetal assessment of sufficient precision to guide intervention.
- In preterm gestations complicated by IUGR, the threshold for delivery is critically influenced by gestational age.

Perinatal Mortality

- Compared with appropriately grown counterparts, perinatal mortality rates in growth-restricted neonates are 6 to 10 times greater; perinatal mortality rates as high as 120 per 1000 for all cases of IUGR and 80 per 1000 after exclusion of anomalous infants have been reported. As many as 53% of preterm stillbirths and 26% of term stillbirths are growth restricted.

Regulation of Fetal Growth

- Of the actively transported primary nutrients, glucose is the predominant oxidative fuel, whereas amino acids are major contributors to protein synthesis and muscle bulk.

- Placental and fetal growth across the three trimesters are characterized by sequential cellular hyperplasia, hyperplasia plus hypertrophy, and lastly, by hypertrophy alone.
- Eighty percent of fetal fat gain is accrued after 28 weeks' gestation, providing essential body stores in preparation for extrauterine life.

Definition and Patterns of Fetal Growth Restriction

- Disturbance of fetal growth dynamics can lead to a reduced cell number, cell size, or both, ultimately resulting in abnormal weight, body mass, or body proportion at birth.
- The currently accepted classification of birthweight is based on percentile: *very small for gestational age* (very SGA; <3rd percentile), *small for gestational age* (SGA; <10th percentile), *average for gestational age* (10th to 90th percentile), or *large for gestational age* (>90th percentile).
- The ponderal index ([birthweight in grams/crown heel length]^3 × 100) has a high accuracy for the identification of SGA.
- Two principal patterns of disturbed fetal growth have been described: asymmetric and symmetric. In the *asymmetric growth pattern,* somatic growth (e.g., the abdominal circumference [AC] and lower body) shows a significant delay, whereas there is relative or absolute sparing of head growth. In the *symmetric growth pattern,* body and head growth are similarly affected.
- The pattern of fetal growth depends on the underlying cause of growth delay and on the timing and duration of the insult. Uteroplacental insufficiency is typically associated with asymmetric fetal growth delay owing to the aforementioned mechanisms. Aneuploidy, nonaneuploid syndromes, and viral infections either disrupt the regulation of growth processes or interfere with growth at the stage of cell hyperplasia. This typically results in a symmetric growth delay.

Etiologies of Intrauterine Growth Restriction

- Maternal causes of FGR include vascular disease such as hypertensive disorders of pregnancy, diabetic vasculopathy, collagen vascular disease, and thrombophilia and chronic renal disease. Abnormalities of the fetus and/or placenta can also result in FGR.
- Genetic and infectious etiologies are of special importance because perinatal and long-term outcomes are ultimately determined by the underlying condition, with little potential impact through perinatal interventions.
- The diagnosis and prognosis of FGR in twin pregnancies is critically determined by the chorionicity (see Chapter 32).

Maternal and Fetal Manifestations of Intrauterine Growth Restriction

- The impact and clinical manifestations of placental insufficiency depend on the gestational age at onset and the severity and type of the placental disease.
- Maternal placental floor infarcts, fetal villous obliteration, and fibrosis each increase placental blood flow resistance, producing a maternal-fetal placental perfusion mismatch that decreases the effective exchange area.
- When uterine oxygen delivery falls below a critical value (0.6 mmol/min/kg fetal body weight in sheep), fetal oxygenation begins to fall and is eventually accompanied by fetal hypoglycemia.
- Fetal hormonal imbalances are believed to have additional negative impacts on linear and growth, bone mineralization, and the potential for postpartum catch-up growth.

- Fetal hematologic responses to placental insufficiency are important because they initially provide a compensatory mechanism for hypoxemia and acidemia but eventually become contributory to the escalation of placental vascular dysfunction.
- Elevated nucleated red blood cell counts correlate with metabolic and cardiovascular status and are independent markers for poor perinatal outcome.
- Increase in whole blood viscosity, decrease in red blood cell membrane fluidity, and platelet aggregation may be important precursors in the acceleration of placental vascular occlusion and dysfunction.
- Growth-restricted fetuses also show evidence of immune dysfunction at the cellular and humoral level.
- *Early* fetal cardiovascular responses are typically adaptive in nature and result in preferential nutrient streaming to essential organs. Shunting of nutrient-rich blood from the ductus venosus (DV) through the foramen ovale to the left side of the heart increases, and left ventricular output rises in relation to the right cardiac output. This relative shift in cardiac output toward the left ventricle that results in increased blood flow to the myocardium and brachiocephalic circulation has been termed *redistribution*, which indicates a compensatory mechanism in response to placental insufficiency.
- *Late* circulatory responses are associated with deterioration of cardiovascular status and are predominantly observed in early-onset growth delay, which requires delivery prior to 34 weeks. Redistribution is effective only as long as adequate forward cardiac function is maintained. Ineffective preload handling and elevation in central venous pressure may result from ineffective redistribution, a measurable decline in cardiac output, and a decline in cardiac forward function.
- Myocardial dysfunction and cardiac dilatation may result in holosystolic tricuspid insufficiency and spontaneous fetal heart rate (FHR) decelerations, followed by fetal demise.
- Fetal organs also have the ability to regulate their individual blood flow through autoregulation.
- Fetal behavioral responses to placental insufficiency and characteristics of the FHR reflect developmental status and undergo changes with advancing gestation. Normally, behavioral milestones progress from the initiation of gross body movements and fetal breathing in the first trimester to coupling of fetal behavior (e.g., heart rate reactivity) and integration of rest-activity cycles into stable behavioral states by 28 to 32 weeks' gestation (see Chapter 11). With the completion of these milestones, heart rate reactivity by traditional criteria is present in 80% of fetuses by 32 weeks' gestation.
- In growth-restricted fetuses with chronic hypoxemia and mild placental dysfunction, the primary central nervous system response is a delay in all aspects of central nervous system maturation. Reduction of global fetal activity and loss of fetal coupling (absence of heart rate reactivity and fetal breathing movements) are typically observed at a mean pH between 7.10 and 7.20.

Diagnostic Tools in Fetal Growth Restriction

FETAL BIOMETRY

- Population-specific formulas have been derived to generate reference limits that generally have 95% confidence limits that deviate approximately 15% around the actual value.
- Measurement of the biparietal diameter alone is a poor tool for the detection of IUGR.
- Using the 10th percentiles as cutoffs, the AC has a higher sensitivity (98% vs. 85%) but lower positive predictive value (PPV) than the sonographically estimated fetal weight (SEFW) (36% vs. 51%).

- Both the sensitivity and the PPV of the head circumference (HC)/AC ratio for growth restriction does not equal either the AC percentile or the SEFW.
- The femur length (FL)/AC ratio is 22 at all gestational ages from 21 weeks to term; therefore this ratio can be applied without knowledge of the gestational age. An FL/AC ratio greater than 23.5 suggests IUGR.
- EFW has become the most common method for characterizing fetal size and thereby growth abnormalities.

REFERENCE RANGES THAT DEFINE FETAL GROWTH

- *SGA* is defined as a birthweight below the population 10th percentile corrected for gestational age
- Approximately 70% of infants with a birthweight below the 10th percentile are normally grown (i.e., constitutionally small) and are not at risk for adverse outcomes because they present one end of the normal spectrum for neonatal size. The remaining 30% consist of infants who are truly growth restricted and are at risk for increased perinatal morbidity and mortality.
- The recommended interval between ultrasound evaluations of fetal growth is 3 weeks because shorter intervals increase the likelihood of a false-positive diagnosis.

AMNIOTIC FLUID ASSESSMENT

- Placental dysfunction and fetal hypoxemia both may result in decreased perfusion of the fetal kidneys with subsequent oliguria and decreasing amniotic fluid volume (AFV).
- If gestational age is unknown, measurements of the FL/AC ratio and a single amniotic fluid pocket have to be used because they are independent of gestational age. Up to 96% of fetuses with fluid pockets less than 1 cm may be growth restricted.
- Oligohydramnios associated with fetal oliguria is associated with a higher rate of intrapartum complications that may be attributed to reduced placental reserve.

DOPPLER VELOCIMETRY

- Doppler velocimetry serves as a diagnostic, as well as a monitoring, tool.
- Arterial Doppler waveforms provide information on downstream vascular resistance, which may be altered because of structural changes in the vasculature or regulatory changes in vascular tone. The systolic/diastolic (S/D) ratio, the resistance index, and the pulsatility index are the three Doppler indices most widely used to analyze arterial blood flow resistance (Table 33.1).
- The vessels that are of primary importance in the differential diagnosis of placental dysfunction are the umbilical artery (UA) and the middle cerebral artery (MCA) (Figs. 33.1 and 33.2). Use of fetal biometry and UA Doppler significantly reduces perinatal mortality and iatrogenic intervention because documentation of placental vascular insufficiency effectively separates growth-restricted fetuses that require surveillance and possible intervention from constitutionally small fetuses.
- Vascular damage that affects approximately 30% of the placenta produces elevations in the Doppler index.
- Milder forms of placental vascular dysfunction, especially near term, may not produce elevation of UA blood flow resistance sufficient to be detectable by traditional Doppler methods.
- Bahado-Singh and coworkers indicated that the predictive accuracy of the cerebroplacental ratio decreased after 34 weeks' gestation. This is presumably attributable to an increasing

TABLE 33.1 ■ Arterial and Venous Doppler Indices

Index	Calculation
Arterial Doppler Indices	
Systolic/diastolic (S/D) ratio	$\dfrac{\text{Systolic peak velocity}}{\text{Diastolic peak velocity}}$
Resistance index (RI)	$\dfrac{\text{Systolic – End-diastolic peak velocity}}{\text{Systolic peak velocity}}$
Pulsatility index (PI)	$\dfrac{\text{Systolic – End-diastolic peak velocity}}{\text{Time averaged maximum velocity}}$
Venous Doppler Indices	
Inferior vena cava preload index	$\dfrac{\text{Peak velocity during atrial contraction}}{\text{Systolic peak velocity}}$
Ductus venosus preload index	$\dfrac{\text{Systolic – Diastolic peak velocity}}{\text{Systolic peak velocity}}$
Inferior vena cava and ductus venosus pulsatility index for veins (PIV)	$\dfrac{\text{Systolic – Diastolic peak velocity}}{\text{Time averaged maximum velocity}}$
Inferior vena cava and ductus venosus peak velocity index for veins (PVIV)	$\dfrac{\text{Systolic – Atrial contraction peak velocity}}{\text{Diastolic peak velocity}}$
Percentage reverse flow	$\dfrac{\text{Systolic time averaged velocity}}{\text{Diastolic time averaged velocity}} \times 100$

number of growth-restricted fetuses who may have normal UA blood flow resistance near term but demonstrate isolated "brain sparing" as the only sign of placental insufficiency of oxygen transfer. These fetuses are at risk for adverse outcomes.

DIAGNOSTIC APPROACH

■ Ultrasound examination is the primary diagnostic tool for the evaluation of fetal growth and should be performed in the first or early second trimester for dating and again at 32 to 34 weeks.
■ If small fetal size is documented, Doppler ultrasound of the umbilical and middle cerebral arteries and invasive tests when indicated are of critical importance to identify fetuses most likely to benefit from antenatal surveillance and perinatal interventions (Fig. 33.3).

Screening and Prevention of Fetal Growth Restriction

■ The maternal history of delivery of a growth-restricted infant in the first pregnancy is associated with a 25% risk of delivering a second infant below the 10th percentile.
■ A single, unexplained elevated maternal serum alpha-fetoprotein or hCG value of 2 to 2.5 multiples of the median raises the risk of growth restriction fivefold to tenfold.
■ A decrease in the pregnancy-associated plasma protein A below 0.8 mOsm is associated with increased risk for placental dysfunction.
■ After 20 weeks' gestation, a lag of the symphyseal-fundal height of 4 cm or more suggests growth restriction.
■ Efforts to prevent FGR have been disappointing.

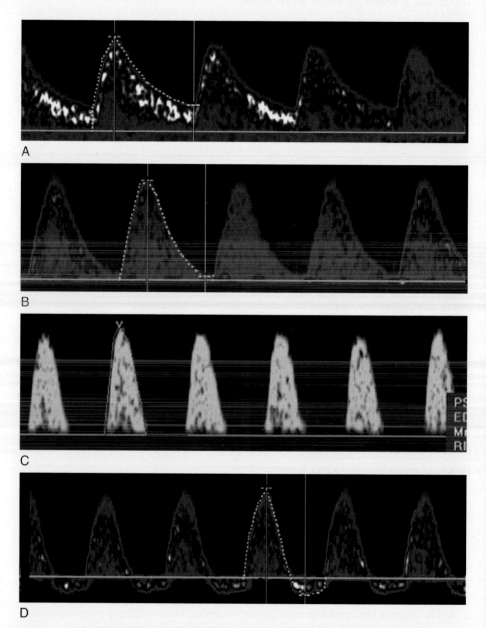

Fig. 33.1 Umbilical artery flow-velocity waveforms. **A,** The normal umbilical artery flow-velocity waveform has positive end-diastolic velocities that increase toward term, reflecting a falling blood flow resistance in the villous vascular tree. **B,** Moderate abnormalities in the villous vascular structure raise the blood flow resistance and are associated with a decline in end-diastolic velocities. When a significant proportion of the villous vascular tree is abnormal, end-diastolic velocities may be absent **(C)** or even reversed **(D)**.

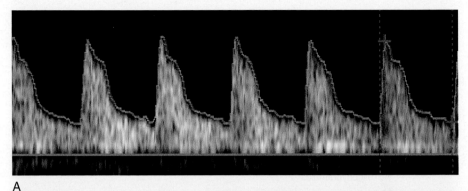

A

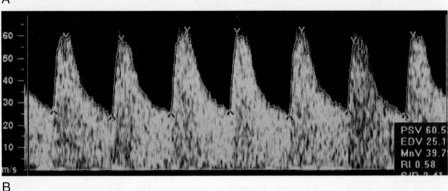

B

Fig. 33.2 Middle cerebral artery flow-velocity waveform. **A,** The normal middle cerebral artery flow pattern has relatively little diastolic flow. With progressive placental dysfunction, an increase in the diastolic velocity results in a decrease in the Doppler index (brain sparing). **B,** With brain sparing, the systolic downslope of the waveform becomes smoother so that the waveform almost resembles that of the umbilical artery. The associated rise in the mean velocity results in a marked decline in the Doppler index.

Management in Clinical Practice

- The majority of fetuses thought to be growth restricted are constitutionally small and require no intervention. Approximately 15% exhibit symmetric growth restriction attributable to an early fetal insult for which there is no effective therapy.
- Approximately 15% of small fetuses have growth restriction as a result of placental disease or reduced uteroplacental blood flow.

THERAPEUTIC OPTIONS

- In 1997, a meta-analysis of the efficacy of low-dose aspirin (50 to 100 mg/day) demonstrated a significant reduction in the frequency of IUGR when low-dose aspirin was used. A dose-dependent relationship is apparent: higher doses (100 to 150 mg/day) were significantly more effective in preventing IUGR than were lower doses (50 to 80 mg/day).
- The therapeutic optimal window to commence aspirin therapy in patients with risk factors for IUGR lies between 12 and 16 weeks' gestation when branching angiogenesis of the placenta is ongoing. We suggest deferral of indicated therapy until completion of organogenesis at 12 weeks' gestation.

DIAGNOSTIC TEST RESULTS   **LIKELY DIAGNOSIS**

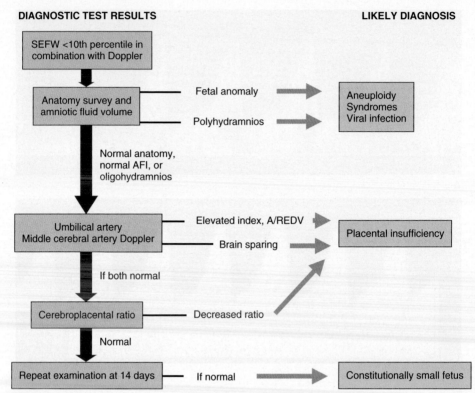

Fig. 33.3 An integrated diagnostic approach to the fetus with suspected fetal growth restriction. This figure displays a decision tree following the evaluation of fetal anatomy, amniotic fluid volume, and umbilical and middle cerebral artery Doppler. The most likely clinical diagnosis based on the test results is presented on the right-hand side. A high index of suspicion for aneuploidy and viral and nonaneuploid syndromes needs to be maintained at all times. AFI, amniotic fluid index; A/REDV, absent/reversed end-diastolic flow; SEFW, sonographically estimated fetal weight. (Data from Unterscheider J, Daly S, Geary MP, et al. Optimizing the definition of intrauterine growth restriction: the multicenter prospective PORTO Study. *Am J Obstet Gynecol.* 2013;208:290.e1-e6.)

- Corticosteroids resulted in a significant reduction in neonatal respiratory distress syndrome, intraventricular hemorrhage, and death when administered. We recommend administration of a complete 48-hour course of antenatal steroids to any growth-restricted fetus when delivery is anticipated before 34 weeks' gestation, if this can be safely accomplished.
- When corticosteroids are administered, it is important to account for their effect on fetal testing parameters when interpreting antenatal surveillance results. Betamethasone, for example, temporarily reduces FHR variation on days 2 and 3 after the first injection, together with a 50% decrease in fetal body movements and a near cessation of fetal breathing movements. Subsequently, the number of fetuses with abnormal biophysical profile scores increases significantly by 48 hours after steroid administration, with a return to the preadministration state at 72 hours.

Assessment of Fetal Well-Being

- Serial ultrasound evaluations of fetal growth are continued every 3 to 4 weeks and should include determinations of the biparietal diameter, HC/AC ratio, fetal weight, and AFV.

- Irrespective of the context, a "reactive" nonstress test (NST) indicates absence of fetal acidemia at the moment of the FHR recording and correlates highly with a fetus not in immediate danger of intrauterine demise.
- Nonreactive NST results are often falsely positive and require further evaluation. The development of repetitive decelerations may reflect fetal hypoxemia or cord compression as a result of the development of oligohydramnios and has been associated with a high perinatal mortality rate.
- A 25% to 50% false-positive rate has been associated with the contraction stress test by some investigators. A possible role for the contraction stress test may be evaluation of placental reserve prior to induction in IUGR fetuses in whom vaginal delivery is attempted.

AMNIOTIC FLUID VOLUME

- AFV provides an indirect measure of vascular status. A relationship between oligohydramnios and progressive deterioration of arterial and venous Doppler studies has been documented in growth-restricted fetuses and prolonged pregnancies.
- If the NST is reactive, a concurrent assessment of the AFV constitutes the *modified biophysical profile* and provides assurance of fetal well-being if both parameters are normal.
- When the FHR is nonreactive, relying on a normal AFV assessment alone is inadequate, and a full biophysical profile should be done (see Chapter 11).

DOPPLER ULTRASOUND

- This utility is greatest for early-onset growth restriction, which is associated with more marked Doppler abnormalities than late-onset disease that requires delivery after 34 weeks, especially in early-onset placental dysfunction.
- The Doppler index is observed when approximately 30% of the fetal villous vessels are abnormal. Absence or even reversal of UA end-diastolic velocity can occur when 60% to 70% of the villous vascular tree is damaged (see Fig. 33.1). Incidences of intrauterine hypoxia that range from 50% to 80% in fetuses with absent end-diastolic flow have been reported.
- Fetal Doppler assessment based on the UA alone is no longer appropriate, particularly in the setting of early-onset IUGR prior to 34 weeks. Incorporation of MCA (see Fig. 33.2) and venous Doppler provide the best prediction of acid-base status, risk of stillbirth, and the anticipated rate of progression.
- In growth-restricted fetuses with an elevated Doppler index in the UA, brain sparing in the presence of normal venous Doppler parameters is typically associated with hypoxemia but a normal pH.
- Abnormal venous Doppler parameters are the strongest Doppler predictors of stillbirth. Even among fetuses with severe arterial Doppler abnormalities (e.g., absent/reversed end-diastolic velocity or reversed end diastolic velocity [REDV]), the risk of stillbirth is largely confined to those fetuses with abnormal venous Dopplers.
- The neonatal mortality rate in fetuses with AEDV or REDV ranges from 5% to 18% when the venous Doppler indices are normal. Elevation of the DV Doppler index greater than 2 standard deviations doubles this mortality rate, although predictive sensitivity is only 38% with a specificity of 98%.
- Advancing Doppler abnormalities indicate acceleration of disease and require increased frequency of fetal monitoring. In growth-restricted fetuses, Doppler evaluation is complementary to all other surveillance modalities.

ANTICIPATING THE PROGRESSION TO FETAL COMPROMISE

- Late-onset FGR (presenting after 34 weeks' gestation) does not typically pose a dilemma for delivery timing because delivery thresholds can be low given the lower neonatal risks but it contributes to over 50% of unanticipated stillbirths at term.
- Studies indicate that 40% of preterm growth-restricted fetuses that deteriorate in utero have an increased DV Doppler index the week prior to delivery.
- Pregnancies at increased risk of adverse outcome were those with an abnormal UA Doppler study and, in particular, those with an EFW below the third percentile with or without oligohydramnios.
- Integrated fetal testing and management protocol is shown in Fig. 33.3, supplemented with maternal assessment of fetal movement ("kick counts") commencing no earlier than 24 weeks' gestation.
- In fetuses with an AFI of less than 5 cm or absent end-diastolic velocity in the umbilical artery, surveillance intervals are shortened to every 3 to 4 days. With elevation of the DV Doppler index to less than 2 standard deviations, testing frequency is increased to every 2 to 3 days. Further escalation of the DV Doppler index may require daily testing, and inpatient admission may be prudent based on local practice. Any change in maternal condition, especially the development of preeclampsia, calls for reassessment of fetal status irrespective of the last examination result (Fig. 33.4).

Timing of Delivery

- The decision for delivery always weighs fetal risks against risks that can be anticipated as a result of delivery. The perinatal mortality with early delivery was associated with a higher rate of neonatal deaths, whereas delaying delivery increased the risk for stillbirth.
- Frigoletto has previously emphasized that the majority of fetal deaths in IUGR occur after the 36th week of gestation and before the onset of labor. The Disproportionate Intrauterine Growth Intervention Trial at Term (DIGITAT) randomized trial illustrates that neonatal morbidity is still a concern until 38 weeks' gestation. For these reasons, a definite delivery indication other than the presence of suspected growth delay is required prior to 38 weeks' gestation. One limitation of the DIGITAT trial was a lack of UA and MCA Doppler assessment or integration in the study.

Delivery

- Because many growth-restricted infants suffer intrapartum asphyxia, intrapartum management demands continuous FHR monitoring. In principle the route of delivery is determined by the severity of the fetal and maternal condition, along with other obstetric factors.
- With late decelerations, the incidence of asphyxia in growth-restricted infants is far greater than in normally grown infants.

SHORT-TERM OUTCOMES

- Meconium aspiration, hypoglycemia, hypocalcemia, polycythemia, hyperbilirubinemia, and hypothermia are more common.

LONG-TERM OUTCOMES

- These infants can be expected to have normal growth curves and a normal, albeit slightly reduced size as adults.

IUGR UNLIKELY		
Normal AC, AC growth rate and HC/AC ratio UA, MCA Doppler, BPS, and AFV normal	Asphyxia extremely rare low risk for intrapartum distress	Deliver for obstetric or maternal factors only, follow growth

IUGR		
AC <5th, low AC growth rate, high HC/AC ratio, abnormal UA and/or CPR, normal MCA and veins, BPS ≥8/10, AFV normal	Asphyxia extremely rare Increased risk for intrapartum distress	Deliver for obstetric or maternal factors only, Every 2 weeks Doppler Weekly BPS

With blood flow redistribution

IUGR diagnosed based on above criteria Low MCA, normal veins BPS ≥8/10, AFV normal	Hypoxemia possible, asphyxia rare Increased risk for intrapartum distress	Deliver for obstetric or maternal factors only, weekly Doppler BPS 2 times/week

With significant blood flow redistribution

UA A/REDV normal veins BPS ≥6/10, oligohydramnios	Hypoxemia common, acidemia or asphyxia possible Onset of fetal compromise	>34 weeks: deliver <32 weeks: antenatal steroids Repeat all testing daily

With proven fetal compromise

Significant redistribution present Increased DV pulsatility BPS ≥6/10, oligohydramnios	Hypoxemia common, acidemia or asphyxia likely	>32 weeks: deliver <32 weeks: admit, Steroids, individualize testing daily vs. tid

With fetal decompensation

Compromise by above criteria Absent or reversed DV a-wave, pulsatile UV BPS <6/10, oligohydramnios	Cardiovascular instability, metabolic compromise, stillbirth imminent, high perinatal mortality irrespective of intervention	Deliver at tertiary care center with the highest level of NICU care

Fig. 33.4 Integrated fetal testing and management protocol. The management algorithm for pregnancies complicated by intrauterine growth restriction (IUGR) is based on the ability to perform arterial and venous Doppler as well as a full five-component biophysical profile score (BPS). AC, abdominal circumference; AFV, amniotic fluid volume; A/REDV, absent/reversed end-diastolic velocity; CPR, cerebroplacental ratio; DV, ductus venosus; HC, head circumference; MCA, middle cerebral artery; NICU, neonatal intensive care unit; tid, three times daily; UA, umbilical artery; UV, umbilical vein. (From Baschat AA, Hecher K. Fetal growth restriction due to placental disease. *Semin Perinatol.* 2004;28:67.)

- The vast majority of children with cerebral palsy were not growth restricted.
- Growth-restricted infants with HCs below the 10th percentile have two to three times the number of serious neurologic sequelae of their normocephalic counterparts.
- Gestational age at delivery, birthweight, and reversal of UA end-diastolic velocity are the main determinants of motor and neurosensory morbidity.

- Neurologic outcome depends on the degree of growth restriction, especially the impact on head growth, its time of onset, the gestational age of the infant at birth, and the postnatal environment.
- The preterm appropriately grown infant has more normal neurologic development and fewer severe neurologic deficits than its preterm growth-restricted counterpart.
- If growth restriction is associated with lagging head growth before 26 weeks, even mature infants have significant developmental delay at 4 years of age.
- Infants born growth restricted have an increased risk of metabolic syndrome, obesity, hypertension, diabetes, and stroke from coronary artery disease (see Chapter 5).

Red Cell Alloimmunization

Kenneth J. Moise Jr

Nomenclature

- Exposure to foreign red cell antigens invariably results in the production of anti–red cell antibodies in a process known as *red cell alloimmunization*, formerly termed *isoimmunization*. The expression *sensitization* can be used interchangeably with *Rhesus alloimmunization*.
- The term *hemolytic disease of the fetus and newborn* (HDFN) would appear more appropriate to describe this disorder.

Historic Perspectives

- The first case of HDFN was probably described in 1609 by a midwife in the French literature.[1] The advent of therapy for HDFN began in 1945 with the description by Wallerstein[2] of the technique of neonatal exchange transfusion and the introduction of the intraperitoneal fetal transfusion by Liley in 1963.

Incidence

- The advent of the routine administration of antenatal and postpartum rhesus immune globulin (RhIG) has resulted in a marked reduction in cases of red cell alloimmunization secondary to the RhD antigen.
- A shift to other red cell antibodies associated with HDFN has occurred as a result of the decreasing incidence of RhD alloimmunization.

Pathophysiology

- In most cases of red cell alloimmunization, a fetomaternal hemorrhage (FMH) occurs in the antenatal period or, more commonly, at the time of delivery. As many as one-fourth of RhD-negative infants have been shown to be immunized in early life as a result of their delivery.[3,4]
- Only 13% of deliveries of RhD-positive fetuses result in RhD alloimmunization in RhD-negative women who do not receive RhIG.
- Anti-D IgG is a nonagglutinating antibody that does not bind complement, resulting in a lack of intravascular hemolysis. Sequestration and subsequent destruction of antibody-coated red cells in the fetal liver and spleen are the mechanism of fetal anemia.
- RhD-positive male fetuses are 13 times more likely than their female counterparts to become hydropic and are 3 times more likely to die of their disease.[5]
- Hydrops fetalis, the accumulation of extracellular fluid in at least two body compartments, is a late finding in cases of fetal anemia. Its exact pathophysiology is complex.

Rhesus Alloimmunization and Fetal/Neonatal Hemolytic Disease of the Newborn

GENETICS

- Only two genes have been identified, an *RHD* gene and an *RHCE* gene.

Prevention of RhD Hemolytic Disease in the Fetus and Newborn

HISTORY

- Recommendations for use during the immediate postpartum period were set forth by the American College of Obstetricians and Gynecologists (ACOG)[6] in 1970. The Food and Drug Administration (FDA) approved the use of antenatal RhIG in 1981. Routine antenatal prophylaxis at 28 to 29 weeks' gestation was proposed by ACOG later that same year.[7]

PREPARATIONS

- Four polyclonal products derived from human plasma are currently available in the United States for the prevention of RhD alloimmunization.

INDICATIONS

- All pregnant patients should undergo determination of blood type and an antibody screen at the first prenatal visit.

- If there is no evidence of anti-D alloimmunization in the RhD-negative woman, the patient should receive 300 μg of RhIG at 28 weeks of gestation.[8]
- Although not well studied, level A (high) scientific evidence has been cited by ACOG to address additional indications for the antepartum administration of RhIG.[8] These include spontaneous miscarriage, elective abortion, ectopic pregnancy, genetic amniocentesis, chorionic villus sampling, and fetal blood sampling.
- The practice of evaluating a persistent maternal anti-D titer as an indication that additional RhIG is not required after an antenatal event is to be discouraged.
- Both ACOG and the American Association of Blood Banks now recommend routine screening of all women at the time of delivery for excessive FMH.
- Should RhIG be inadvertently omitted after delivery, some protection has been proven with administration within 13 days. Recommendations have been made to administer it as late as 28 days after delivery.[9]
- If delivery occurs less than 3 weeks from the administration of RhIG used for antenatal indications such as external cephalic version, a repeat dose is unnecessary unless a large FMH is detected at the time of delivery.[10]
- In others with a weak D phenotype, the individual has inherited a gene that results in a variant expression of the D antigen. In these cases, one or more of the D antigen epitopes are missing, and the patient can become alloimmunized to these missing portions of the D antigen. Severe HDFN has been reported in these cases when a maternal antibody develops to the missing epitope.[11] Although clinical trials have not been undertaken, the current recommendation is that these patients should receive RhIG.

DIAGNOSTIC METHODS

Maternal Antibody Determination

- Once a maternal antibody screen reveals the presence of an anti-D antibody, a titer is the first step in the evaluation of the RhD-sensitized patient during the first affected pregnancy.
- The human antiglobulin titer (indirect Coombs test) is used to determine the degree of alloimmunization because it measures the maternal IgG response.
- A *critical titer* is defined as the anti–red cell titer associated with a significant risk for hydrops fetalis.
- In most centers, a critical titer for anti-D between 8 and 32 is usually used.

Fetal Blood Typing

- The initial step in determining the fetal RhD type involves an assessment of paternity and paternal zygosity.
- Several techniques have been used to determine the fetal blood type if the patient's partner is determined to be heterozygous for the involved red cell antigen. In 50% of cases in which the fetus is found to be antigen negative, further maternal and fetal testing is unnecessary. This method has now been replaced in many countries, including the United States, by the use of fetal *RHD* determination using circulating cell-free fetal DNA (ccffDNA).
- In a recent series of more than 1000 patients, ccffDNA testing for *RHD* was found to be accurate in 99% of cases.[12]
- In the cases with an inconclusive result, a repeat maternal sample can be submitted or amniocentesis can be undertaken to determine the fetal *RHD* status.

Amniocentesis to Follow the Severity of Hemolytic Disease of the Fetus and Newborn

- The advent of noninvasive testing for fetal anemia with middle cerebral artery (MCA) Doppler has now replaced serial amniocenteses for amniotic fluid delta OD 450 (ΔOD_{450}).

Fetal Blood Sampling

- Fetal blood sampling is reserved for patients with elevated peak systolic MCA Doppler velocities.

Ultrasound

- Perhaps the greatest advance in the management of the alloimmunized pregnancy has been the use of ultrasound.
- When hydrops is present, fetal hemoglobin deficits of 7 to 10 g/dL from the mean hemoglobin value for the corresponding gestational age can be expected.[13]
- The early second-trimester fetus can be severely anemic without obvious signs of hydrops.[14]
- The severely anemic fetus exhibits an increased cardiac output in an effort to enhance oxygen delivery to peripheral tissues.[15]
- Doppler ultrasound has been used to study the peak systolic velocity in the fetal MCA to predict fetal anemia. A value of greater than 1.5 multiples of the median for the corresponding gestational age predicts moderate to severe fetal anemia with a sensitivity of 88% and a negative predictive rate of 89%.[16]
- Serial MCA Doppler studies are now the mainstay of surveillance for fetal anemia in the red cell–alloimmunized pregnancy.

Clinical Management

- As a general rule, the patient's first RhD-sensitized pregnancy involves minimal fetal/neonatal disease but subsequent gestations are associated with worsening degrees of anemia.

FIRST AFFECTED PREGNANCY

- Once sensitization to the RhD antigen is detected, maternal titers are repeated every month until approximately 24 weeks. Titers should be repeated every 2 weeks thereafter (Fig. 34.1).

PREVIOUSLY AFFECTED FETUS OR INFANT

- If the patient has a history of a previous perinatal loss related to HDFN, a previous need for intrauterine transfusion (IUT), or a previous need for neonatal exchange transfusion, she should be referred to a tertiary care center with experience in the management of the severely alloimmunized pregnancy.
- Amniocentesis can be used after 15 weeks' gestation to determine the status of the fetal red cell antigen in cases of other maternal antibodies such as anti-Kell.

Intrauterine Transfusion

TECHNIQUE

- IUTs today are performed under continuous ultrasound guidance with direct infusions of red blood cells into the umbilical cord vessels or into the intrahepatic portion of the umbilical vein of the fetus.[17]
- The peak systolic velocity in the MCA has been shown to be useful in timing the second IUT.
- Severely anemic fetuses in the early second trimester do not tolerate the acute correction of their hematocrit to normal values.[18]

COMPLICATIONS AND OUTCOME

- Complications from IUT are uncommon.
- An overall survival rate of 91% has been reported in one series of over 1400 procedures.[19]

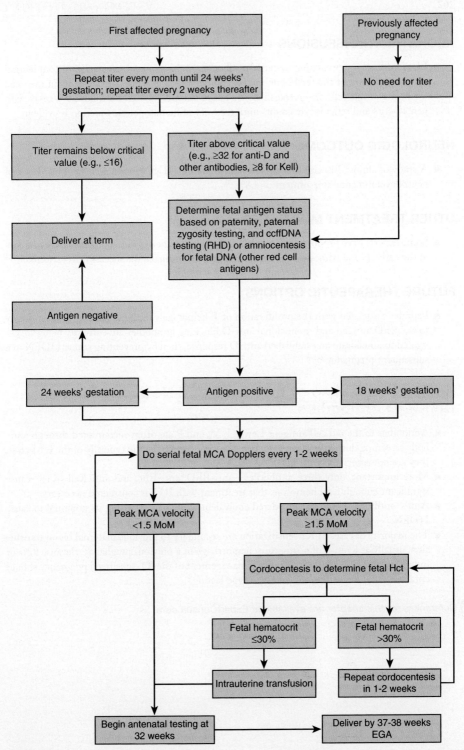

Fig. 34.1 Algorithm for clinical management of a patient with red cell alloimmunization. ccffDNA, circulating cell-free fetal DNA; EGA, estimated gestational age; Hct, hematocrit; MCA, middle cerebral artery; MoM, multiples of the median.

NEONATAL TRANSFUSIONS

- Elevated levels of circulating maternal antibodies in the neonatal circulation in conjunction with suppression of the fetal bone marrow production of red cells often results in the need for neonatal red cell *top-up* transfusions. These children should be followed weekly with hematocrits and reticulocyte counts until recovery of hematopoietic function is evident.

NEUROLOGIC OUTCOME

- A study of almost 300 children treated with IUTs for HDFN found an overall incidence of neurodevelopmental impairment of 4.8%.[20]

OTHER TREATMENT MODALITIES

- Some experts have proposed a combined approach in patients with a previous perinatal loss in the early second trimester when technical limitations make the success of IUT unlikely.[21]

FUTURE THERAPEUTIC OPTIONS

- Peptides associated with the proliferation of T-helper cells in the development of antibody to the RhD antigen and monoclonal anti-D blocking antibodies are currently being investigated to ameliorate an established anti-D response, thereby preventing severe HDFN in a subsequent pregnancy.[22,23]

Hemolytic Disease of the Fetus and Newborn Due to Non-RhD Antibodies

- Antibodies to the red cell antigens Lewis, I, M, and P are often encountered through antibody screening during prenatal care. Because these antibodies are typically of the IgM class, they are not associated with HDFN.[24]
- More important, only three antibodies—anti-RhD, anti-Rhc, and anti-Kell (K1)—cause significant enough fetal hemolysis that treatment with IUT is considered necessary.
- Anti-c antibody should be considered equivalent to anti-D regarding its potential to cause HDFN.
- The majority of cases of K1 sensitization are secondary to previous maternal blood transfusion, usually as a result of postpartum hemorrhage in a previous pregnancy. Because 92% of individuals are Kell negative, the initial management of the K1-sensitized pregnancy should entail paternal red cell typing and genotype testing.

🔗 *References for this chapter are available at ExpertConsult.com.*

CHAPTER 35

Amniotic Fluid Disorders

William M. Gilbert

KEY POINTS

- AF is dynamic, with large volume flows into and out of the amniotic compartment each day.
- Clinical estimates of actual AFV based on ultrasound measurements of the AFI or MVP are not accurate in predicting true volume.
- In the presence of intrauterine growth restriction or a prolonged gestation, oligohydramnios is associated with significant increases in perinatal morbidity and mortality.
- Preterm or term isolated oligohydramnios is not associated with an increase in perinatal morbidity or mortality with an otherwise normal fetus.
- Early-onset or severe polyhydramnios is associated with aneuploidy, congenital malformations, preterm delivery, and an increased perinatal mortality rate.
- The cause of mild polyhydramnios, especially in the latter part of the third trimester, is usually idiopathic or related to diabetes mellitus and has little impact on perinatal survival.
- AFV as estimated by the AFI may be expanded with increased maternal oral ingestion of water and/or bed rest in the left lateral recumbent position.
- Short-term use of indomethacin decreases fetal urine production and can reduce AFV within 24 hours of administration; prolonged use should be avoided because of the risk of premature closure of the ductus arteriosus and renal abnormalities in the newborn.

Overview

- Abnormalities of amniotic fluid volume (AFV) raise the concern for an underlying fetal or maternal complication during pregnancy or fetal/neonatal compromise. The perinatal mortality rate approaches 90% to 100% with severe oligohydramnios in the second trimester and can exceed 50% with significant polyhydramnios in midpregnancy.

Amniotic Fluid Volume

- From 22 through 39 weeks of gestation, the average volume of amniotic fluid (AF) (Fig. 35.1) remains unchanged despite an increase in fetal weight from about 500 g to 3500 g, a sevenfold increase.

ULTRASOUND ASSESSMENT OF AMNIOTIC FLUID VOLUME

- Polyhydramnios may be present if the maternal uterus is large for gestational age or if the fetus cannot be easily palpated or is ballotable. The diagnosis of oligohydramnios is a consideration when the fundal height is small for gestational age or the fetus is easily palpated.

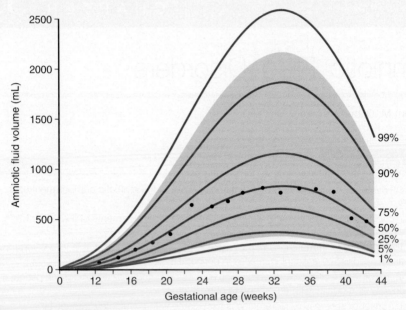

Fig. 35.1 Nomogram showing amniotic fluid volume as a function of gestational age. The black dots are the mean for each 2-week interval. Percentiles are calculated from a polynomial regression equation and standard deviation of residuals. (*From Brace RA, Wolf EJ. Normal amniotic fluid volume throughout pregnancy. Am J Obstet Gynecol. 1989;161:382.*)

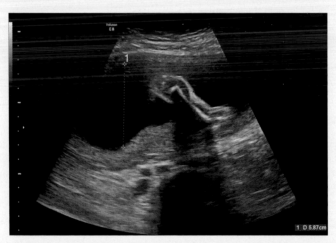

Fig. 35.2 Ultrasound image demonstrates measurement of the maximum vertical pocket (MVP) within the uterus by holding the transducer perpendicular to the floor and determining the MVP of amniotic fluid in centimeters.

- Early ultrasound estimations of AFV were made by measuring the maximum vertical pocket (MVP) of AF (Fig. 35.2).
- Subsequently, a four-quadrant assessment of AF referred to as the *amniotic fluid index* (AFI) was introduced into practice (Fig. 35.3). The sum of the MVP in each quadrant equals the AFI.

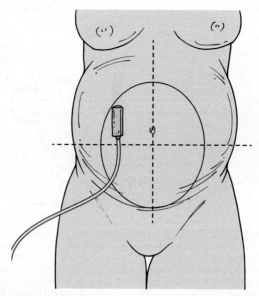

Fig. 35.3 Schematic diagram of the technique for measuring the four-quadrant amniotic fluid index.

■ Although the MVP appears to be the preferred method to diagnose oligohydramnios near term, the vast majority of research on ultrasound measurement of AFV utilizes the AFI.
■ When the MVP is less than 1 cm, a marked increase in perinatal morbidity and mortality has been reported that persisted even after correcting for birth defects.

Amniotic Fluid Formation

■ The main source of amniotic fluid is fetal urination. Human fetal urine-production rate appears to be approximately 1000 to 1200 mL/day at term, which suggests that the entire AFV is replaced more frequently than every 24 hours (Fig. 35.4).
■ Fetal lung liquid also plays an important role in amniotic fluid formation.

Amniotic Fluid Removal

■ In the human, fetal swallowing begins early in gestation and contributes to the removal of amniotic fluid. Fetal swallowing does not remove the entire volume of fluid that enters the amniotic compartment from fetal urine production and lung liquid; therefore other mechanisms of amniotic fluid removal such as intramembranous absorption must occur.
■ Researchers have noted that 200 to 500 mL/day leaves the amniotic compartment under normal physiologic conditions. Intramembranous absorption could easily explain this movement.

Oligohydramnios

■ In clinical practice, an MVP less than 1 to 2 cm or an AFI less than 5 cm are commonly used as criteria for the diagnosis of oligohydramnios.
■ AF is required for fetal lung development during certain periods of early and mid-gestation.
■ Although the evidence for induction in the prolonged pregnancy is solid (see Chapter 36), the term or preterm patient with isolated oligohydramnios may not need immediate delivery.

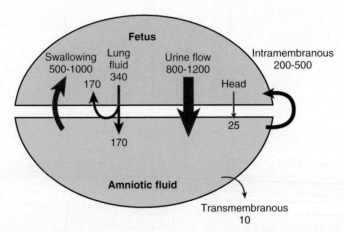

Fig. 35.4 All known pathways for fluid and solute entry and exit from the amniotic fluid in the fetus near term. Arrow size is relative to associated flow rate. Brown arrows represent directly measured flows, whereas the blue arrows represent estimated flows. The numbers represent volume flow in milliliters per day. The curved portion of the double arrow represents lung fluid that is directly swallowed after leaving the trachea, whereas the straight portion represents lung fluid that enters the amniotic cavity from the mouth and nose. (*From Gilbert WM, Moore TR, Brace RA. Amniotic fluid volume dynamics. Fetal Med Review. 1991;3:89.*)

BOX 35.1 ■ Fetal and Maternal Causes of Oligohydramnios

Fetal Conditions

- Renal agenesis
- Obstructed uropathy
- Spontaneous rupture of the membranes
- Premature rupture of the membranes
- Abnormal placentation
- Prolonged pregnancy
- Severe intrauterine growth restriction

Maternal Conditions

- Dehydration-hypovolemia
- Hypertensive disorders
- Uteroplacental insufficiency
- Antiphospholipid syndrome

- All cases with oligohydramnios should be evaluated for evidence of intrauterine growth restriction and should be followed with antepartum testing.

EVALUATION AND TREATMENT OF OLIGOHYDRAMNIOS

- When the diagnosis of oligohydramnios is made in the second trimester, it is vitally important to obtain a complete history and physical exam and to perform a targeted ultrasound to help identify a cause (Box 35.1).
- Several investigators have attempted to treat oligohydramnios with the oral administration of water in the hope of "hydrating" the fetus through the mother.
- Groups have demonstrated that the AFI can be influenced by increasing or decreasing water intake orally.

BOX 35.2 ■ Fetal and Maternal Causes of Polyhydramnios

Fetal Conditions

Congenital anomalies
■ Gastrointestinal obstruction, central nervous system abnormalities, cystic hygroma, nonimmune hydrops, sacrococcygeal teratoma, cystic adenoid malformations of lung

Aneuploidy

Genetic disorders
■ Achondrogenesis type 1-B
■ Muscular dystrophies
■ Bartter syndrome

Twin-to-twin transfusion syndrome

Infections
■ Parvovirus B-19

Placental abnormalities
■ Chorioangioma

Maternal Conditions

Idiopathic

Poorly controlled diabetes mellitus

Fetomaternal hemorrhage

OLIGOHYDRAMNIOS IN LABOR

- Although most report a decrease in the frequency of variable decelerations with amnioinfusion in the setting of oligohydramnios, few have demonstrated any decrease in perinatal morbidity or mortality or in the cesarean delivery rate.
- Based on a large multicenter trial, ACOG recommends against routine prophylactic amnioinfusion for the dilution of meconium-stained amniotic fluid.

Polyhydramnios

- Many authors define polyhydramnios as an MVP of greater than 8 cm, whereas others use an AFI of 25 cm or greater.
- Severe polyhydramnios in the second trimester has a significant perinatal mortality rate due to prematurity or aneuploidy.

EVALUATION AND TREATMENT OF POLYHYDRAMNIOS

- The pregnant woman who presents with a rapidly enlarging uterus in mid pregnancy, with or without preterm labor, needs to be evaluated to identify a cause (Box 35.2). Ultrasound examination should be performed to measure the AFV and assess fetal anatomy.
- When polyhydramnios occurs in the third trimester of pregnancy, it is usually mild and is not associated with a structural defect.
- With severe polyhydramnios associated with preterm labor, one medical treatment option involves the administration of a prostaglandin inhibitor such as indomethacin, which decreases fetal urine production.

PART VI

Pregnancy and Coexisting Disease

CHAPTER 36

Prolonged and Postterm Pregnancy

Roxane Rampersad ■ George A. Macones

KEY POINTS

- Ultrasonography, preferably done in the first trimester, is the most accurate method with which to establish the EDD.
- No gestational cutoff has been established by which to define a prolonged pregnancy in multiple gestations. The risk for stillbirth increases after 38 weeks in twins and after 35 weeks in triplets.
- Late-term and postterm pregnancies are associated with an increased risk for perinatal morbidity and mortality, oligohydramnios, macrosomia, postmaturity, and maternal morbidity.
- It seems prudent to initiate antenatal fetal surveillance at 41 weeks in a normal, uncomplicated pregnancy in the absence of intrauterine growth restriction.
- Antenatal fetal surveillance at 41 weeks should include a modified biophysical profile at least once a week.
- If the cervix is favorable at 41 weeks, induction of labor can be considered.
- Delivery after $42^{0/7}$ weeks and by $42^{6/7}$ weeks is recommended based on the small but increased risk of perinatal morbidity and mortality.
- Either prostaglandin preparation, PGE_1 or PGE_2, can be used for induction of the postterm pregnancy.

Definition

- *Postterm pregnancy* is a gestation that has completed or gone beyond 42 weeks or 294 days, from the first day of the last menstrual period (LMP).
- Pregnancies are designated as "late term" at $41^{0/7}$ weeks through $41^{6/7}$ weeks.

Incidence

- According to the vital statistics reported by the Centers for Disease Control and Prevention, the overall incidence of postterm pregnancies was 5.6% in 2012 and has not significantly changed compared with previous years.

Etiology

- The etiology of the majority of pregnancies that are late term or postterm is unknown. Some pregnancies may be defined as late term or postterm as the result of an error in dating.
- A number of observational studies have identified risk factors for postterm pregnancy, including primigravidity, prior postterm pregnancy, male fetus, obesity, and a genetic predisposition.

Diagnosis

- The diagnosis of truly late term and postterm pregnancy is based on accurate gestational dating.
- The use of ultrasound to determine the accuracy of gestational dating based on the LMP is superior to the use of the LMP alone. The estimated date of delivery (EDD) is most accurately determined if the crown-rump length is measured in the first trimester with an error of ± 5 to 7 days.

Perinatal Morbidity and Mortality

- More recent observational studies that have evaluated the risk of perinatal mortality at each gestational week show an increased risk as gestational age advances beyond the EDD (Fig. 36.1).
- Clausson and colleagues evaluated a large Swedish database of term and postterm (defined as ≥294 days) singleton, normal neonates and showed that postterm pregnancies were associated with an increased frequency of neonatal convulsions, meconium aspiration syndrome, and Apgar scores of less than 4 at 5 minutes (Table 36.1).

OLIGOHYDRAMNIOS

- In a setting of oligohydramnios, the risk of perinatal morbidity and mortality is increased, regardless of the pathophysiology.

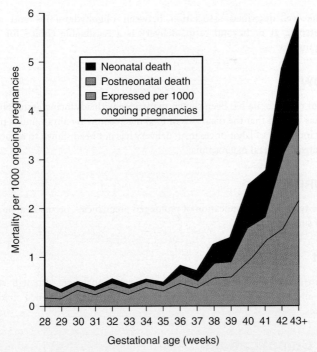

Fig. 36.1 The summed mortality at each gestation for the rate of stillbirth (*red*), neonatal death (*blue*), and postneonatal death (*green*) expressed per 1000 ongoing pregnancies. (*Modified from Hilder L, Costeloe K, Thilaganathan B. Prolonged pregnancy: evaluating gestation specific risks of fetal and infant mortality. BJOG. 1998;105:169.*)

TABLE 36.1 ■ Neonatal Morbidity in Postterm Average and SGA Infants

Complications	Term Aga Neonates*
Convulsions	
Term SGA	2. 3 (1.6–3.4)
Postterm AGA	1. 5 (1.2–2.0)
Postterm SGA	3. 4 (1.5–7.6)
Meconium Aspiration	
Term SGA	2. 4 (1.6–3.4)
Postterm AGA	3. 0 (2.6–3.7)
Postterm SGA	1. 6 (0.5–5.0)
Apgar Score <4 at 5 min	
Term SGA	2. 2 (1.4–3.4)
Postterm AGA	2. 0 (1.5–2.5)
Postterm SGA	3. 6 (1.5–8.7)

Modified from Clausson B, Cnattinguis S, Axelsson O. Outcomes of post-term births: the role of fetal growth restriction and malformations. Obstet Gynecol. 1999;94:758.
*Values are presented as odds ratios (confidence interval).
AGA, average for gestational age; SGA, small for gestational age.

- Given the well-described association between oligohydramnios and adverse pregnancy outcome at or beyond term, delivery is a reasonable choice for patients with oligohydramnios.

FETAL GROWTH

- The risk of macrosomia has been shown to increase with advancing gestational age.
- ACOG has warned that the diagnosis of fetal macrosomia by ultrasound is not precise and that early induction of labor or cesarean delivery has not been shown to reduce the morbidity associated with fetal macrosomia.

POSTMATURITY

- Postmaturity, another complication of prolonged pregnancies, occurs in approximately 10% to 20% of such pregnancies.

MECONIUM

- Meconium-stained fluid can be seen at any gestational age, although several studies have documented a significantly increased risk of meconium-stained fluid in postterm pregnancies.

Maternal Complications

- Prolonged pregnancies are also associated with significant risk to the mother (perineal lacerations, chorioamnionitis, postpartum hemorrhage, emdomyometritis, cesarean delivery).

Management

- Accurate assessment of gestational age is paramount in the management of late-term and postterm pregnancies.

ANTENATAL SURVEILLANCE

- Given the increased risk of stillbirth, antenatal surveillance is recommended in the management of prolonged and postterm pregnancies.
- Based on the studies of perinatal morbidity and mortality, it would seem prudent to initiate fetal testing no later than 41 weeks of gestation.
- ACOG proposed that amniotic fluid volume should be assessed when surveillance is initiated for late-term pregnancies because oligohydramnios has been associated with abnormal fetal heart tracings, umbilical cord compression, and meconium-stained fluid.
- ACOG currently recommends the initiation of fetal surveillance at 41 weeks or beyond with assessment of amniotic fluid volume.

EXPECTANT MANAGEMENT VERSUS INDUCTION OF LABOR

- New evidence supports the induction of labor after $42^{0/7}$ weeks and by $42^{6/7}$ weeks to decrease the risk of perinatal morbidity and mortality,
- A Cochrane meta-analysis suggests that induction may yield slightly improved perinatal outcomes.
- Studies show a small but significantly increased risk in perinatal morbidity and mortality in postterm pregnancies, and hence, postterm pregnancy is one of the most common reasons for induction of labor in the United States.

Long-Term Neonatal Outcomes

- Several small and older studies show no apparent difference in long-term neonatal outcome for neonates born at 42 weeks and later.

Multiple Gestation

- No defined gestational age cutoff has been established to define a prolonged pregnancy in twin, triplet, or higher-order multiples.
- It would seem reasonable to utilize antenatal testing as these gestational ages approach and to accomplish delivery at the nadir of stillbirth risk (see Chapter 32).

CHAPTER 37

Heart Disease in Pregnancy

Jason Deen ■ Suchitra Chandrasekaran ■ Karen Stout ■ Thomas Easterling

KEY POINTS

- Hemodynamic changes in pregnancy may adversely affect maternal cardiac performance.
- Intercurrent events (e.g., infection) in pregnancy are usually the cause of decompensation.
- Women with heart disease in pregnancy frequently have unique psychosocial needs.
- Labor, delivery, and postpartum are periods of hemodynamic instability.
- The postpartum period can be characterized as a "perfect storm" of volume loading, tachycardia, and increased afterload; each of these may contribute to the destabilization of a pregnant woman with heart disease.
- Invasive hemodynamic monitoring should be used to address specific clinical questions.
- Many maternal heart conditions can be medically managed during pregnancy.
- Management of anticoagulation in women with mechanical valves requires an experienced team and careful consideration of the balance between maternal and fetal risk followed by appropriate counseling. Very aggressive therapeutic monitoring is required.
- Mothers with cyanotic heart disease are at particular risk for adverse fetal and neonatal outcomes.
- Eisenmenger syndrome, Marfan syndrome with a dilated aorta, and pulmonary hypertension with right heart dysfunction are associated with a very high risk for maternal mortality.
- Many women with congenital heart disease can successfully complete a pregnancy.
- Preconceptual counseling is based on achieving a balance between medical information and the patient's value system.
- Cardiovascular adaptations to pregnancy are well tolerated by healthy young women.

Maternal Hemodynamics

- In the supine position, a pregnant woman in the third trimester may experience significant hypotension as a result of venocaval occlusion by the gravid uterus.
- Heart rate (HR), blood pressure, and cardiac output (CO) all increase with uterine contractions, and the magnitude of the change increases as labor advances.
- In the context of cardiac disease, acute centralization of blood may increase pulmonary pressures and pulmonary congestion.[1]
- Three key features of the maternal hemodynamic changes in pregnancy are particularly relevant to the management of women with cardiac disease: (1) increased CO, (2) increased HR, and (3) reduced vascular resistance. The features change across the course of pregnancy and in the postpartum period (Fig. 37.1).

BLOOD VOLUME

- The pregnant woman will expand her blood volume by 40% to 50%. As a result, serum oncotic pressure falls in parallel by 20% to about 19 mm Hg.

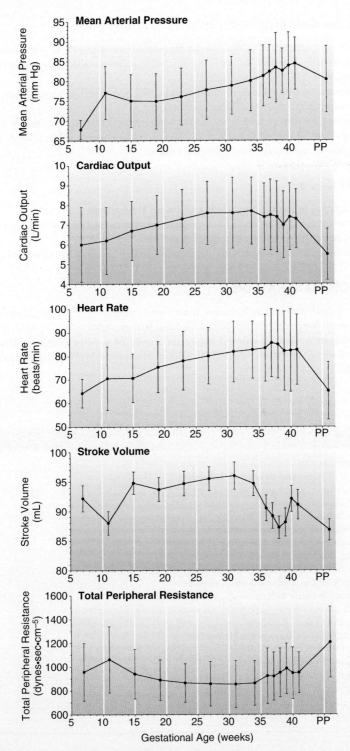

Fig. 37.1 Changes in hemodynamic parameters throughout pregnancy (mean ± standard deviation). PP, postpartum.

Diagnosis and Evaluation of Heart Disease

- The classic symptoms of cardiac disease are palpitations, shortness of breath with exertion, and chest pain. A careful history is needed to determine whether the symptoms are out of proportion to the stage of pregnancy.
- Any diastolic murmur and any systolic murmur that is loud (grade 3/6 or higher) or radiates to the carotids should be considered pathologic.
- Indications for further cardiac diagnostic testing in pregnant women include a history of known cardiac disease, symptoms, a pathologic murmur, evidence of heart failure on physical, or oxygen desaturation without pulmonary disease.

General Care

- Deterioration in cardiac status during pregnancy is frequently insidious.
- Intercurrent events superimposed on pregnancy in the context of maternal heart disease are usually responsible for acute decompensation.
- The ideal labor for a woman with heart disease is short and pain free (Box 37.1).

RISK-SCORING STRATEGIES

- Risks include maternal arrhythmias, heart failure, preterm birth, fetal growth restriction, and a small but significant risk of maternal and fetal mortality.
- Quantification of maternal and fetal risks should be used to counsel patients and to direct care. CARPREG, ZAHARA I, and the modified WHO are described risk models.

BOX 37.1 ■ Standard Cardiac Care for Labor and Delivery

1. Accurate diagnosis
2. Mode of delivery based on obstetric indications
3. Medical management initiated early in labor
   - Prolonged labor avoided
   - Induction with a *favorable* cervix
4. Maintenance of hemodynamic stability
   - Invasive hemodynamic monitoring when required
   - Initial, compensated hemodynamic reference point
   - Specific emphasis based on particular cardiac condition
5. Avoidance of pain and hemodynamic responses
   - Epidural analgesia with narcotic/low-dose local technique
6. Consideration for prophylactic antibiotics when at risk for endocarditis
7. Avoidance of maternal pushing
   - Caudal block for dense perineal anesthesia
   - Low forceps or vacuum delivery
8. Avoidance of maternal blood loss
   - Proactive management of the third stage
   - Early but appropriate fluid replacement
9. Early volume management postpartum
   - Often careful but aggressive diuresis

VALVULAR DISEASE

- The American College of Cardiology and the American Heart Association have published guidelines for the management of valvular heart disease

MITRAL STENOSIS

- CO is limited by the relatively passive flow of blood through the valve during diastole; increased venous return results in pulmonary congestion rather than increased CO.
- Elevated pulmonary pressures may be due to hydrostatic forces associated with elevated left atrial pressures or, in more advanced disease, may result from pathologic elevations of pulmonary vascular resistance.
- Pregnancy does not negatively affect the natural history of mitral stenosis.
- The goal of antepartum care is to achieve a balance between the drive to increase CO and the limitations of flow across the stenotic valve.
- Aggressive, anticipatory diuresis reduces pulmonary congestion and risk for oxygen desaturation. Aggressive medical management, including hospital bed rest in selected cases, is sufficient to manage women with mitral stenosis.

MITRAL REGURGITATION

- Acute mitral regurgitation in young patients is uncommon and is associated with ruptured chordae tendineae as a result of endocarditis or myxomatous valve disease.
- Excessive preload results in pulmonary congestion, and insufficient preload will not fill the enlarged left ventricle and will result in insufficient forward flow.
- In the absence of conditions of abnormal connective tissue, women with mitral prolapse can be expected to have uncomplicated pregnancies.

AORTIC STENOSIS

- The natural history of aortic stenosis is characterized by a long, asymptomatic period. The murmur can easily be distinguished from a physiologic murmur of pregnancy by its harshness and radiation into the carotid arteries.
- Consideration for valve replacement or valvotomy during pregnancy should be reserved for patients who remain clinically symptomatic despite hospital care.
- Given a hypertrophied ventricle and some degree of diastolic dysfunction, the volume-pressure relationship is very steep. A small loss of left ventricular (LV) filling results in a proportionately large fall in LV pressure and a large fall in forward flow and CO.
- In general, pulmonary edema associated with excess preload is much easier to manage than hypotension due to hypovolemia.

AORTIC REGURGITATION

- The reduction in vascular resistance associated with pregnancy tends to improve cardiac performance.

PROSTHETIC VALVES

- Delay in valve replacement until childbearing is completed is appropriate when the severity of heart disease is believed to be manageable in pregnancy.

- Accelerated deterioration of bioprosthetic valves in the setting of pregnancy has been confirmed by several studies.[2]
- Outcomes are better when clinical care teams are experienced with monitoring and dosing anticoagulation and work to achieve compliance.

Congenital Heart Disease

- Congenital heart disease is present in 0.7% to 1% of live births and accounts for as many as 30% of infants with birth anomalies.
- Major risks in pregnancy include (1) cyanosis; (2) left (or systemic) ventricular dysfunction and poor functional status; (3) pulmonary hypertension and Eisenmenger syndrome, particularly with right ventricular (RV) dysfunction; and (4) severe left (or systemic) outflow tract obstruction.
- Specific parental defects are not usually associated with the same defect in the child.
- All women who have congestive heart disease (CHD) should undergo fetal echocardiographic examination at approximately 18 to 22 weeks' gestation.
- Contraceptive education should probably be initiated as part of general health care education before the overt need for birth control.

ISOLATED SEPTAL DEFECTS

- Ventricular septal defects (VSDs) and atrial septal defects (ASDs) represent greater than 40% of cases of CHD identified in childhood.
- The patient with a significant VSD or ASD shunt can be expected to normally expand her CO during pregnancy.

PATENT DUCTUS ARTERIOSUS

- In the absence of Eisenmenger syndrome, pregnancy is not usually complicated.

TETRALOGY OF FALLOT

- Tetralogy of Fallot is the most common cyanotic CHD and is often well tolerated during pregnancy. Preconception evaluation should include assessment of right and left ventricular size and function along with the severity of the pulmonary insufficiency or stenosis, with consideration given to repair of severe pulmonary insufficiency before pregnancy if appropriate.

TRANSPOSITION OF THE GREAT ARTERIES

- In complete transposition of the great arteries (TGA), systemic venous blood returns to the right atrium and passes through the tricuspid valve, into the RV, and directly into the transposed aorta. Although this is an adequate circulation for fetal life, infants decompensate at birth owing to ineffective systemic circulation.
- The RV, as the systemic ventricle, must work against systemic resistance, and the tricuspid valve is exposed to systemic pressures. Long-term complications are associated with failure of the systemic RV and arrhythmia.
- Young women with surgically or congenitally corrected TGA can successfully complete pregnancy.

FONTAN PROCEDURE

- The Fontan procedure and subsequent modifications are currently used to correct a variety of complex congenital heart conditions characterized by a single functional ventricle.

EISENMENGER SYNDROME

- Eisenmenger syndrome may develop from any intracardiac shunt that results in blood from the high-pressure systemic circulation being directed into the pulmonary circulation.
- Reversal of flow from the pulmonary to the systemic circulation and the development of hypoxemia with increasing hematocrit herald the development of Eisenmenger syndrome. The fall in systemic vascular resistance associated with pregnancy may initiate right-to-left shunting in a patient not previously cyanotic.
- A more modern review[3] of cases in the United Kingdom between 1991 and 1995 confirms the poor prognosis for pregnant women with Eisenmenger syndrome.
- Cesarean delivery is reserved for obstetric indications. Unlike many cardiac conditions in pregnancy, meticulous care frequently fails to prevent maternal death.

COARCTATION OF THE AORTA

- β-Blockade may serve to protect against dissection and may promote diastolic flow through the aortic narrowing.

Summary

- Cyanotic heart disease in the absence of pulmonary hypertension is associated with increased rates of miscarriage and preterm birth.
- Arrhythmias may become worse in pregnancy and may precipitate cardiac decompensation.

Cardiomyopathy

- Dilated cardiomyopathy is characterized by the development of pulmonary edema in the context of LV dysfunction and dilation (Box 37.2)
- The mortality rate for peripartum cardiomyopathy is 25% to 50%.
- Women with a diagnosis of peripartum cardiomyopathy in a previous pregnancy are at risk for heart failure in a subsequent pregnancy.
- The postpartum period represents a time of particular risk. Women have received exogenous volume loading from IV fluids during labor; blood volume is centralized with uterine contractions, extravascular fluid is mobilized, tachycardia persists, and systemic vascular resistance increases.
- Preemptive HR control, diuresis, and afterload reduction should be used.

BOX 37.2 ■ Diagnostic Criteria for Peripartum Cardiomyopathy

1. Heart failure within the last month of pregnancy or within 5 months postpartum
2. Absence of prior heart disease
3. No determinable cause
4. Echocardiographic indication of left ventricle dysfunction
   - Ejection fraction of <45% or fractional shortening of <30%
   - Left ventricle end-diastolic dimension of >2.7 cm/m^2

Myocardial Infarction

- An increased risk for myocardial infarction (MI) in pregnancy is consistently associated with maternal age greater than 40 years, chronic hypertension, diabetes, smoking, migraine headache, transfusion, and postpartum infection.[4]
- Coronary dissection and normal coronary arteries are observed in approximately 50% of cases.
- ST-segment elevation is not a normal finding.
- Acute therapy is based on rapid coronary reperfusion.
- Elective delivery within 2 weeks of infarction should be avoided.
- The experience with pregnancy after a remote MI is limited. Of 33 reported cases, recurrent infarction and significant complications have not been reported.[5]

Marfan Syndrome

- Marfan syndrome is an autosomal-dominant disorder with a maternal mortality rate in pregnancy of greater than 50%.
- A precise risk for death from aortic dissection or rupture cannot be quantified.
- A prior aortic dissection or an aortic diameter greater than 4.5 cm likely are at higher risk. For these women, prophylactic aortic graft and valve replacement is recommended before pregnancy.[6]

Pulmonary Hypertension

- The maternal mortality is reported to be as high as 50%.[7]
- Sudden, irreversible deterioration in the postpartum period is common, and as many as 75% of deaths will occur postpartum.
- Pulmonary hypertension with RV dysfunction is poorly tolerated in pregnancy.
- Women with pulmonary hypertension and RV dysfunction should be strongly discouraged from becoming pregnant.

Other Conditions

- **Malignant ventricular arrhythmias.** Due to idiopathic ventricular fibrillation, cardiomyopathy, long-QT syndrome, CHD, or hypertrophic cardiomyopathy. An implantable cardioverter-defibrillator can effectively protect these patients from sudden death.
- **Hypertrophic cardiomyopathy.** Excessive volume loading may reveal a stiff ventricle and diastolic dysfunction.

Critical Care: Hemodynamic Monitoring and Management

- Obstetricians must be familiar with basic principles and techniques of critical care medicine to manage these patients or serve as critical care team consultants.

HEMODYNAMIC MONITORING

- Provides continuous assessment of systemic and intracardiac pressures and the means to determine CO and calculate systemic and pulmonary resistances.

HEMODYNAMIC MANAGEMENT

- Hemodynamic monitoring permits the physician to choose an intervention and subsequently assess the positive and negative effects.
- Reduction in serum oncotic pressure is rarely a primary cause of pulmonary edema.
- Fetal decompensation is usually encountered before a significant reduction in maternal perfusion and hypotension.

References for this chapter are available at ExpertConsult.com.

CHAPTER 38

Respiratory Disease in Pregnancy

Janice E. Whitty ■ Mitchell P. Dombrowski

KEY POINTS

- Pneumonia is the most common nonobstetric infectious cause of maternal mortality, and more than 40% of pneumonia cases are complicated by preterm delivery. *Streptococcus pneumoniae* is the most common bacterial pathogen associated with pneumonia during pregnancy.
- To treat pneumonia, empiric antibiotic coverage should be started that includes a third-generation cephalosporin and a macrolide, such as azithromycin, to cover atypical pathogens. If CA-MRSA is suspected, add vancomycin or linezolid.
- The HIV-infected gravida with a CD4+ count of less than 200 cells/mm^3 should receive prophylaxis with trimethoprim-sulfamethoxazole, as well as highly active antiretroviral therapy, to prevent secondary PJP.
- High-risk gravidae should be screened for TB and treated appropriately with INH prophylaxis for infection without overt disease and with dual anti-TB therapy for active disease. If resistant TB is identified, ethambutol, 2.5 g/day, should be added to therapy, and the treatment period should be extended to 18 months.
- It is safer for pregnant women with asthma to be treated with asthma medications than it is for them to have asthma symptoms and exacerbations. Inhaled corticosteroids are the preferred treatment for persistent asthma in pregnancy.
- Step-care therapy uses the principle of tailoring medical therapy according to asthma severity. Inhaled albuterol is recommended for rescue therapy during pregnancy.
- The interstitial lung diseases include idiopathic pulmonary fibrosis, sarcoidosis, hypersensitivity pneumonitis, drug-induced lung disease, and connective tissue disease. Restrictive lung disease is generally well tolerated in pregnancy; however, exercise intolerance and need for oxygen supplementation may develop.
- An increasing number of women with cystic fibrosis are surviving to the reproductive years. Close attention to nutrition is required secondary to maldigestion, malabsorption, and malnutrition, which can complicate cystic fibrosis during pregnancy. Fetal growth should be monitored closely.

Pneumonia in Pregnancy

- Pneumonia contributes to considerable maternal mortality and is reportedly the most common nonobstetric infectious cause of maternal mortality in the peripartum period.[1]
- With modern management and antibiotic therapy, the maternal mortality rate currently ranges from 0% to 4%.[1-3] Maternal complications of pneumonia include respiratory failure and mechanical ventilation in 10% to 20%, bacteremia in 16%, and empyema in 8%.[2,3]
- Those infected with HIV are 7.8 times more likely to develop pneumonia.

- Pneumonia can complicate pregnancy at any time during gestation and may be associated with preterm birth, poor fetal growth, and perinatal loss. Preterm labor occurs in around half, with a third delivering prematurely. Preterm labor is more likely in those women who experience bacteremia, require mechanical ventilation, or have a serious underlying maternal disease.

Bacteriology

- *Streptococcus pneumoniae* and *Haemophilus influenzae* remain the most common identifiable causes of pneumonia in pregnancy.[1,2]
- Several unusual pathogens have been reported to cause pneumonia in pregnancy, including mumps, infectious mononucleosis, swine flu, influenza A, varicella, coccidioidomycosis, and other fungi.[4]
- Varicella pneumonia complicates primary varicella infections in 9% of infections in pregnancy, compared with 0.3% to 1.8% in the nonpregnant population.[5] The increase in virulence of viral infections reported in pregnancy may be secondary to the changes in maternal immune status that characterize pregnancy, including reduced lymphocyte proliferative response, reduced cell-mediated cytotoxicity, and a decrease in the number of helper T lymphocytes (see Chapter 4).[6,7]
- Recent reports have been made of community-acquired methicillin-resistant *Staphylococcus aureus* (CA-MRSA) causing necrotizing pneumonia in pregnancy and postpartum.[6–8]

Bacterial Pneumonia

- *Streptococcus pneumoniae* (*pneumococcus*) is the most common bacterial pathogen to cause pneumonia in pregnancy, and *H. influenzae* is the next most common. Less frequent bacterial pathogens include *Klebsiella pneumoniae and Staphylococcus aureus* pneumonia.
- Streptococcal pneumonia produces a "rusty" sputum, and gram-positive diplococci appear on Gram stain with asymmetric consolidation and air bronchograms on chest radiograph.
- *Klebsiella pneumoniae* causes extensive tissue destruction with air bronchograms, pleural effusion, and cavitation noted on chest radiograph.
- Patients with *Staphylococcus aureus* pneumonia present with pleuritis, chest pain, purulent sputum, and consolidation without air bronchograms noted on chest radiograph. Community-acquired methicillin-resistant *Staphylococcus aureus* (CA-MRSA) can present with a viral-like prodrome that progresses to severe pneumonia with high fever, hypotension, and hemoptysis followed by septic shock and need for ventilator support.[6] Severe cases of CA-MRSA have been reported during influenza seasons or associated with a preceding influenza illness in 33% to 71% patients.[6] Leukopenia can be observed and has been found to be a predictor of poor outcome.[6] Mortality from CA-MRSA pneumonia in the United States and Europe is reportedly greater than 50%.
- Patients with *Mycoplasma pneumoniae, Legionella pneumophila,* and *Chlamydia pneumoniae* (Taiwan acute respiratory agent) present with gradual onset and a lower fever, appear less ill, and have a mucoid sputum and a patchy or interstitial infiltrate on chest radiograph. *M. pneumoniae* is the most common organism responsible for atypical pneumonia and is best detected by the presence of cold agglutinins, which are present in 70% of cases. Any gravida suspected of having pneumonia should be managed aggressively. Hospital admission is generally recommended until additional information is available.
- Workup should include physical examination, arterial blood gases, chest radiograph, sputum for Gram stain and culture, and blood cultures.

- An assay approved by the U.S. Food and Drug Administration (FDA) for pneumococcal urinary antigen has been assessed in several studies.[11] The sensitivity for identifying pneumococcal disease in adults is reportedly 60% to 90% with specificity close to 100%.[11]
- 10% of samples from patients with pneumonia caused by other agents are positive for the pneumococcal assay, which indicates a potential problem with specificity.[12] Therefore if the response to therapy directed at pneumococcus (*S. pneumoniae*) is inadequate, coverage for other potential pathogens should be added.
- A test is available for *Legionella* urinary antigen as well, with a sensitivity of 70% and specificity of 90% for serogroup 1.[13]
- Current U.S. federal standards require that the first dose of antibiotics be administered within 4 hours of arrival to the hospital.[14] Empiric antibiotic coverage should be started, usually with a macrolide for mild illness with addition of a β-lactam for severe illness.
- A macrolide combined with a β-lactam is safe and will provide adequate coverage for most community-acquired bacterial pneumoniae, including *Legionella*.
- The use of macrolides to treat community-acquired pneumonia should be limited when possible because their use has also been associated with increased penicillin resistance among patients with *S. pneumoniae*.[15]
- Respiratory quinolones including levofloxacin, gatifloxacin, and moxifloxacin should be avoided in pregnancy because they may damage developing fetal cartilage. However, with the emergence of highly resistant bacterial pneumonia, their use may be life saving and therefore justified in specific circumstances. There ideal agents for community-acquired pneumonia because they are highly active against penicillin-resistant strains of *S. pneumoniae*. They are also active against *Legionella* and the other atypical pulmonary pathogens.
- If CA-MRSA pneumonia is suspected, vancomycin or linezolid should be added to empiric therapy.[6] CA-MRSA is susceptible to fluoroquinolones and trimethoprim-sulfamethoxazole and often are only resistant to β-lactams.[6]
- Arterial saturation should be monitored with pulse oximetry with a goal of maintaining the Po_2 at 70 mm Hg, a level necessary to ensure adequate fetal oxygenation. When the gravida is afebrile for 48 hours and has signs of clinical improvement, an oral cephalosporin or macrolide, or both, can be initiated and IV therapy discontinued. A total of 10 to 14 days of treatment should be completed.
- Pneumococcal polysaccharide vaccination prevents pneumococcal pneumonia in otherwise healthy populations with an efficacy of 65% to 84%.[16] The vaccine is safe in pregnancy.
- After in utero exposure to the vaccine, significantly high concentrations of pneumococcal antibodies are present in infants at birth and at 2 months of age.[17] In addition, colostrum and breast milk antibodies are significantly increased in women who have received the pneumococcal vaccine.[18]
- The potentially viable fetus should be monitored with continuous fetal monitoring. Serial ultrasound examinations for amniotic fluid index and growth will help to guide clinical management.
- No evidence suggests that elective delivery results in an overall improvement in respiratory function.[19] However, if clear evidence of fetal compromise or profound maternal compromise and impending demise is apparent, delivery should be accomplished.

Viral Pneumonia

INFLUENZA VIRUS

- Every year in the United States, an estimated 4 million cases of pneumonia occur that complicate influenza. This represents the sixth leading cause of death in this country.[20]

- Most epidemic infections are due to influenza A,[4] which typically has an acute onset after a 1- to 4-day incubation period and first manifests as high fever, coryza, headache, malaise, and cough. In uncomplicated cases, the chest examination and chest radiograph remain clear.[4] If symptoms persist longer than 5 days, especially in a pregnancy, complications should be suspected.
- In the epidemic of 1957, autopsies demonstrated that pregnant women most commonly died of fulminant viral pneumonia, whereas nonpregnant patients died most often of secondary bacterial infection.[21]
- A more recent matched cohort study using the administrative database of pregnant women enrolled in the Tennessee Medicaid population examined pregnant women aged 25 to 44 years with respiratory hospitalization during influenza seasons in 1985 to 1993.[22] In this population of pregnant women, those with asthma accounted for half of all respiratory hospitalizations during influenza season.
- Early data on pandemic 2009 influenza A (H1N1) suggest pregnant women had an increased risk for hospitalization and death.[23]
- When pneumonia complicates influenza in pregnancy, antibiotics should be started, directed at the likely pathogens that can cause secondary infection: *S. aureus*, *S. pneumoniae* (pneumococcus), *H. influenzae*, and certain enteric gram-negative bacteria.
- It has been recommended that the influenza vaccine be given routinely to gravidae during the flu season. Prospective studies have demonstrated higher cord blood antibody levels to influenza in infants born to mothers immunized during pregnancy.

VARICELLA VIRUS

- Varicella infection occurs in 0.7 of every 1000 pregnancies.[24] Women with varicella pneumonia are significantly more likely to be current smokers and to have 100 or more skin lesions.[25]
- Varicella pneumonia occurs most often in the third trimester, and the infection is likely to be severe.[24,26] With modern management, mortality has decreased dramatically.
- All gravidae with varicella pneumonia should be aggressively treated with antiviral therapy and admitted to the ICU for close observation. The early use of acyclovir has been associated with an improved hospital course after the fifth day and a lower mean temperature, lower respiratory rate, and improved oxygenation and survival.[27] Treatment with acyclovir is safe in pregnancy. A dose of 7.5 mg/kg IV every 8 hours has been recommended.
- Varicella vaccine was added to the universal childhood immunization schedule in the United States in 1995. It has resulted in a sharp decline in the rate of death from varicella.[28] This vaccine is not recommended for use in pregnancy.[29]
- As of 1995, more than 80% of women with AIDS were of reproductive age. Pneumocystis jiroveci pneumonia (PJP) remains the most prevalent opportunistic infection in patients infected with HIV.[30] It is an AIDS-defining illness that occurs more frequently when the helper T-cell count (CD4+) is less than 200 cells/mm³.[30] When AIDS is complicated by PJP, the mortality rate is 10% to 20% during the initial infection.
- Trimethoprim-sulfamethoxazole is the preferred treatment for PJP. Thus far, resistance to this therapeutic agent has not been identified[30] and is associated with an increased survival rate.[31]

Tuberculosis in Pregnancy

- From 1985 through 1991, reported cases of tuberculosis (TB) increased by 18%, representing about 39,000 more cases than expected had the previous downward trend continued.

This increase is due to many factors, including the HIV epidemic, deterioration in the health care infrastructure, and significantly more cases among immigrants.[33] The emergence of drug-resistant TB has also become a serious concern.

DIAGNOSIS

- Those at risk include people who have had recent infection with TB and those who have clinical conditions associated with an increased risk for progression of latent TB infection (LTBI) to active TB (Boxes 38.1 and 38.2).
- All gravidae at high risk for TB should be screened with tuberculin skin testing (TST). This is usually done with subcutaneous administration of intermediate-strength purified protein derivative (PPD).[35] The sensitivity of the PPD is 90% to 99% for exposure to TB. The tine test is not recommended for screening because of its low sensitivity.
- Three cut off levels have been recommended for defining a positive tuberculin reaction: Induration of greater than 5 mm is a positive reaction in individuals with highest risk for conversion to active TB (see Box 38.2).
- Interferon-γ release assays (IGRAs), an alternative diagnostic tool for LTBI, have specificity of greater than 95% for diagnosis of LTBI.[36] Because IGRAs are not affected by Bacille Calmette-Guérin (BCG) vaccination status, they are useful for evaluation of LTBI in BCG-vaccinated individuals. CDC 2012 guidelines indicate that IGRAs can be used in place of, but not in addition to, TST in all situations—including pregnancy—in which the CDC recommends TST as an aid in diagnosing *Mycobacterium tuberculosis* infection.

BOX 38.1 ■ High-Risk Factors for Tuberculosis

- Close contact with people known or suspected to have tuberculosis
- Medical risk factors known to increase risk for disease if infected
- Birth in a country with a high tuberculosis prevalence
- Medically underserved status
- Low income
- Alcohol addiction
- Intravenous drug use
- Residency in a long-term care facility (e.g., correctional institution, mental institution, nursing home or facility)
- Health professionals working in high-risk health care facilities

---

BOX 38.2 ■ Clinical Risk Factors for Developing Active Tuberculosis

- Human immunodeficiency virus infection
- Recent tuberculosis infection
- Injection drug use
- Silicosis
- Solid organ transplantation
- Chronic renal failure
- Jejunoileal bypass
- Diabetes mellitus
- Carcinoma of the head or neck
- Underweight by >15%

- Immigrants from areas where TB is endemic may have received the BCG vaccine. If the BCG vaccine was given 10 years earlier and the PPD is positive with a skin test reaction of 10 mm or more, that individual should be considered infected with TB and should be managed accordingly.[37]
- Symptoms of active TB include cough (74%), weight loss (41%), fever (30%), malaise and fatigue (30%), and hemoptysis (19%).[38]
- Extrapulmonary TB occurs in up to 16% of cases in the United States; however, in patients with AIDS, the pattern may occur in 60% to 70%.[41] Extrapulmonary TB that is confined to the lymph nodes has no effect on obstetric outcome, but TB at other extrapulmonary sites does adversely affect the outcome of pregnancy.[42]
- The diagnosis of congenital TB is based on one of the following factors: (1) demonstration of primary hepatic complex or cavitating hepatic granuloma by percutaneous liver biopsy at birth; (2) infection of the maternal genital tract or placenta; (3) lesions noted in the first week of life; or (4) exclusion of the possibility of postnatal transmission by a thorough investigation of all contacts, including attendants.[43]

PREVENTION

- Most gravidae with a positive PPD in pregnancy are asymptomatic with no evidence of active disease and are therefore classified as having LTBI. The risk for progression to active disease is highest in the first 2 years of conversion.
- Known recent conversion (2 years) to a positive PPD and no evidence of active disease, the recommended prophylaxis is INH, 300 mg/day, starting after the first trimester and continuing for 6 to 9 months. INH should be accompanied by pyridoxine (vitamin B_6) supplementation, 50 mg/day, to prevent the peripheral neuropathy associated with INH treatment.
- INH prophylaxis is not recommended for women older than 35 years who have an unknown or prolonged PPD positivity in the absence of active disease. INH is associated with hepatitis in both pregnant and nonpregnant adults.[37] Monthly monitoring of liver function tests may prevent this adverse outcome.

TREATMENT

- Untreated TB has been associated with higher morbidity and mortality among pregnant women. The gravida with active TB should be treated initially with INH, 300 mg/day, combined with RIF, 600 mg/day.[44]
- If resistance to INH is identified or anticipated, ethambutol should be added, 2.5 g/day, and the treatment period should be extended to 18 months.[44] Ethambutol is teratogenic in animals; however, this has not been demonstrated in humans. The most common side effect of ethambutol therapy is optic neuritis. Streptomycin should be avoided during pregnancy because it is associated with eighth nerve damage in neonates.[45]
- The risk for postpartum transmission of TB to the infant may be higher among infants born to mothers with drug-resistant TB.[46,47] Therefore in patients with active disease at the time of delivery, separation of the mother and newborn should be accomplished to prevent infection of the newborn.
- Women who are being treated with antituberculous drugs may breastfeed. Ethambutol excretion into breast milk is also minimal.
- Breastfed infants of women receiving INH therapy should receive a multivitamin supplement that includes pyridoxine.[48] Neonates of women receiving antituberculous therapy should have a PPD skin test at birth and again at 3 months of age.
- Infants and children at high risk for intimate and prolonged exposure to untreated or ineffectively treated individuals should receive the BCG vaccine.

Asthma in Pregnancy

- Current medical management for asthma emphasizes treatment of airway inflammation to decrease airway responsiveness and prevent asthma symptoms. The National Asthma Education and Prevention Program (NAEPP) Working Group has found that "it is safer for pregnant women with asthma to be treated with asthma medications than it is for them to have asthma symptoms and exacerbations."[49]

DIAGNOSIS

- Diagnosis of asthma in pregnancy is no different than for a nonpregnant patient. Asthma typically includes characteristic symptoms (wheezing, chest cough, shortness of breath, chest tightness), temporal relationships (fluctuating intensity, worse at night), and triggers (e.g., allergens, exercise, infections).
- The NAEPP defined *mild intermittent, mild persistent, moderate persistent,* and *severe persistent asthma* according to daytime and nighttime symptoms—wheezing, cough, or dyspnea—and objective tests of pulmonary function.[49]

EFFECTS OF PREGNANCY ON ASTHMA

- Asthma during pregnancy has been associated with considerable maternal morbidity. Compared with women without a history of asthma, women with asthma have been reported to have higher risks for complications of pregnancy even after adjustment for potential confounders.[50]
- Prospective studies that actively managed asthma during pregnancy have generally had excellent perinatal outcomes.[51–57]

ASTHMA MANAGEMENT

- Effective management of asthma during pregnancy relies on four integral components: (1) objective measures for assessment and monitoring, (2) patient education, (3) avoidance or control of asthma triggers, and (4) pharmacologic therapy.

OBJECTIVE MEASURES FOR ASSESSMENT AND MONITORING

- Forced expiratory volume in 1 second (FEV_1) is the single best measure of pulmonary function.
- The peak expiratory flow rate correlates well with the FEV_1 and has the advantage that it can be measured reliably with inexpensive, disposable, portable peak flowmeters.

PATIENT EDUCATION

- The importance of adherence to treatment should be stressed.

AVOIDANCE OR CONTROL OF ASTHMA TRIGGERS

- Limiting adverse environmental exposures during pregnancy is important for controlling asthma. Irritants and allergens that provoke acute symptoms also increase airway inflammation and hyperresponsiveness. Avoiding or controlling such triggers can reduce asthma symptoms, airway hyperresponsiveness, and the need for medical therapy.[58]

PHARMACOLOGIC THERAPY

- Medications for asthma are divided into *long-term controllers* that prevent asthma manifestations: inhaled corticosteroids, long-acting β-agonists, leukotriene modifiers, and theophylline and *rescue therapy*, such as with albuterol, to provide quick relief of symptoms.
- Use of asthma medication has been reported to significantly decline in the first trimester according to the number of prescriptions filled: a 23% decrease in inhaled corticosteroids, a 13% decrease in β-agonist, and a 54% decrease in rescue corticosteroids has been noted.[59]
- It is safer for pregnant women with asthma to be treated with asthma medications than it is for them to have asthma symptoms and exacerbations.[49]

Step Therapy

- The step-care therapeutic approach increases the number and frequency of medications with increasing asthma severity.[49,58] Based on clinical trials in patients with varying degrees of disease severity, medications (Table 38.1) are considered to be "preferred" or "alternative" at each step of therapy.
- Patients who do not respond optimally to treatment should be stepped up to more intensive medical therapy.

Inhaled Corticosteroids

- Inhaled corticosteroids are the preferred treatment for the management of all levels of persistent asthma during pregnancy.[49]
- No consistent evidence links inhaled corticosteroid use to increases in congenital malformations or adverse perinatal outcomes (See Chapter 8).[49,60]

Inhaled β₂-Agonists

- As-needed use of inhaled β₂-agonists is currently recommended for all levels of asthma during pregnancy.[49]
- An increased frequency of bronchodilator use could be an indicator of the need for additional antiinflammatory therapy.

TABLE 38.1 ■ Step Therapy Medical Management of Asthma During Pregnancy

Step	Asthma Severity
1. No daily medications; albuterol as needed	Mild intermittent
2. Low-dose inhaled corticosteroid (alternatives: LTRA or theophylline*)	Mild persistent
3. Medium-dose inhaled corticosteroid† (alternatives: low-dose inhaled corticosteroid and LABA, LTRA, or theophylline*)	Moderate persistent
4. Medium-dose inhaled corticosteroid and LABA (alternatives: medium-dose inhaled corticosteroid plus LTRA or theophylline*)	Moderate persistent
5. High-dose inhaled corticosteroid and LABA	Severe persistent
6. High-dose inhaled corticosteroid and LABA and oral prednisone	Severe persistent

Modified from Quick Reference NAEPP Expert Panel Report: Managing asthma during pregnancy: Recommendations for pharmacologic treatment—2004 update. *J Allergy Clin Immunol.* 2005;115:34-36.
LABA, long-acting β-agonist; *LTRA*, leukotriene-receptor agonist.
*Theophylline (serum level, 5-12 µg/mL).
†We have modified step 3 to reflect the choice of a medium-dose inhaled corticosteroid over a low-dose inhaled corticosteroid plus a LABA because of the lack of safety data on the use of a LABA during pregnancy.

Omalizumab

■ Because of the paucity of data on omalizumab (humanized monoclonal antibody to immunoglobulin E) side effect, its use should not be initiated in pregnancy.

Theophylline

■ Dosing guidelines have recommended that serum theophylline concentrations be maintained at 5 to 12 μg/mL during pregnancy.[49]

Leukotriene Moderators

■ Leukotriene modifiers are less effective as single agents than inhaled corticosteroids and are less effective than long-acting β_2-agonists as add-on therapy.[58]

Oral Corticosteroids

■ The NAEPP recommends the use of oral corticosteroids when indicated for the long-term management of severe persistent asthma or for exacerbations during pregnancy.[49]

MANAGEMENT OF ALLERGIC RHINITIS AND GASTROESOPHAGEAL REFLUX

■ Rhinitis, sinusitis, and gastroesophageal reflux may exacerbate asthma symptoms, and their management should be considered an integral aspect of asthma care.

ANTENATAL ASTHMA MANAGEMENT

■ Women with asthma that is not well controlled, or those who have an exacerbation, may benefit from additional fetal surveillance in the form of ultrasound examinations and antenatal fetal testing.[49]
■ The response is considered good if symptoms are resolved or if they become subjectively mild, normal activities can be resumed, and the peak expiratory flow rate is more than 80% of the personal best.

Hospital and Emergency Department Management of Asthma Exacerbations

■ The principal goal should be the prevention of maternal hypoxia.
■ Continuous electronic fetal monitoring should be initiated if gestation has advanced to the point of potential fetal viability. Albuterol (2.5 to 5 mg every 20 minutes for 3 doses, then 2.5 to 10 mg every 1 to 4 hours as needed, or 10 to 15 mg/h continuously) should be delivered by a nebulizer driven with oxygen.[49]

Labor and Delivery Management of Asthma

■ Asthma medications should not be discontinued during labor and delivery.
■ Methylergonovine and especially carboprost (15-methyl $PGF_{2\alpha}$) can cause bronchospasm.[61]

BREASTFEEDING

■ Only a small amount of asthma medications enters the breast milk and thus is not contraindicated during breastfeeding.

Restrictive Lung Disease

- Restrictive ventilatory defects occur when lung expansion is limited because of alterations in the lung parenchyma or because of abnormalities in the pleura, chest wall, or the neuromuscular apparatus.
- Additional conditions that cause a restrictive ventilatory defect include pleural and chest wall diseases and extrathoracic conditions such as obesity, peritonitis, and ascites.[62]

SARCOIDOSIS

- Sarcoidosis is a systemic granulomatosis disease of undetermined etiology that often affects young adults. Pregnancy outcome for most women with sarcoidosis is good.[63,64] The overall cesarean delivery rate is around 40% and a quarter of infants weigh less than 2500 g.
- Patients with pulmonary hypertension complicating restrictive lung disease may suffer a mortality rate as high as 50% during gestation. These patients need close monitoring during labor and delivery and postpartum. Close fetal surveillance throughout gestation is also warranted because chronic impaired oxygenation may compromise fetal growth.
- Gravidae with restrictive lung disease, including pulmonary sarcoidosis, may benefit from early institution of steroid therapy for evidence of worsening pulmonary status.
- During labor, consideration should be given to early use of epidural anesthesia, if it is not contraindicated. The use of general anesthesia should be avoided, if possible.

CYSTIC FIBROSIS

- Cystic fibrosis (CF) is a genetically transmitted disease with an autosomal-recessive pattern of inheritance. In the United States, about 4% of the white population are heterozygous carriers of the CF gene, and the disease occurs in 1 in 3000 live white births.
- Survival for patients with CF has increased dramatically since 1940. According to the Cystic Fibrosis Foundation's patient registry, mean survival in 2008 had increased to 39.6 years. Today, more than 45% of individuals with CF in the United States are older than 18 years. Therefore more women with CF are now entering reproductive age.
- In contrast to men with CF, who for the most part are infertile, women with CF are more often fertile. Because the number of women with CF who achieve pregnancy is steadily increasing, it is important that the obstetrician be familiar with the disease. Liberal consultation with a CF specialist should be obtained because a team effort will increase the chance for an improved pregnancy outcome.

Effect of Pregnancy on Cystic Fibrosis

- Women with CF and advanced lung disease may suffer from pulmonary hypertension with high pulmonary artery pressures. Regardless of the etiology, pulmonary hypertension is associated with unacceptable maternal risk during pregnancy and is considered to be a contraindication to pregnancy.
- Pulmonary involvement in CF includes chronic infection of the airways and bronchiectasis. Selective infection with certain microorganisms occurs, and *P. aeruginosa* is the most frequent pathogen.
- Women with pulmonary hypertension may not be able to adequately increase cardiac output during pregnancy. Most patients with CF also have pancreatic exocrine insufficiency. As a result, digestive enzymes and bicarbonate ions are diminished, which results in maldigestion, malabsorption, and malnutrition. Women with CF are therefore at risk of uteroplacental

insufficiency that leads to intrauterine growth restriction and stillbirth. Poor outcomes are associated with a maternal weight gain of less than 4.5 kg and a forced vital capacity of less than 50% of predicted.

- Patients who have mild CF, good prepregnancy nutritional status, and less impairment of lung function tolerate pregnancy well. Those with moderate to severe lung disease—an FEV_1 less than 60% of predicted—more often had preterm infants and had increased loss of lung function compared with those with milder disease.[65] Prepregnancy FEV_1 was found to be the most useful predictor of outcome in pregnant women with CF.[65,66] In addition, a positive correlation has been was found between prepregnancy FEV_1 and maternal survival.

Counseling Patients With Cystic Fibrosis in Pregnancy

- When the mother has CF and the proposed father is a white individual of unknown genotype, the risk for the fetus having CF is 1 in 50, compared with 1 in 3000 in the general white population. If the prospective father is a known carrier of a CF mutation, the risk to the fetus increases to 1 in 2.
- Gravidae with poor nutritional status, pulmonary hypertension (cor pulmonale), and deteriorating pulmonary function early in gestation should consider therapeutic abortion because the risk for maternal mortality may be unacceptably high.
- The woman with CF who is considering pregnancy should also give consideration to the need for strong psychosocial and physical support after delivery. The need for care of a potentially preterm growth-restricted neonate with all of its attendant morbidities and potential mortality should be discussed.
- Overall, 20% of mothers with CF succumb to the disease before the child's 10th birthday, and this number increases to 40% if the FEV_1 is less than 40% of predicted.[67]

Management of the Pregnancy Complicated by Cystic Fibrosis

- Care of the gravida with CF should be a coordinated team effort. Physicians familiar with CF, its complications, and management should be included as well as a maternal-fetal medicine specialist and neonatal team.
- Gravidae should be advised to be 90% of ideal body weight before conception if possible. A weight gain in pregnancy of 11 to 12 kg is recommended.[68] Frequent monitoring of weight, blood glucose, hemoglobin, total protein, serum albumin, prothrombin time, and fat-soluble vitamins A and E is suggested.[68]
- Patients who are unable to achieve adequate weight gain through oral nutritional supplements may be given nocturnal enteral nasogastric tube feedings. In this situation, the risk for aspiration should be considered, especially in patients with a history of gastroesophageal reflux, which is common in CF. If malnutrition is severe, parenteral hyperalimentation may be necessary for successful completion of the pregnancy. Baseline pulmonary function should be assessed, preferably before conception.
- Forced vital capacity, FEV_1, lung volumes, pulse oximetry, and arterial blood gases should be serially monitored during gestation, and deterioration in pulmonary function should be addressed immediately. An echocardiogram can assess the patient for pulmonary hypertension and cor pulmonale.
- Early recognition and prompt treatment of pulmonary infections are important. Treatment includes IV antibiotics in the appropriate dose, keeping in mind the increased clearance of these drugs secondary to pregnancy and CF.
- Chest physical therapy and bronchial drainage are also important components of the management of pulmonary infections in CF. Because *P. aeruginosa* is the most frequently isolated bacterium associated with chronic endobronchitis and bronchiectasis, antibiotic regimens should include coverage for this organism.

- Because of malabsorption of fats and frequent use of antibiotics, the patient with CF is prone to vitamin K deficiency. Therefore prothrombin time should be checked regularly, and parenteral vitamin K should be administered if the prothrombin time is elevated.
- Fundal height should be measured routinely, and serial ultrasound evaluations of fetal growth and amniotic fluid volume should be made. If fetal compromise is evident, nonstress testing should be started at 32 weeks or sooner.
- Evidence of profound maternal deterioration such as a marked and sustained decline in pulmonary function, development of right-sided heart failure, refractory hypoxemia, and progressive hypercapnia and respiratory acidosis may be indications for early delivery.
- If general anesthesia is needed, preoperative anticholinergic agents should be avoided because they tend to promote drying and inspissation of airway secretions.

References for this chapter are available at ExpertConsult.com.

CHAPTER 39

Renal Disease in Pregnancy

David F. Colombo

KEY POINTS

- Asymptomatic bacteriuria complicates 5% to 7% of pregnancies. If left untreated, it will result in symptomatic urinary tract infections in 40% of women.
- Pyelonephritis complicates 1% to 2% of pregnancies and generally requires inpatient treatment.
- Women with glomerular disease can have successful pregnancies, but pregnancy loss rates increase greatly if the patient has preexisting hypertension.
- Creatinine clearance can decline 70% before significant increases are seen in the BUN or serum creatinine level. Therefore a 24-hour urine specimen for creatinine clearance should be collected from any pregnant woman with underlying renal disease.
- The chance of a successful pregnancy outcome is reduced if the creatinine clearance is less than 50 mL/min or if the serum creatinine level is more than 1.5 mg/dL.
- Severe hypertension poses the greatest threat to the pregnant woman with chronic renal disease.
- Growth restriction and preeclampsia are common complications in women with chronic renal disease. Frequent sonograms and antepartum fetal surveillance at 28 weeks' gestation are recommended in affected pregnancies.
- Women with chronic renal disease are often anovulatory. Following transplantation, ovulation may resume, which can result in an unplanned pregnancy.
- Women should wait 2 years after receiving a cadaver renal allograft and 1 year after receiving a living allograft before attempting conception. Furthermore, no signs of allograft rejection should be apparent.
- Renal transplant patients may continue with cyclosporine or azathioprine throughout gestation, although levels may need to be adjusted during pregnancy. Other immunosuppressive medications such as mycophenolate mofetil and sirolimus are contraindicated.
- Renal function may decline as a result of pregnancy among patients with renal disease. An increased risk for this decline is observed in women with an elevated serum creatinine level (above 1.5 mg/dL) and hypertension.

Altered Renal Physiology in Pregnancy

- Marked dilation of the collecting system, including both the renal pelvis and ureters, occurs during pregnancy. This dilation is most pronounced on the right side and is most likely due to hormonal changes (i.e., from progesterone, endothelin, relaxin) and mechanical obstruction by the gravid uterus.
- Renal plasma flow increases greatly during pregnancy.[1]

- The glomerular filtration rate increases by 50% during a normal gestation.
- Glycosuria can be a feature of normal pregnancy.
- Serum urate levels are elevated in women with preeclampsia.

Asymptomatic Bacteriuria

- The prevalence of asymptomatic bacteriuria (ASB) in sexually active women has been reported to be as high as 5% to 6%.
- To secure a diagnosis, the urine culture should reveal greater than 100,000 colonies/mL of a single organism.
- The smooth muscle relaxation and subsequent ureteral dilation that accompany pregnancy are believed to facilitate the ascent of bacteria from the bladder to the kidney. As a result, untreated bacteriuria during pregnancy has a greater propensity to progress to pyelonephritis (up to 40%) than in nonpregnant women.
- Recognition and therapy for ASB can eliminate 70% of urinary tract infections in pregnancy.
- The American College of Obstetricians and Gynecologists recommends routine screening of all women for ASB at their first prenatal visit.
- *Escherichia coli* is the organism responsible for most cases of ASB and urinary tract infection during pregnancy.
- Therapy for ASB is recommended for 7 days, and a follow-up culture should be performed 1 to 2 weeks after discontinuing therapy.

Pyelonephritis

- Acute pyelonephritis during pregnancy is most often treated on an inpatient basis with IV antibiotics. Empiric therapy should be begun as soon as the presumptive diagnosis is established.
- Generally, a broad-spectrum first-generation cephalosporin is the initial therapy of choice.
- IV antibiotic therapy should be continued for 24 to 48 hours after the patient becomes afebrile and costovertebral angle tenderness subsides. After the cessation of IV therapy, treatment with appropriate oral antibiotics is recommended for 10 to 14 days.
- After an episode of acute pyelonephritis, antibiotic suppression should also be implemented and should be continued for the remainder of the pregnancy.
- Pulmonary injury that resembles acute respiratory distress syndrome can occur in pregnant women with acute pyelonephritis. Clinical manifestations of this complication usually occur 24 to 48 hours after the patient is admitted for pyelonephritis. Some of these women will require intubation, mechanical ventilation, and positive end-expiratory pressure. Acute respiratory distress syndrome is believed to result from endotoxin-induced alveolar capillary membrane injury.

Acute Renal Disease in Pregnancy
UROLITHIASIS

- Urolithiasis affects 0.03% of all pregnancies, a frequency similar to that of the general population.
- Because of the physiologic hydroureter of pregnancy, 75% to 85% of women with symptomatic urolithiasis will spontaneously pass their stones. Treatment should therefore be conservative and should consist of hydration and narcotic analgesia.
- Ureteral stenting to relieve obstruction is an option for managing pregnant women with renal stones. For refractory cases, nephrostomy tubes can also be used.
- Lithotripsy is contraindicated during pregnancy.

GLOMERULAR DISEASE

- Acute glomerulonephritis is an uncommon complication of pregnancy, with a reported incidence of 1 per 40,000 pregnancies.
- Acute glomerulonephritis can be difficult to distinguish from preeclampsia. Periorbital edema, a striking clinical feature of acute glomerulonephritis, is often seen in preeclampsia. However, hematuria, red blood cell (RBC) casts in the urine sediment, and depressed serum complement levels support the diagnosis of glomerulonephritis.
- Treatment of acute glomerulonephritis in pregnancy is similar to that for the nonpregnant individual.
- The highest incidence of fetal and maternal complications in women with glomerular disease occurred in those with primary focal and segmental hyalinosis and sclerosis, whereas the lowest incidence was observed in non–immunoglobulin A diffuse mesangial proliferative glomerulonephritis.
- The overall perinatal mortality is 13% among women with preexisting glomerular disease. Hypertension, azotemia, and nephrotic-range proteinuria are the strongest predictive factors for a poor pregnancy outcome.

ACUTE RENAL FAILURE IN PREGNANCY

- *Acute renal failure* (ARF) is defined as a urine output of less than 400 mL in 24 hours.
- Renal ischemia is a common phenomenon in cases of ARF. With mild ischemia, quickly reversible prerenal failure results; with more prolonged ischemia, acute tubular necrosis occurs. This process is also reversible because glomeruli are not affected. Severe ischemia, however, may produce acute cortical necrosis.
- The only significant risk factor associated with cortical necrosis is placental abruption.
- Individuals with reversible ARF experience a period of oliguria of variable duration followed by polyuria, or a high-output phase. It is important to recognize that blood urea nitrogen (BUN) and serum creatinine levels continue to rise early in the polyuric phase.
- Acidosis must be treated promptly because it can exacerbate hyperkalemia.
- The main indications for dialysis in ARF of pregnancy are hypernatremia, hyperkalemia, severe acidosis, volume overload, and worsening uremia.

HEMOLYTIC-UREMIC SYNDROME

- The hemolytic-uremic syndrome (HUS) is a rare idiopathic disorder that must be considered when a patient exhibits signs of hemolysis and decreasing renal function, particularly during the third trimester and in the postpartum period.
- Disseminated intravascular coagulation with hemolysis usually accompanies HUS. However, it is not the cause of the syndrome. Microscopically, the kidney shows thrombotic microangiopathy. The glomerular capillary wall is thick, and biopsy specimens taken later in the course of the disease show severe nephrosclerosis and deposition of the third component of complement (C_3).
- Plasma exchange is employed in cases of ARF caused by postpartum HUS.

POLYCYSTIC KIDNEY DISEASE

- Polycystic kidney disease is an autosomal dominant disorder that usually manifests during the fifth decade. Reproductive age women may occasionally display symptoms including hypertension.

VESICOURETERAL REFLUX

- Reflux may be exacerbated by pregnancy but usually does not cause morbidity unless it becomes severe.

RENAL ARTERY STENOSIS

- This disorder is rarely discovered during pregnancy but may be a cause of underlying hypertension.

NEPHROTIC SYNDROME

- The nephrotic syndrome was initially described as a 24-hour urine protein excretion equal to or in excess of 3.5 g, reduced serum albumin, edema, and hyperlipidemia.[2] Currently, the syndrome is defined by proteinuria alone, which is often the result of glomerular damage. These cases require close monitoring and may complicate the diagnosis of preeclampsia.

Chronic Renal Disease in Pregnancy

- Chronic renal disease can be silent until its advanced stages. Because obstetricians routinely test women's urine for the presence of protein, glucose, and ketones, they may be the first to detect chronic renal disease.
- Microscopic examination of the urine can aid in detection. renal More RBCs than 1 to 2 per high-power field or RBC casts are indicative of glomerular disease.
- The obstetrician can easily be misled when relying solely on BUN and serum creatinine levels to assess renal function. A 70% decline in creatinine clearance, an indirect measure of glomerular filtration rate, can be seen before a significant rise in serum BUN or serum creatinine occurs.
- A single creatinine clearance value less than 100 mL/min is therefore not diagnostic of renal disease. An incomplete 24-hour urine collection is the most frequent cause of this finding. An abnormal clearance rate should prompt a repeat assay.
- Excretion of uric acid is dependent not only on glomerular filtration but also on tubular secretion.

EFFECT OF PREGNANCY ON RENAL FUNCTION

- Although baseline creatinine clearance is decreased in women with chronic renal insufficiency, a physiologic rise will often occur in pregnancy. A moderate fall in creatinine clearance may then be observed during late gestation in patients with renal disease. This decline is typically more severe in women with diffuse glomerular disease and typically reverses after delivery.
- The long-term effect of pregnancy on renal disease remains controversial. If the serum creatinine is less than 1.5 mg/dL, pregnancy appears to have little effect on the long-term prognosis.
- Occasionally, some women with a baseline serum creatinine of more than 1.5 mg/dL will experience a significant decrease in renal function during gestation that does not improve during the postpartum period.
- Severe hypertension remains the most significant complication for a pregnant patient with chronic renal disease.
- Worsening proteinuria is common during pregnancy complicated by chronic renal disease and often reaches the nephrotic range.

■ In late pregnancy, it can be particularly difficult to differentiate preeclampsia from worsening chronic renal disease. For this reason, an evaluation in the first trimester to establish a baseline for creatinine clearance and total protein is essential.

EFFECT OF CHRONIC RENAL DISEASE ON PREGNANCY

■ More than 85% of women with chronic renal disease will have a surviving infant if renal function is well preserved.
■ The outlook for pregnancies complicated by severe renal insufficiency with a baseline serum creatinine level more than 1.5 mg/dL is less certain. This is due in part to the limited number of pregnancies reported in these women.
■ Preterm birth and IUGR remain important complications, with the reported incidence of preterm birth ranging from 20% to 50%.

MANAGEMENT OF CHRONIC RENAL DISEASE IN PREGNANCY

■ A 24-hour urine collection for creatinine clearance and total protein excretion should be obtained in women with known renal disease as soon as the pregnancy is confirmed.
■ Control of hypertension is critical in managing patients with chronic renal disease. Home blood pressure monitoring is advised for women with underlying hypertension, and β-blockers, calcium channel blockers, and hydralazine can be used to treat blood pressure effectively as long as the dosages are monitored carefully.
■ The use of diuretics in pregnancy is controversial. For massive debilitating edema, a short course of diuretics can be helpful, although electrolytes must be monitored carefully. Salt restriction does not appear to be beneficial once edema has developed; however, it should be instituted without hesitation in pregnant women with true renal insufficiency.
■ The timing of delivery should be individualized. Maternal indications for delivery include uncontrollable hypertension, the development of superimposed preeclampsia, fetal growth restriction, and decreasing renal function after fetal viability has been reached.
■ Renal biopsy is rarely indicated during pregnancy, and it is not advised after 34 weeks' gestation, when delivery of the fetus and subsequent biopsy would prove a safer alternative.

HEMODIALYSIS IN PREGNANCY

■ Women with chronic hemodialysis can have successful pregnancies. However, many women with chronic renal failure experience oligomenorrhea, and their fertility is often impaired.
■ As in all patients with impaired renal function, the most important aspect of care is meticulous control of blood pressure.
■ Women should be counseled that a successful pregnancy will often require longer and more frequent periods of dialysis[3] and a dose response to dialysis and pregnancy outcome exists.
■ Criteria for initiating hemodialysis during pregnancy are controversial. Some investigators believe that beginning regular hemodialysis in patients with moderate renal insufficiency may improve pregnancy outcome.
■ Preterm birth occurs more frequently in women undergoing dialysis.

RENAL TRANSPLANT

■ Pregnancy following renal transplantation has become increasingly common. Many previously anovulatory patients begin ovulating postoperatively and regain fertility as renal function normalizes.

- Many transplant recipients will discontinue all medications after discovering they are pregnant. Immunosuppressive therapy should be continued.
- Cyclosporine A appears to be relatively safe for use during gestation but does hold some risks. Women may develop arterial hypertension secondary to its interference with the normal hemodynamic adaptation to pregnancy.
- Mycophenolate mofetil has been shown to cause adverse effects on fetal development and is associated with first-trimester loss and congenital defects and is contraindicated during pregnancy.
- Sirolimus is also contraindicated in pregnancy. This medication has been shown to be embryotoxic and is associated with increased fetal mortality.
- Tacrolimus has been poorly studied in pregnancy.
- Preeclampsia complicates 30% of these pregnancies, but as previously noted, the diagnosis is difficult to make in a patient who may already have hypertension and proteinuria. The allograft rejection rate in these women is approximately 9%, a rate no different from that expected in a nonpregnant population. The long-term rejection rate was also the same as for women who had not experienced a pregnancy.
- The clinical hallmarks of rejection—fever, oliguria, tenderness, and decreasing renal function—are not always exhibited by the pregnant patient. Occasionally, rejection may mimic pyelonephritis or preeclampsia, which occurs in approximately one-third of renal transplant patients.
- Infection can be disastrous for the renal allograft; therefore urine cultures should be obtained at least monthly during pregnancy, and any bacteriuria should be aggressively treated. It is crucial to recognize that the allograft is denervated, and pain may not accompany pyelonephritis; the only symptoms may be fever and nausea.
- Similar to women with chronic renal disease, serial ultrasonography should be used to assess fetal growth. Approximately 50% of renal allograft recipients will deliver preterm.

References for this chapter are available at ExpertConsult.com.

CHAPTER 40

Diabetes Mellitus Complicating Pregnancy

Mark B. Landon ■ Patrick M. Catalano ■ Steven G. Gabbe

KEY POINTS

- Pregnancy has been characterized as a diabetogenic state because of increased postprandial glucose levels in late gestation.
- Both hepatic and peripheral (tissue) insulin sensitivity are reduced in normal pregnancy. As a result, a progressive increase in insulin secretion follows a glucose challenge.
- In women with GDM, the hormonal milieu of pregnancy may represent an unmasking of a susceptibility to the development of type 2 DM.
- According to the Pedersen hypothesis, maternal hyperglycemia results in fetal hyperglycemia and hyperinsulinemia, which results in excessive fetal growth and perinatal morbidities. Tight maternal glycemic control is associated with a reduced risk for fetal macrosomia.
- Congenital malformations occur with a twofold to sixfold increased rate in offspring of women with pregestational diabetes compared with that of the normal population. Impaired glycemic control and associated derangement in maternal metabolism appear to contribute to abnormal embryogenesis.
- Women with class F (nephropathic) diabetes have an increased risk for preeclampsia and preterm delivery that correlates with their degree of renal impairment.
- Diabetic retinopathy may worsen during pregnancy, yet for women optimally treated with laser photocoagulation *before* pregnancy, significant deterioration of vision is uncommon.
- Screening for GDM is generally performed between 24 and 28 weeks' gestation. A two-step method that consists of a 50-g screen and a diagnostic 100-g oral glucose tolerance test is commonly performed in the United States.
- Treatment of women with type 1 and type 2 DM during pregnancy requires intensive therapy that consists of frequent self-monitoring of blood glucose and aggressive insulin dosing by multiple injections or continuous subcutaneous insulin infusion (insulin pump).
- The cornerstone of treatment for GDM is dietary therapy. Insulin and oral agents are reserved for individuals who manifest significant fasting hyperglycemia or postprandial glucose elevations despite dietary intervention.
- Antepartum fetal assessment for women with both pregestational diabetes or GDM is based on the degree of risk believed to be present in each case. Glycemic control, prior obstetric history, and the presence of vascular disease or hypertension are important considerations.
- Delivery should generally be delayed in patients whose glucose is well controlled until 39 weeks' gestation. The mode of delivery for the suspected large fetus remains controversial. In cases of suspected macrosomia, cesarean delivery has been recommended to prevent a traumatic birth.
- Women with type 1 and type 2 DM should seek prepregnancy consultation. Efforts to improve glycemic control before conception have been associated with a significant reduction in the rate of congenital malformations in the offspring of such women.

Perinatal Morbidity and Mortality

- Diabetes in pregnancy is associated with an increase in perinatal morbidity, including congenital malformations, macrosomia, hypoglycemia, hypocalcemia, hyperbilirubinemia and polycythemia, and a transient form of cardiomyopathy.
- Excessive stillbirth rates in pregnancies complicated by diabetes have been linked to chronic intrauterine hypoxia.

CONGENITAL MALFORMATIONS

- Most studies have documented a twofold to sixfold increase in major malformations in infants of type 1 and type 2 diabetic mothers.
- Central nervous system malformations (anencephaly, open spina bifida, and holoprosencephaly) are increased tenfold. Cardiac anomalies are the most common malformations, with ventricular septal defects and complex lesions such as transposition of the great vessels increased fivefold.
- Maternal hyperglycemia has been proposed as the primary teratogenic factor.

FETAL MACROSOMIA

- *Macrosomia* has been defined as birthweight greater than 4000 to 4500 g, as well as meeting the criteria for large for gestational age, in which birthweight is above the 90th percentile for population and sex-specific growth curves. Fetal macrosomia complicates as many as 50% of pregnancies in women with gestational diabetes mellitus (GDM) and 40% of pregnancies complicated by type 1 and type 2 diabetes, which includes some women treated with intensive glycemic control.
- Infants of mothers with GDM have an increase in fat mass, compared with fat-free mass. The growth is disproportionate, with chest-to-head and shoulder-to-head ratios larger than those of infants of women with normal glucose tolerance.

HYPOGLYCEMIA

- *Neonatal hypoglycemia,* a blood glucose level less than 35 to 40 mg/dL during the first 12 hours of life, results from a rapid drop in plasma glucose concentrations following clamping of the umbilical cord. Hypoglycemia, a byproduct of hyperinsulinemia, is particularly common in macrosomic newborns, in whom rates exceed 50%.

RESPIRATORY DISTRESS SYNDROME

- Several studies suggest that in women with well-controlled diabetes whose fetus is delivered at 38 to 39 weeks' gestation, the risk for respiratory distress syndrome is no higher than that observed in the general population.

Maternal Classification and Risk Assessment

- Priscilla White first noted that the patient's age at onset of diabetes, the duration of the disease, and the presence of vasculopathy significantly influenced perinatal outcome. Her classification system has been widely applied to pregnant women with diabetes (Table 40.1).
- Class A₁ DM includes those women who have demonstrated carbohydrate intolerance during an oral glucose tolerance test (GTT); however, their fasting and postprandial glucose

TABLE 40.1 ■ Modified White Classification of Pregnant Diabetic Women

Class	Diabetes Onset Age (yr)	Duration (yr)	Vascular Disease	Need for Insulin or Oral Agent
Gestational Diabetes				
A$_1$	Any	Any	–	–
A$_2$	Any	Any	–	+
Pregestational Diabetes				
B	>20	<10	–	+
C	10 to 19	or 10 to 19	–	+
D	<10	or >20	+	+
F	Any	Any	+	+
R	Any	Any	+	+
T	Any	Any	+	+
H	Any	Any	+	+

Modified from White P. Pregnancy complicating diabetes. *Am J Med*. 1949;7:609.

levels are maintained within physiologic range by dietary regulation alone. Class A$_2$ includes women with GDM who require medical management.

■ Diabetes first identified in early pregnancy most likely represents cases of "overt diabetes."

NEPHROPATHY

■ Overt diabetic nephropathy is diagnosed in women with type 1 or type 2 DM when persistent proteinuria exists in the absence of infection or other urinary tract disease.

■ Class F describes pregnant women with underlying renal disease. This includes those with reduced creatinine clearance or proteinuria of at least 500 mg in 24 hours measured during the first 20 weeks of gestation.

■ Control of hypertension in pregnant women with diabetic nephropathy is crucial to prevent further deterioration of kidney function and to optimize pregnancy outcome. Some have recommended instituting antihypertensive therapy to maintain blood pressure less than 135/85 mm Hg in pregnant women with nephropathy.

■ Calcium channel blockers are our first choice for treatment of hypertension in pregnant women with diabetic nephropathy because of the renoprotective effects similar to those of angiotensin-converting enzyme inhibitors and do not appear to be teratogenic. Angiotensin-converting enzyme inhibitors and angiotensin II receptor blockers are contraindicated during pregnancy.

■ Changes in creatinine clearance are variable during pregnancy in women with diabetic nephropathy. Most will not exhibit a normal rise in creatinine clearance. Protein excretion will frequently rise during gestation to levels that can reach the nephrotic range.

RETINOPATHY

■ Class R diabetes designates women with proliferative retinopathy, which represents neovascularization or growth of new retinal capillaries. These vessels may cause vitreous hemorrhage with scarring and retinal detachment, which results in vision loss.

TABLE 40.2 ▪ **Detection of GDM**

Screening Test (50 g, 1 h)		Plasma (mg/dL, 130-140)
Oral GTT*	NDDG	Carpenter & Coustan
Fasting glucose	105	95
1-hr glucose	190	180
2-hr glucose	165	155
3-hr glucose	145	110

*Diagnosis of gestational diabetes is made when any two values are met or exceeded in a 100-g, 3-hour test.
GDM, gestational diabetes mellitus; GTT, glucose tolerance test; NDDG, National Diabetes Data Group.

- For women with proliferative changes, laser photocoagulation is indicated, and most will respond to this therapy. However, women who demonstrate severe florid disc neovascularization that is unresponsive to laser therapy during early pregnancy may be at great risk for deterioration of their vision.

CORONARY ARTERY DISEASE

- Class H diabetes refers to the presence of diabetes of any duration associated with ischemic myocardial disease.

Early Screening for Overt Diabetes and Detection of Gestational Diabetes Mellitus

- The frequency of diabetes complicating pregnancy has been estimated to be as high as 6% to 7% with approximately 90% of these cases representing women with GDM.
- At the present time, most practitioners in the United States continue to perform glucose-challenge screening (50-g) followed by a diagnostic 100-g oral GTT (two-step approach) (Table 40.2).
- A plasma value between 130 and 140 mg/dL is commonly used as a threshold for performing a 3-hour oral GTT.

Treatment of the Patient With Type 1 or Type 2 Diabetes Mellitus

- Insulin therapy is recommended by the American Diabetes Association as the primary medication to achieve optimal glycemic control in pregnant women with both type 1 and type 2 diabetes (Table 40.3). Women with type 2 diabetes may present in early pregnancy on an oral agent for treatment of their diabetes. Our approach is to continue metformin therapy in well-controlled type 2 diabetic women, whereas those receiving other agents are generally switched to insulin therapy. Many type 2 diabetic women who enter pregnancy with their disease controlled with metformin will eventually require the addition of insulin to their regimen.
- To achieve the best glycemic control possible for each patient, intensive insulin therapy is recommended to simulate physiologic insulin requirements. Insulin administration is provided for both basal needs and meals, and rapid adjustments are made in response to glucose measurements. The treatment regimen generally involves three to four daily injections or the use of continuous subcutaneous insulin infusion (CSII) devices.

TABLE 40.3 ■ **Target Plasma Glucose Levels in Pregnancy**

Time	Glucose Level (mg/dL)
Before breakfast	60-90
Before lunch, supper, bedtime snack	60-105
One hour after meals	≤140
Two hours after meals	≤120
2 AM to 6 AM	>60

TABLE 40.4 ■ **Type of Human Insulin and Insulin Analogues**

	Source	Onset (h)	Peak (h)	Duration (h)
Short Acting				
Humulin R (Lilly)	Human	0.5	2-4	5-7
Velosulin H (Novo Nordisk)	Human	0.5	1-3	8
Novolin R (Novo Nordisk)	Human	0.5	2.5-5	6-8
Rapid Acting				
Lispro (Humalog, Lilly)	Analogue	0.25	0.5-1.5	4-5
Aspart (NovoLog, Nordisk)	Analogue	0.25	1-3	3-5
Intermediate Acting				
Humulin Lente (Lilly)	Human	1-3	6-12	18-24
Humulin NPH (Lilly)	Human	1-2	6-12	18-24
Novolin I (Novo Nordisk)	Human	2.5	7-15	22
Novolin N (Novo Nordisk)	Human	1.5	4-20	24
Long Acting				
Glargine (Lantus, Sanofi)	Analogue	1	—	24
Detemir (Levemir, Novo Nordisk)	Analogue	1-2	—	24

- Semisynthetic human insulin preparations and newer insulin analogues (Table 40.4) are preferred for use during pregnancy. Insulin lispro and insulin aspart are rapid-acting insulin preparations that have replaced regular insulin.
- The flat profile of glargine may be undesirable during pregnancy when variation in basal insulin needs are likely. For this reason, we frequently suggest that women who receive glargine change to a twice-daily regimen of NPH insulin.
- Our approach is to maintain patients on insulin detemir if their blood glucose is well controlled.
- Open-loop CSII pump therapy is preferred by many women with type 1 diabetes during pregnancy. A systematic review that compared randomized trials of CSII versus multiple-injection regimens revealed no difference in measures of glycemic control or pregnancy outcome.
- Diet therapy is critical to successful regulation of maternal diabetes. A program that consists of three meals and several snacks is used for most patients (Box 40.1).

BOX 40.1 ■ Dietary Recommendations

- Three meals, three snacks
- Diet: 30-35 kcal/kg normal body weight, 2000 to 2400 kcal/day
- Composition: carbohydrate 40%-50% complex, high fiber; protein 20%; fat 30%-40% (<10% saturated)
- Weight gain: per Institute of Medicine guidelines

- The presence of maternal vasculopathy should be thoroughly assessed early in pregnancy. Ophthalmologic examinations are performed during each trimester and are repeated more often if retinopathy is detected.

KETOACIDOSIS

- With strict metabolic control of blood glucose levels for women who require insulin, diabetic ketoacidosis (DKA) has fortunately become a less common occurrence (between 0.5% and 3.0% of diabetic pregnancies).
- DKA can occur in the newly diagnosed diabetic patient, and the hormonal milieu of pregnancy may become the background for this phenomenon. Because pregnancy is a state of insulin resistance marked by enhanced lipolysis and ketogenesis, DKA may develop in a pregnant woman with glucose levels that barely exceed 200 mg/dL (11.1 mmol/L). This phenomenon has been referred to as *euglycemic ketoacidosis.*
- A pregnant diabetic woman with poor fluid intake and persistent vomiting over 8 to 12 hours should be evaluated for potential DKA.
- Fluid resuscitation and insulin infusion should be maintained even in the face of normoglycemia until bicarbonate levels return to normal, indicating that acidemia has cleared (Box 40.2).
- Successful fetal resuscitation often accompanies correction of maternal acidosis.

Antepartum Fetal Evaluation

- Recommended antepartum surveillance for low-risk and high-risk insulin-dependent diabetics is shown in Tables 40.5 and 40.6.
- It is important not only to include the results of antepartum fetal testing but also to weigh all of the clinical features that involve the mother and fetus before deciding to intervene for suspected fetal compromise, especially if this decision may result in a preterm delivery.
- A comprehensive ultrasound examination at 18 to 20 weeks, as well as fetal echocardiography performed at 20 to 22 weeks, is undertaken to diagnose fetal anomalies. We prefer to use fetal echocardiography as a screening tool in all type 1 and type 2 diabetic pregnancies.
- An increased rate of cephalopelvic disproportion and shoulder dystocia, accompanied by significant risk for traumatic birth injury and asphyxia, has been consistently associated with vaginal delivery of large infants. The risk for such complications rises exponentially when birthweight exceeds 4 kg, and it is greater for the fetus of a diabetic mother when compared with a fetus with similar weight whose mother does not have diabetes.

Timing and Mode of Delivery

- Delivery should be delayed until fetal maturation has taken place, provided diabetes is well controlled and antepartum surveillance remains normal.

BOX 40.2 ■ Management of Diabetic Ketoacidosis During Pregnancy

Intravenous Fluids

- Isotonic sodium chloride is used, with total replacement of 4-6 L in the first 12 hours.
- Insert intravenous catheters: Maintain hourly flow sheet for fluids and electrolytes, potassium, insulin, and laboratory results.
- Administer normal saline (0.9% NaCl) at 1-2 L/h for the first hour.
- Infuse normal saline at 250 to 500 mL/h depending on hydration state (8 hours). If serum sodium is elevated, use half-normal saline (0.45% NaCl).
- When plasma or serum glucose reaches 200 mg/dL, change to 5% dextrose with 0.45% NaCl at 150-250 mL/h.
- After 8 hours, use half-normal saline at 125 mL/h.

Potassium

- Establish adequate renal function (urine output ~50 mL/h).
- If serum potassium is <3.3 mEq/L, hold insulin and give 20-30 mEq K$^+$/h until K$^+$ is >3.3 mEq/L or is being corrected.
- If serum K$^+$ is >3.3 mEq/L but <5.3 mEq/L, give 20-30 mEq K$^+$ in each liter of IV fluid to keep serum K$^+$ between 4 and 5 mEq/L.
- If serum K$^+$ is >5.3 mEq/L, do not give K$^+$ but check serum K$^+$ every 2 hours.

Insulin

- Use regular insulin intravenously.
- Consider a loading dose of 0.1-0.2 U/kg as an IV bolus depending on plasma glucose.
- Begin continuous insulin infusion at 0.1 U/kg/h.
- If plasma or serum glucose does not fall by 50-70 mg/dL in the first hour, double the insulin infusion every hour until a steady glucose decline is achieved.
- When plasma or serum glucose reaches 200 mg/dL, reduce insulin infusion to 0.05-0.1 U/kg/h.
- Keep plasma or serum glucose between 100 and 150 mg/dL until resolution of diabetic ketoacidosis.

Bicarbonate

- Assess need, and provide based on pH.
- pH >7.0: No HCO$_3$ is needed.
- pH is 6.9-7.0: Dilute NaHCO$_3$ (50 mmol) in 200 mL H$_2$O with 10 mEq KCl and infuse over 1 hour. Repeat NaHCO$_3$ administration every 2 hours until pH is 7.0. Monitor serum K$^+$.
- pH <6.9-7.0: Dilute NaHCO$_3$ (100 mmol) in 400 mL H$_2$O with 20 mEq KCl and infuse for 2 hours. Repeat NaHCO$_3$ administration every 2 hours until pH is 7.0. Monitor serum K$^+$.

TABLE 40.5 ■ Antepartum Fetal Surveillance in Low-Risk Insulin-Dependent Diabetes Mellitus*

Study	Indicated
Ultrasonography at 4- to 6-wk intervals	Yes
Maternal assessment of fetal activity, daily at 28 wk	Yes
NST at 32 wk; BPP or CST if NST is nonreactive	Yes
Amniocentesis for lung profile	Yes, if elective delivery is planned before 39 wk

*Excellent control, no vasculopathy (classes B, C), no stillbirth.
BPP, biophysical profile; CST, contraction stress test; NST, nonstress test.

TABLE 40.6 ■ **Antepartum Fetal Surveillance in High-Risk Insulin-Dependent Diabetes Mellitus***

Study	Indicated
Ultrasonography at 4- to 6-wk intervals	Yes
Maternal assessment of fetal activity daily at 28 wk	Yes
NST; BPP or CST if NST is nonreactive	Initiate at 28-30 wk
Consider amniocentesis for lung profile prior to 38 wk	

*Poor control (macrosomia, hydramnios), vasculopathy (classes D, F, R), prior stillbirth.
BPP, biophysical profile; *CST,* contraction stress test; *NST,* nonstress test.

- Tests of fetal lung maturity appear to have the same predictive value in diabetic pregnancies as in the normal population.
- When antepartum testing suggests fetal compromise, delivery must be considered. In the presence of presumed lung immaturity, the decision to proceed with delivery should be based on confirmation of deteriorating fetal condition by several tests that show abnormal values.
- Choosing the route of delivery for the diabetic patient remains controversial.
- The increased rate of shoulder dystocia and brachial plexus injury in the offspring of diabetic women has prompted adoption of early induction strategies, as well as selection of patients for cesarean delivery, based on ultrasound estimation of fetal size.

Glucoregulation During Labor and Delivery

- Because neonatal hypoglycemia is in part related to maternal glucose levels during labor, it is important to maintain maternal plasma glucose levels within the physiologic normal range (Box 40.3).

Management of Gestational Diabetes

IS THERE A BENEFIT TO THE TREATMENT OF GESTATIONAL DIABETES MELLITUS?

- The National Institute of Child Health and Human Development Maternal-Fetal Medicine Unit Network trial demonstrated that although treatment of mild GDM did not reduce the frequency of several neonatal morbidities characteristic of diabetic pregnancy, it did lower the risk for fetal overgrowth, neonatal fat mass, shoulder dystocia, cesarean delivery, and hypertensive disorders of pregnancy. These findings, along with those reported in the Australian Carbohydrate Intolerace Study in Pregnant Women study, have confirmed a benefit to treatment of even mild carbohydrate intolerance of pregnancy.

TREATMENT OF GESTATIONAL DIABETES MELLITUS

- The mainstay of treatment of GDM remains nutritional counseling and dietary intervention (see Box 40.1). The optimal diet should provide caloric and nutrient needs to sustain pregnancy without resulting in significant postprandial hyperglycemia.
- During the past 15 years, oral hypoglycemic therapy has become a suitable alternative to insulin treatment in women with GDM.

BOX 40.3 ■ Insulin Management During Labor and Delivery

- Usual dose of intermediate-acting insulin is given at bedtime.
- Morning dose of insulin is withheld.
- Intravenous infusion of normal saline is begun.
- Once active labor begins or glucose levels fall to <70 mg/dL, the infusion is changed from saline to 5% dextrose and is delivered at a rate of 2.5 mg/kg/min.
- Glucose levels are checked hourly using a portable reflectance meter allowing for adjustment in the infusion rate.
- Regular (short-acting) insulin is administered by intravenous infusion if glucose levels exceed 140 mg/dL.

From Jovanovic L, Peterson CM. Management of the pregnant, insulin-dependent diabetic woman. Diabetes Care. _1980;3:63._

BOX 40.4 ■ Summary of Glyburide Versus Insulin Treatment in Gestational Diabetes Mellitus

- Maternal fasting and postprandial glycemia comparable to that with insulin treatment
- Glyburide failure rate of 15%-20%
- Glyburide failures associated with earlier diagnosis of gestational diabetes and fasting glucose levels >110-115 mg/dL
- Comparable neonatal outcomes
- Significant cost savings

- Metformin has also been used for treatment of GDM. Although metformin clearly crosses the placenta, it does not appear to be teratogenic.
- It appears that glyburide may be superior to metformin in achieving satisfactory glucose control in women with GDM. Observational data suggest that glyburide may be less successful in obese women and in those with marked hyperglycemia discovered early in gestation (Box 40.4).
- Women with GDM that is well controlled are at low risk for intrauterine fetal demise. For this reason, we do not routinely institute antepartum fetal heart rate testing in uncomplicated diet-controlled GDM. Women with a hypertensive disorder, a history of a prior stillbirth, or suspected macrosomia do undergo fetal testing.

Postpartum Follow-up in Gestational Diabetes Mellitus

- Women with GDM have a sevenfold increased risk for developing type 2 diabetes compared with women who do not have diabetes during pregnancy.
- ACOG recommends using either a fasting plasma glucose or a 75-g 2-hour oral GTT at 6 to 12 weeks' postpartum. The American Diabetes Association recommends repeat testing at least every 3 years for women with prior GDM and normal results of postpartum screening.
- Women with GDM are at high risk for recurrence in future pregnancies; therefore we recommend early pregnancy screening or testing, followed by screening at 24 to 28 weeks, or testing in those not found to have GDM earlier in pregnancy.

Prepregnancy Counseling in Preexisting Diabetes Mellitus

- Management and counseling of women with diabetes in the reproductive age group should begin before conception to reduced risk of congenital anomalies (Box 40.5).

BOX 40.5 ■ Prepregnancy Care for Diabetic Women

- Multidisciplinary care team: obstetrician, endocrinologist, diabetes educator, nutritionist
- Evaluation for vascular complications
  - Retinal examination
  - Assess renal function: serum creatinine and evaluation for proteinuria
- Evaluation for cardiovascular status
  - Hypertension
  - Ischemic cardiac disease: electrocardiogram if long-standing diabetes, hypertension, or symptoms
- Review medications
  - Angiotensin-converting enzyme inhibitors, angiotensin II receptor blockers, and statins best avoided if planning conception
  - Folate supplementation recommended
- Assessment of glycemic control
  - Measure hemoglobin A1c every 2 months
  - Target hemoglobin A1c should be ≤7.0%
  - Contraception not advised until glucose is well controlled
- Promote healthy lifestyle
  - Regular exercise
  - Nutrition counseling and weight loss for obese women
  - Smoking cessation

Contraception

- Because no risks are inherent to the diaphragm and other barrier methods, and these methods do not affect carbohydrate metabolism, they have become the preferred interim method of contraception for women with DM.
- The serious side effects of oral contraceptive use, including thromboembolic disease and myocardial infarction, may be increased in diabetic women who use combined oral contraceptives.
- At present, little information is available concerning long-acting progestins in women with diabetes or previous GDM.

CHAPTER 41

Obesity in Pregnancy

Patrick M. Catalano

KEY POINTS

- Behavioral modification of diet or diet plus exercise can decrease excessive gestational weight gain in obese women.
- Weight gain in pregnancy should be based on pregravid BMI and should follow the Institute of Medicine recommendations.
- Obese women should be counseled as to the limitation of ultrasound in identifying structural anomalies.
- At the first prenatal visit, obese women should be screened for glucose intolerance.
- Antenatal fetal surveillance is not recommended for obese women without other maternal or fetal indications.
- Obese women should be counseled about the increased risk of CD for obese, compared with normal-weight, women.
- Closure of subcutaneous tissue greater than 2 cm, but not placement of subcutaneous drains, decreases the risk of postpartum cesarean wound complications.
- Excessive gestational weight gain is a significant risk factor for postpartum weight retention.
- Behavioral interventions that use diet and/or diet and exercise, but not those that use exercise alone, can improve postpartum weight reduction.
- Because of the increase in plasma volume in obese women, consideration should be given to increase the bolus of preepidural intravenous fluid and dosage of prophylactic antibiotics for CD.

Prevalence of Obesity in Women of Reproductive Age

- Obesity is commonly classified by the body mass index (BMI), which is weight in kilograms divided by height in meters squared (kg/m^2) using the World Health Organization criteria. Underweight is less than 18.5, normal weight is 18.5 to 24.9, overweight is 25.0 to 29.9; obese class I, is 30.0 to 34.9, obese class II is 35.0 to 39.9, and obese class III is 40 or more.
- Based on the 2011 to 2012 National Health and Nutrition Examination Survey, the prevalence of obesity in women of reproductive age (20 to 39 years) in the United States was 31.8% (95% confidence interval [CI], 28.5 to 35.5), whereas overweight plus obesity was 58.5% (95% CI, 51.4 to 65.2) of that population.[1]

GESTATIONAL WEIGHT GAIN IN OBESE WOMEN

- Excessive gestational weight gain is a significant factor for postpartum weight retention and hence is a significant contributor to the obesity epidemic.

- During pregnancy, medications for weight management are not recommended because of safety concerns and side effects.
- There is not enough evidence to recommend any specific intervention for preventing excessive weight gain in pregnancy,
- Nutritional strategies, rather than exercise, appear to be more useful in avoiding excessive gestational weight gain in pregnancy.

Pregnancy Complications in Obese Women

EARLY PREGNANCY

- The risk of spontaneous abortion (odds ratio [OR], 1.2; 95% confidence interval [CI], 1.01 to 1.46) and recurrent miscarriage (OR, 3.5; 95% CI, 1.03 to 12.01) is increased in obese women.
- The risk of congenital anomalies is also increased in obese mothers, who are at increased risk for pregnancies affected by neural tube, cardiovascular, orofacial, and limb-reduction anomalies.
- Based on one study, routine ultrasound detected 46.2% (1146 of 2483) of structural anomalies in fetuses with a normal karyotype.[2] Detection rates decreased significantly with increasing maternal BMI, and the odds of detection of any anomaly were significantly lower in obese women than in those with a normal BMI (adjusted OR, 0.77; 95% CI, 0.60 to 0.99).[2]

MID TO LATE PREGNANCY

- The risk of gestational diabetes mellitus and preeclampsia is increased, as is the risk of cardiac dysfunction, proteinuria, sleep apnea, and nonalcoholic fatty liver disease in obese as compared with normal-weight pregnant women.
- Not only is the risk of indicated preterm deliveries increased, the risk of idiopathic preterm birth is also increased in overweight and obese pregnant women. The risk of stillbirth also increases with progressive degrees of maternal obesity.
- Although obese women are at increased risk for adverse perinatal outcomes, data are insufficient to recommend antenatal surveillance in this population without additional clinical indications.

INTRAPARTUM COMPLICATIONS

- At delivery, obese women are at increased risk of CD, endometritis, wound rupture/dehiscence, and venous thrombosis, and they have an almost twofold increased risk of composite maternal morbidity and a fivefold risk of neonatal injury.
- The length of labor in nulliparous women is proportional to maternal BMI.
- In a mixed nulliparous and multiparous cohort, the second stage of labor was not significantly different among normal, overweight, and obese women.
- Maternal obesity significantly increases the risk of anesthetic complications.
- The optimal type of skin incision for primary cesarean delivery in order to decrease morbidity in obese class II and III patients has not been resolved.

Postpartum Considerations

MATERNAL

- Because CD increases the risk of venous thromboembolism, placement of pneumatic compression devices has been recommended for all patients before and after cesarean delivery by the American College of Obstetricians and Gynecologists.[3]

- An open wound can be managed in any of three ways: with secondary closure, closure by secondary intention with dressings, and closure by secondary intention using negative-pressure wound therapy.
- Weight loss between pregnancies in obese women has been shown to decrease the risk of a large-for-gestational-age infant, whereas an interpregnancy weight gain was associated with an increased risk of delivering a large-for-gestational-age infant.

Neonate/Child

- The infants of obese women are at increased risk for fetal macrosomia and, more specifically, for increased body fat compared with infants of normal-weight women.

Other Considerations

FACILITIES

- In the outpatient setting, common requirements include large chairs and examining tables capable of supporting weights up to 500 to 750 lb, large blood pressure cuffs capable of extending around 80% of the arm circumference, and large wheelchairs.
- Because of the increased possibility of emergency CD in obese women, doorways and hallways require enough space to accommodate large beds and additional staff moving patients safely.
- Operating tables need to be strong enough to safely support patients with weights up to 500 to 750 lb and should have attachments to increase the width of tables.
- Long instruments are also necessary to facilitate the surgeon's access to the proper tissue planes.

References for this chapter are available at ExpertConsult.com.

CHAPTER 42

Thyroid and Parathyroid Diseases in Pregnancy

Jorge H. Mestman

KEY POINTS

- Hyperthyroidism due to Graves disease needs to be differentiated in the first trimester of pregnancy from the syndrome of gestational thyrotoxicosis.
- Recent reports indicate increased risk for liver failure with the use of PTU; it is recommended that PTU be used in the first trimester of pregnancy and MMI after 13 weeks' gestation. MMI is not indicated in the first trimester because of the potential risk for the syndrome of MMI embryopathy. PTU may also be teratogenic, but the risk is much less than that associated with MMI.
- The dose of antithyroid medications should be adjusted frequently, aiming to use the minimal amount of drug that will keep the FT_4 at the upper limit of normal.
- Hypothyroid women on thyroid replacement therapy should have their thyroid tests checked at the time of planning their pregnancy, and they should have their serum TSH adjusted to close to 1 mIU/L.
- Women on suppressive T_4 therapy for thyroid cancer before pregnancy must continue with therapy. The levothyroxine dose should be adjusted to keep serum TSH at the same level before pregnancy and to keep FT_4 within the normal reference range.
- Women with risk factors for thyroid disease—such as a family history of thyroid disease, the presence of a goiter, or a history of PPT—should be studied before or early in pregnancy.
- Postpartum thyroiditis affects up to 16.7% of all women in the postpartum period. Women with chronic thyroiditis are at higher risk for developing the syndrome. Long-term follow-up is strongly advised because up to 50% of these patients will develop permanent hypothyroidism in 5 to 10 years.

Parathyroid Disorders

HYPERPARATHYROIDISM

- The most common cause of primary parahyperthyroidism (PHPT) in pregnancy is a single parathyroid adenoma, which is present in about 80% of all cases.
- Hyperparathyroidism should be considered in the differential diagnosis of acute pancreatitis during pregnancy.
- Serum calcium should be obtained in any pregnant woman with persistent significant nausea, vomiting, and abdominal pain.
- The two most common causes of neonatal morbidity are prematurity and neonatal hypocalcemia; the latter is related to levels of maternal hypercalcemia.
- The diagnosis of PHPT is based on persistent hypercalcemia in the presence of increased PTH or a PTH level inappropriate for the level of serum calcium.

- Ultrasonography of the neck is the current first-line investigation during pregnancy for localization of parathyroid diseases, with a sensitivity of 69% and a specificity of 94% in experienced hands. Parathyroid contrast imaging studies are contraindicated in pregnancy.
- Although most young women with hypercalcemia have PHPT, other unusual causes should be ruled out, mainly endocrine disorders, vitamin D or A overdose, the use of thiazide diuretics, or granulomatous diseases.

Therapy

- Surgery is the only effective treatment for PHPT.
- It is preferable to perform the surgery in the second trimester of pregnancy.
- Medical therapy is reserved for patients with significant hypercalcemia who are not surgical candidates.
- In patients undergoing surgical treatment, hypocalcemia—albeit transient—may occur after surgery in some cases.

HYPOPARATHYROIDISM

- The most common etiology of hypoparathyroidism is damage to or removal of the parathyroid glands in the course of surgery for thyroid gland pathology.
- Typical symptoms of hypocalcemia are numbness and tingling of the fingers and toes and around the lips.
- The diagnosis of hypoparathyroidism is confirmed by the presence of persistent low serum calcium and high serum phosphate levels.
- Treatment of hypoparathyroidism in pregnancy does not differ from that in the nonpregnant state, including a normal high-calcium diet and vitamin D supplementation.

Thyroid Diseases

OVERALL

- The suggested total daily iodine ingestion for pregnant women is 229 μg/day, and for lactating women, it is 289 μg/day; prenatal vitamins should contain 150 μg of iodine in the form of potassium iodine.
- The normal thyroid gland is able to compensate for the increase in thyroid hormone demands by increasing its secretion of thyroid hormones and maintaining them within normal limits throughout gestation.
- Active secretion of thyroid hormones by the fetal thyroid gland commences at about 18 weeks' gestation, although iodine uptake by the fetal gland occurs between 10 and 14 weeks. Transfer of thyroxine (T_4) from mother to embryo occurs from early pregnancy.
- The serum free fractions of both T_4 and total triiodothyronine remain within normal limits during pregnancy.
- The detection of a goiter in pregnancy is an abnormal finding that needs careful evaluation.

HYPERTHYROIDISM
Graves Disease

- The natural course of hyperthyroidism due to Graves disease in pregnancy is characterized by an exacerbation of symptoms in the first trimester and during the postpartum period and an amelioration of symptoms in the second half of pregnancy.
- On physical examination, the thyroid gland is enlarged in almost every pregnant woman with Graves disease.

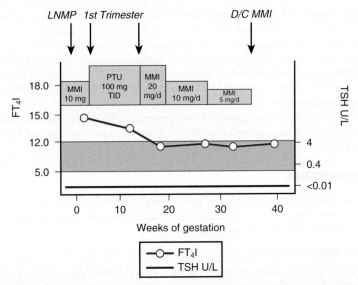

Fig. 42.1 A representative example of management of hyperthyroidism in pregnancy. The patient is hyperthyroid at time of conception on methimazole (MMI) 10 mg daily. When pregnancy is diagnosed, MMI is discontinued, and propylthiouracil (PTU) is added at a dosage of 150 mg three times daily. By the end of the first trimester, PTU is discontinued and MMI is given at a dosage of 20 mg daily. By week 20, the free thyroxine index (FT₄I) is almost normal, and the MMI dosage is reduced to 10 mg. By week 26, the FT₄I is in the upper reference range and thyrotropin remains suppressed; the MMI dosage is reduced to 5 mg daily. The FT₄I remains in the upper reference range, and by week 34 MMI is discontinued (D/C), and the patient remains euthyroid until delivery. The orange band indicates the reference range. LNMP, last normal menstrual period; TSH, thyroid-stimulating hormone.

- An undetected thyroid-stimulating hormone (TSH) value in the presence of a high FT₄, or FT₄ index or total thyroxine adjusted for pregnancy confirms the diagnosis of hyperthyroidism.[1]
- Left ventricular decompensation in hyperthyroid pregnant women may develop in the presence of superimposed preeclampsia, at the time of delivery, or with undercurrent complications such as anemia or infection.
- The goal of treatment is normalization of thyroid tests as soon as possible and maintenance of euthyroidism with the minimal amount of antithyroid medication.
- Although the incidence of both liver toxicity with propylthiouracil (PTU) and embryopathy from methimazole (MMI) are very low, a panel convened by the U.S. Food and Drug Administration and the American Thyroid Association recommended the use of PTU only in the first trimester of pregnancy with a change to MMI in the second trimester (Fig. 42.1).[2]
- In our experience, 20 mg/day of MMI or 100 to 150 mg of PTU three times a day is an effective initial dose in most patients.
- Once clinical improvement occurs, mainly weight gain and reduction in tachycardia, the dose of antithyroid medication may be reduced by half of the initial dose.
- The main concerns of maternal drug therapy are the potential side effects in the fetus, mainly goiter and hypothyroidism, as well as birth defects.
- The most common complications of both PTU and MMI are pruritus and skin rash.
- β-Adrenergic blocking agents (propranolol 20 to 40 mg every 6 hours or atenolol 25 to 50 mg/day) are very effective in controlling hyperdynamic symptoms and are indicated for the first few weeks in patients who have symptoms.

- Thyroid storm is a life-threatening condition with a mortality rate of 20% to 30%; it requires early recognition and aggressive therapy in an intensive unit care setting.
- Iodine 131 therapy is contraindicated in pregnancy because when given after 12 weeks' gestation, it could produce fetal hypothyroidism. A pregnancy test is mandatory in any woman of childbearing age before a therapeutic or diagnostic dose of ^{131}I is administered.
- Breastfeeding should be permitted if the daily dose of PTU or MMI is less than 300 mg/day or 20 mg/day, respectively.
- Fetal hyperthyroidism is diagnosed in the presence of persistent fetal tachycardia (>160 beats/min), intrauterine growth restriction, oligohydramnios, hydrops, and occasionally a goiter identified on ultrasonography.

HYPOTHYROIDISM

- The two most common etiologies of primary hypothyroidism in countries with sufficient dietary iodine supply are autoimmune (Hashimoto) thyroiditis and post–thyroid ablation therapy, either surgical or ^{131}I induced.

Subclinical Hypothyroidism

- Subclinical hypothyroidism diagnosed in the first trimester of pregnancy has been associated with maternal, fetal, and neonatal complications in some but not all studies.
- One laboratory test diagnostic of subclinical hypothyroidism is an elevated serum TSH in the presence of normal trimester-specific FT_4 levels.

Clinical Hypothyroidism

- The diagnosis of clinical or overt hypothyroidism in pregnancy is confirmed by the presence of an elevated serum TSH and an FT_4 below the trimester-specific reference range or a serum TSH greater than 10 mIU/L irrespective of the serum thyroxine level.
- Serum thyroid antibodies—thyroid peroxidase antibodies, also known as *antimicrosomal antibodies*—are elevated in almost 95% of patients with autoimmune hypothyroidism.
- One of the most common obstetric complications of overt hypothyroidism is preeclampsia, with an incidence of 21% in one study.
- It is important to normalize thyroid tests as early as possible before conception or soon after the diagnosis of pregnancy.
- Women planning their pregnancies should have a serum TSH below 2.5 mIU/L, ideally closer to 1 mIU/L.

SINGLE NODULE OF THE THYROID GLAND

- It is estimated that nodular thyroid disease is clinically detectable in 10% of pregnant women. The size of the thyroid nodule clinically detectable is 1.0 to 1.5 cm.
- It is estimated that as many as 14 of every 100,000 pregnancies in the United States are complicated by a new diagnosis of thyroid cancer.
- When advising pregnant women on the evaluation of a thyroid nodule, it must be kept in mind that the incidence of malignancy is between 5% and 10%, and in most cases, the tumors are slow growing.

PATIENTS WITH KNOWN THYROID CANCER BEFORE PREGNANCY

- Pregnancy does not appear to be a risk factor for recurrences in women with a previous history of treated thyroid cancer and no evidence of residual disease.
- No evidence suggests that exposure to radioiodine affects the outcome of subsequent pregnancies and offspring.

BOX 42.2 ■ Postpartum Thyroid Dysfunction

Chronic Thyroiditis

Transient hyperthyroidism (low RAIU)
Transient hypothyroidism
Permanent hypothyroidism

Graves Disease

Exacerbation of hyperthyroidism (high RAIU, positive TRAb)
Transient hyperthyroidism of chronic thyroiditis (low RAIU, negative TRAb)

Hypothalamic-Pituitary Disease

Sheehan syndrome
Lymphocytic hypophysitis

RAIU, radioactive iodine uptake; *TRAb,* thyroid-blocking antibody.
From Mestman JH. Endocrine diseases in pregnancy. In Sciarra JJ, editor. *Gynecology and Obstetrics.*
Philadelphia: Lippincott-Raven; 1997:34.

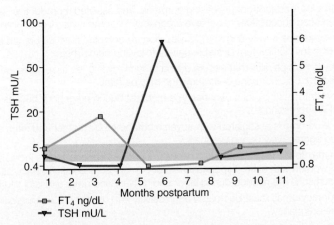

Fig. 42.2 Clinical course of postpartum thyroiditis. The green band indicates the reference range. FT₄, free thyroxine; TSH, thyroid-stimulating hormone.

POSTPARTUM THYROID DYSFUNCTION

- *Postpartum thyroiditis* (PPT) is defined as transient thyroid dysfunction in the first year after delivery in women who were euthyroid before pregnancy on no thyroid therapy.
- The etiology in most cases is autoimmune chronic (Hashimoto) thyroiditis, with a few cases due to hypothalamic or pituitary lesions (Box 42.2).
- The clinical course of PPT is not uniform (Fig. 42.2).
- It is recommended that a diagnosis of PPT be considered for any thyroid abnormality that occurs within 1 year after a delivery or miscarriage.

✪ *References for this chapter are available at ExpertConsult.com.*

CHAPTER 43

Pituitary and Adrenal Disorders in Pregnancy

Mark E. Molitch

KEY POINTS

- About 30% of prolactin-secreting macroadenomas enlarge significantly during pregnancy.
- Dopamine agonists can be used safely for the treatment of prolactinomas if stopped when pregnancy is diagnosed.
- In patients with acromegaly, the risks of gestational diabetes and hypertension are increased.
- Gonadotropins, gonadotropin-releasing hormone, and assisted reproductive technology have been used successfully to achieve pregnancy in women with hypopituitarism.
- Sheehan syndrome is very uncommon with modern obstetric practice but still must be thought of in the postpartum unstable patient following hemorrhage.
- Lymphocytic hypophysitis that occurs during pregnancy is often associated with adrenocorticotropic hormone deficiency and may be fatal.
- Subclinical diabetes insipidus may become manifest during pregnancy because of placental vasopressinase.
- Cushing syndrome is associated with adverse outcomes for mother and fetus and should be treated aggressively during pregnancy.
- Although maintenance glucocorticoid replacement does not need to be increased in pregnant women with either hypopituitarism or primary adrenal insufficiency, stress doses of hydrocortisone are needed during labor and delivery and other stressful situations.
- Pheochromocytomas must be treated aggressively and usually require surgical resection during the pregnancy.

Anterior Pituitary

ANTERIOR PITUITARY HORMONE CHANGES IN PREGNANCY

- Cortisol levels rise progressively over the course of a normal gestation and result in a twofold to threefold increase by term due both to the estrogen-induced increase in corticosteroid-binding globulin levels and an increase in cortisol production, so that the bioactive "free" fraction, urinary free cortisol levels, and salivary cortisol levels are also increased.[1,2]

PITUITARY TUMORS

Prolactinoma

- Transsphenoidal surgery for *microadenomas* is curative in 50% to 60% of prolactinomas after accounting for recurrences, and it rarely causes hypopituitarism when it is performed by experienced neurosurgeons on women with tumors less than 10 mm in diameter.[3]

- The dopamine agonists bromocriptine and cabergoline are the primary mode of medical therapy, restoring ovulatory menses in about 80% and 90% of cases, respectively,[3,4] and reducing *macroadenoma size.*
- When a dopamine agonist is stopped once a woman has missed her menstrual period and pregnancy is diagnosed, no increase in spontaneous abortions, ectopic pregnancies, trophoblastic disease, multiple pregnancies, or malformations were found in over 6000 pregnancies in which bromocriptine was used and in 822 pregnancies in which cabergoline was used.[5-9]
- Patients with large macroadenomas should be assessed monthly for symptoms of tumor enlargement, and visual fields should be tested each trimester.

Acromegaly

- Most patients with acromegaly are treated with surgery as primary therapy; those not cured by surgery are usually treated medically with the somatostatin analogues octreotide and lanreotide.[10]

Clinically Nonfunctioning Adenomas

- Pregnancy would not be expected to influence tumor size in patients with clinically nonfunctioning adenomas. Indeed, only two cases have been reported in which tumor enlargement during pregnancy resulted in a visual field defect.[11,12]

HYPOPITUITARISM

Hypopituitarism

- Because of increased thyroxine turnover and volume of distribution in pregnancy, thyroxine levels usually fall and thyroid-stimulating hormone levels rise with a fixed thyroxine dose over the course of gestation.[13]
- The dose of chronic glucocorticoid replacement does not usually need to be increased during pregnancy.[2] Hydrocortisone is metabolized by the placental enzyme 11β-hydroxysteroid dehydrogenase 2; thus the fetus is generally protected from any overdose of hydrocortisone. The usual dose is in the range of 12 to 15 mg/m^2 given in 2 or 3 divided doses; 10 mg in the morning and 5 mg in the afternoon is a common regimen.[2]

SHEEHAN SYNDROME

- Sheehan syndrome consists of pituitary necrosis secondary to ischemia that occurs within hours of delivery,[14]
- If acute necrosis is suspected, treatment with saline and stress doses of corticosteroids should be instituted immediately after drawing the blood for testing.

LYMPHOCYTIC HYPOPHYSITIS

- Lymphocytic hypophysitis is thought to be autoimmune, with infiltration and destruction of the parenchyma of the pituitary and infundibulum by lymphocytes and plasma cells.[15-17]
- Treatment of lymphocytic hypophysitis is generally conservative and involves identification and correction of any pituitary deficits, especially of adrenocorticotropic hormone secretion, which is particularly common in this condition.[15-17]

Posterior Pituitary

- The set point for plasma osmolality at which arginine vasopressin (AVP) is secreted and thirst is stimulated is reduced approximately 5 to 10 mOsm/kg in pregnancy.[18] The placenta produces vasopressinase, an enzyme that rapidly inactivates AVP, thereby greatly increasing its clearance.[19,20]
- Standard water deprivation tests, which require 5% weight loss, should be avoided during pregnancy because they can cause uterine irritability and can alter placental perfusion. Instead, desmopressin is used to assess urinary concentrating ability.[19]

DIABETES INSIPIDUS

- Central diabetes insipidus (DI) may develop in pregnancy because of an enlarging pituitary lesion, lymphocytic hypophysitis, or hypothalamic disease. Because of the increased clearance of AVP by placental vasopressinase, DI usually worsens during gestation, and subclinical DI may become manifest.[19-21]

Adrenals

CUSHING SYNDROME

- A persistent circadian variation in the elevated levels of total and free serum cortisol during normal pregnancy may be most helpful in distinguishing Cushing syndrome from the hypercortisolism of pregnancy, because this finding is characteristically absent in all forms of Cushing syndrome.[1,2]
- Cushing syndrome is associated with a pregnancy loss rate of 25% due to spontaneous abortion, stillbirth, and early neonatal death because of extreme prematurity.[22-25]
- Medical therapy for Cushing syndrome during pregnancy with metyrapone and ketoconazole is not very effective.[23-25]
- The U.S. Food and Drug Administration has issued a black box warning for ketoconazole with respect to severe liver toxicity; therefore its use cannot be recommended.
- Pasireotide is a new somatostatin analogue with modest efficacy in patients with Cushing disease.[26] It has the adverse effect of hyperglycemia, and there is no experience with its use during pregnancy.
- Although any surgery poses risks for the mother and fetus,[27] it appears that with Cushing syndrome, the risks of not operating are considerably higher than those of proceeding with surgery.

ADRENAL INSUFFICIENCY

- In developed countries, the most common etiology for primary adrenal insufficiency is autoimmune adrenalitis.
- Tuberculosis or fungal infection may be etiologic.
- If unrecognized, maternal adrenal crisis may ensue at times of stress, such as a urinary tract infection or labor.[28-30] The fetoplacental unit largely controls its own steroid milieu, so maternal adrenal insufficiency generally causes no problems with fetal development.
- Patients who have received glucocorticoids as antiinflammatory therapy are presumed to have adrenal axis suppression for at least 1 year following cessation of such therapy.[31] These patients should be treated with stress doses of glucocorticoids during labor and delivery.

PRIMARY HYPERALDOSTERONISM

- Primary hyperaldosteronism rarely has been reported in pregnancy and is most often caused by an adrenal adenoma.[32-35]
- Hypertension
- Spironolactone, the usual nonpregnant therapy for hyperaldosteronism, is contraindicated in pregnancy because it crosses the placenta and is a potent antiandrogen, which can cause ambiguous genitalia in a male fetus.[32]

PHEOCHROMOCYTOMA

- Exacerbation of hypertension is the typical presentation of pheochromocytoma, which can often be mistaken for pregnancy-induced hypertension or preeclampsia.[36-39] As the uterus enlarges and an actively moving fetus compresses the neoplasm, maternal complications such as severe hypertension, hemorrhage into the neoplasm, hemodynamic collapse, myocardial infarction, cardiac arrhythmias, congestive heart failure, and cerebral hemorrhage may occur.
- Adverse fetal effects such as hypoxia are a result of catecholamine-induced uteroplacental vasoconstriction and placental insufficiency[36,37] and of maternal hypertension, hypotension, or vascular collapse.
- The diagnosis should be considered in pregnant women with severe or paroxysmal hypertension, particularly in the first half of pregnancy or in association with orthostatic hypotension or episodic symptoms of pallor, anxiety, headaches, palpitations, chest pain, or diaphoresis.
- Laboratory diagnosis of pheochromocytoma relies on measuring urine metanephrines and catecholamines and plasma metanephrines.[36-39] This is unchanged from the nonpregnant state because catecholamine metabolism is not altered by pregnancy per se.
- Initial medical management involves α-blockade with phenoxybenzamine, phentolamine, prazosin, or labetalol.
- β-Blockade is reserved for treating maternal tachycardia or arrhythmias that persist after full α-blockade and volume repletion.[36-39]
- Pressure from the uterus, motion of the fetus, and labor contractions are all stimuli that may cause an acute crisis.

References for this chapter are available at ExpertConsult.com.

CHAPTER 44

Hematologic Complications of Pregnancy

Philip Samuels

KEY POINTS

- Four percent of pregnancies will be complicated by maternal platelet counts of less than 150,000/mm^3. The vast majority of these patients have gestational thrombocytopenia with a benign course and need no intervention.
- Surgical bleeding occurs if the platelet count falls below 50,000/mm^3, and spontaneous bleeding occurs if the platelet count falls below 20,000/mm^3. Platelet counts below 30,000/mm^3 warrant therapy during pregnancy.
- In the second and third trimesters of pregnancy, intravenous immunoglobulin is an effective initial treatment, although glucocorticoids can also be utilized.
- Iron deficiency anemia is the most common cause of anemia in pregnancy, and serum ferritin is the single best test to diagnose it.
- If a patient with presumed iron deficiency does not increase her reticulocyte count with iron therapy, she may also have a concomitant folic acid deficiency.
- Patients pregnant with twins, those on anticonvulsant therapy, those with a hemoglobinopathy, and those who conceive frequently need supplemental folic acid during gestation.
- Most hereditary hemoglobinopathies can be detected in utero, and prenatal diagnosis should be offered to the patient early in pregnancy. Early testing can be done using DNA analysis from the chorionic villus sampling specimen.
- As in the nonpregnant patient, analgesia, hydration, and oxygen are the key factors in treating pregnant women with sickle cell crisis.
- Women with sickle cell disease are at high risk for maternal complications during the puerperium and should be closely monitored.
- Patients with sickle cell disease are at increased risk for a fetus with growth restriction and adverse fetal outcomes; therefore they warrant frequent sonography and antepartum fetal evaluation.
- Any woman with a low mean corpuscular volume without evidence of iron deficiency should be screened for thalassemia.
- In the pregnant patient with von Willebrand disease, the normal increase in the factor VIII clotting complex reduces the risk of bleeding, but levels can fall postpartum and can place the patient at risk for delayed postpartum hemorrhage.

Hematologic conditions during pregnancy require a multidisciplinary approach to treatment. The differential diagnosis of thrombocytopenia during pregnancy includes idiopathic thrombocytopenic purpura (ITP), gestational thrombocytopenia, preeclampsia, and thrombotic thrombocytopenic purpura (TTP). Glucocorticoids are the mainstay of treatment for ITP, whereas gestational thrombocytopenia does not require any specific therapy. Iron deficiency is the most common anemia of pregnancy. Sickle cell anemia complicating pregnancy increases the risk for preterm delivery, preeclampsia, and maternal morbidity as a result of vasoocclusive episodes.

Pregnancy-Associated Thrombocytopenia

- In pregnancy, the vast majority of cases of mild to moderate thrombocytopenia are caused by gestational thrombocytopenia. This form of thrombocytopenia is unlikely to result in maternal or neonatal complications.

GESTATIONAL THROMBOCYTOPENIA

- These patients require no therapy, and the fetus appears to be at negligible risk of being born with clinically significant thrombocytopenia or a bleeding diathesis.
- There is little risk to the mother or neonate in cases of gestational thrombocytopenia.
- The obstetrician must use judgment in giving this diagnosis because no test exists for this disorder. If platelet counts continue to fall to levels below 50,000/mm^3, other diagnoses should be considered.

IMMUNE THROMBOCYTOPENIC PURPURA

- Pregnancy has not been determined to cause ITP or to change its severity.
- Approximately 90% of women with ITP have platelet-associated immunoglobulin G. Unfortunately, this is not specific for ITP, because studies have shown that these tests are also positive in women with gestational thrombocytopenia and preeclampsia.
- ITP has a predisposition for women aged 18 to 40 years, with an overall female/male ratio of 1.7.

THROMBOTIC THROMBOCYTOPENIC PURPURA AND HEMOLYTIC UREMIC SYNDROME

- The complete pentad occurs only in approximately 40% of patients, but approximately 75% have a triad of microangiopathic hemolytic anemia, thrombocytopenia, and neurologic changes.
- TTP/hemolytic-uremic syndrome (HUS) may mimic preeclampsia.
- Delay in diagnosing TTP/HUS can have fatal consequences.
- To diagnose the hemolytic anemia associated with TTP, the indirect antiglobulin (Coombs) test must be negative.
- The neurologic findings in TTP are usually nonspecific. They include headache, confusion, and lethargy.
- If untreated, TTP carries a 90% mortality rate, whereas treatment with plasma exchange decreases the mortality rate to 20%.
- A decrease of ADAMTS13 (the von Willebrand cleaving enzyme) activity is strongly associated with TTP.
- All four immunoglobulin subclasses of anti-ADAMTS13 antibodies are associated with TTP, but the IgG4 subclass is most common.
- The mean gestational age at onset of symptoms is 23.4 weeks.
- In preeclampsia, antithrombin III levels are frequently low; this is not the case with TTP.

- The majority of cases of HUS that occur in pregnancy develop at least 2 days after delivery.
- It is not important to make the distinction between TTP and HUS because the initial therapy for both disorders is plasmapheresis.

Evaluation of Thrombocytopenia During Pregnancy and the Puerperium

- Excessive bleeding from an episiotomy site or cesarean delivery (CD) incision site or bleeding from IV sites during labor should alert the physician to the possibility of thrombocytopenia.
- It is imperative that a peripheral blood smear be examined by an experienced physician or technologist whenever a case of pregnancy-associated thrombocytopenia is diagnosed.

Therapy of Thrombocytopenia During Pregnancy

GESTATIONAL THROMBOCYTOPENIA

- Gestational thrombocytopenia, the most common form of thrombocytopenia encountered in the third trimester, requires no special intervention or therapy.

IMMUNE THROMBOCYTOPENIC PURPURA

- Surgical bleeding does not usually occur until the platelet count is less than $50,000/mm^3$. Hospital admission is not necessary unless the platelet count falls to below $20,000/mm^3$ or if clinical bleeding is present.
- Methylprednisolone is commonly used to treat ITP. This medication can be given intravenously and has very little mineralocorticoid effect.
- If a woman has been taking glucocorticoids for a period of at least 2 to 3 weeks, she may have adrenal suppression and should undergo increased doses of steroids during labor and delivery to avoid an adrenal crisis. Tapering should be done slowly thereafter.
- Although glucocorticoids are the mainstays of treating maternal thrombocytopenia, up to 30% of patients do not respond to these medications. In such cases, IV immunoglobulin is used.
- No pharmacologic treatment in the first or second trimesters is recommended unless the platelet count is less than $30,000/mm^3$ or if clinically significant bleeding is evident. If the count is between $10,000/mm^3$ and $30,000/mm^3$ in the second or third trimester, IV immunoglobulin is recommended. Platelet transfusion is not undertaken unless the platelet count falls below $10,000/mm^3$.
- In an emergent situation, platelets can be transfused during CD if significant clinical bleeding is evident.
- Each "pack" of platelets increases the platelet count by approximately $10,000/mm^3$. The half-life of these platelets is extremely short because the same antibodies and reticuloendothelial cell clearance rates that affect the mother's endogenous platelets also affect the transfused platelets.

Management of Thrombotic Thrombocytopenic Purpura and Hemolytic-Uremic Syndrome

- The prognosis has improved greatly with plasma infusion and plasma exchange.
- Supportive therapy remains the mainstay in cases of HUS.

Fetal/Neonatal Alloimmune Thrombocytopenia

- In neonatal alloimmune thrombocytopenia, a rare disorder, the mother lacks a specific platelet antigen and develops antibodies to this antigen.
- The most common antibodies noted in these patients is anti–human platelet antigen–1a antibodies, although several other antibodies have been identified.
- These patients should be managed in a tertiary care center with experience caring for mothers and infants with this rare disorder.
- Transfusion of maternal or donor platelets (lacking the antigen) into the fetus and neonate has improved outcomes in these cases.

Iron Deficiency Anemia

- Hemoglobin and hematocrit levels usually fall during gestation. These changes are not necessarily pathologic but usually represent a physiologic alteration of pregnancy.
- Most clinicians diagnose anemia when the hemoglobin concentration is less than 11 g/dL or the hematocrit is less than 32%. Using these criteria, 50% of pregnant women are anemic.
- Approximately 75% of anemia that occurs during pregnancy is secondary to iron deficiency.
- If the dietary iron intake is poor, the interval between pregnancies is short, or the delivery is complicated by hemorrhage, iron deficiency anemia readily and rapidly develops.
- Care must be taken when using laboratory parameters to establish the diagnosis of iron deficiency anemia during gestation.
- The ferritin level indicates the total status of a woman's iron stores.
- Most women do need some iron supplementation.
- One 325 mg tablet of ferrous sulfate daily provides adequate prophylaxis. It contains 60 mg of elemental iron, 10% of which is absorbed.
- For those patients who are noncompliant or unable to take oral iron and are severely anemic, IV iron can be given.
- Parenteral iron is indicated in those who cannot or will not take oral iron therapy and are not anemic enough to require transfusion.
- Iron dextran can result in anaphylaxis caused by dissociation of the iron and carbohydrate components.
- In developing nations, severe anemia is alarmingly common and is a major cause of maternal morbidity and mortality.

Megaloblastic Anemia

- During pregnancy, folate deficiency is the most common cause of megaloblastic anemia. The daily folate requirement in the nonpregnant state is approximately 50 μg, but this rises at least fourfold during gestation. Fetal demands increase the requirement, as does the decrease in the gastrointestinal absorption of folate during pregnancy.
- Clinical megaloblastic anemia seldom occurs before the third trimester of pregnancy.
- Red blood cell folate levels give a better idea of folate status at the tissue level.
- Prenatal vitamins that require physician prescription contain 1 mg of folic acid, and most nonprescription prenatal vitamins contain 0.8 mg of folic acid. These amounts are more than adequate to prevent and treat folate deficiency. Women with significant hemoglobinopathies, those taking anticonvulsant medications, women carrying a multiple gestation, and women with frequent conception may require more than 1 mg of supplemental folate daily. Often, 4 mg of folic acid is recommended daily because this is the dose that has been shown to reduce the risk of recurrent neural tube defects.

- Folic acid deficiency should be considered when a patient has unexplained thrombocytopenia.
- The hematocrit level may rise as much as 1% per day after 1 week of folate replacement.
- Vitamin B_{12} deficiency is not uncommon following bariatric surgery.
- Because of the abundant vitamin B_{12} stores in the body, it takes several years for a clinical vitamin B_{12} deficiency to develop.
- In addition to bariatric surgery, gastrointestinal diseases such as Crohn disease may lead to an inability to absorb vitamin B_{12}.
- Megaloblastic anemia usually leads to a suspicion of folate or vitamin B_{12} deficiency. As noted earlier, if an associated iron deficiency is present, the red blood cell indexes may be normocytic normochromic.
- Evaluation of methylmalonate and homocysteine levels can be used to distinguish folate deficiency from vitamin B_{12} deficiency.

Hemoglobinopathies

HEMOGLOBIN S

- These individuals generally have 35% to 45% hemoglobin (Hb) S and are asymptomatic. The offspring of two individuals with sickle cell trait have a 50% probability of inheriting the trait and a 25% probability of actually having sickle cell disease.
- All at-risk patients should undergo hemoglobin electrophoresis.
- If a patient has HbAS, the spouse/partner should be tested, and if both are carriers of a hemoglobinopathy, prenatal diagnosis should be offered.
- Painful vasoocclusive episodes that involve multiple organs are the clinical hallmark of sickle cell disease.
- Analgesia, oxygen, and hydration are the clinical foundations for treating these painful crises, and physicians often underestimate the associated pain.
- It is important to treat this pain, which may require significant doses of narcotic medication.
- Osteomyelitis is common in individuals with sickle cell disease.
- Pyelonephritis is increased in women with sickle cell disease.
- Cholelithiasis is seen in 30% of cases.
- High-output cardiac failure may occur as a result of chronic anemia.
- Pregnancies complicated by sickle cell disease are at risk for poor perinatal outcomes. The rate of spontaneous abortion may be as high as 25%, and the perinatal mortality rate can approach 15%.
- Approximately 30% of infants born to mothers with sickle cell disease have birthweights less than 2500 g.
- Women with SS disease with high HbF levels have a significantly lower perinatal mortality rate.
- Careful antepartum fetal surveillance is recommended that includes serial ultrasonography to assess fetal growth.
- Although maternal mortality is rare in patients with sickle cell anemia, maternal morbidity is significant. Infections are common and occur in 50% to 67% of women with HbSS.
- Women with sickle cell disease should receive pneumococcal vaccine before pregnancy.
- The presence of infection demands prompt attention, because fever, dehydration, and acidosis results in further sickling and painful crises.
- Pregnancy-induced hypertension is increased in women with sickle cell disease.
- Thromboembolic phenomena are more common in these individuals, especially during sickle cell crisis and in episodes of pneumonia.
- No role exists for prophylactic transfusions in these patients.

- No significant difference has been observed in perinatal outcome between sickle cell women receiving prophylactic exchange transfusion and those managed without this intervention. However, prophylactic transfusion does appear to significantly decrease the incidence of painful crises.
- Vaginal delivery is preferred for women with sickle cell disease, and CD should be reserved for obstetric indications.

HEMOGLOBIN SC DISEASE

- Women with both S and C hemoglobin suffer less morbidity in pregnancy than do women with with HbSS.
- Crises in patients with HbSC may be marked by sequestration of a large volume of red blood cells in the spleen accompanied by a dramatic fall in hematocrit. Because these patients have increased splenic activity, they may be mildly thrombocytopenic throughout pregnancy and may become profoundly thrombocytopenic during a crisis.

THALASSEMIA

- Thalassemia is due to a defect in the rate of globin chain synthesis.
- Thalassemia screening is recommended for pregnant women with a low mean corpuscular volume and no evidence of iron deficiency.
- Homozygous α-thalassemia results in the formation of tetramers of β-chains known as *hemoglobin Bart*. This hemoglobinopathy can result in hydrops fetalis.
- β-Thalassemia is the most common form of thalassemia.
- The homozygous state of β-thalassemia is known as *thalassemia major* (formerly known as *Cooley anemia*). These individuals rarely become pregnant.
- As in the case of sickle hemoglobinopathies, iron supplementation should be given only if necessary, because indiscriminate use of iron can lead to hemosiderosis and hemochromatosis.
- Folic acid supplementation appears important in β-thalassemia carriers.
- Antepartum fetal evaluation is essential in patients with thalassemia who are anemic.
- A stepwise approach to the workup of anemia is recommended for pregnant women (Fig. 44.1).

von Willebrand Disease

- The most common congenital bleeding disorder in humans is von Willebrand disease (vWD), which affects up to 1% of the population.
- Quantitative or qualitative abnormalities of von Willebrand factor (vWF) may complicate this disorder.
- Distinct abnormalities of vWF are responsible for the three types of vWD.
- In type 2B, the only clinical symptom in pregnancy may be thrombocytopenia.
- The clinical severity of vWD is variable. Menorrhagia, easy bruising, gingival bleeding, and epistaxis are common.
- von Willebrand disease does not appear to affect fetal growth or development.
- In pregnancy, clotting factors that include the factor VIII complex increase, and the patient's bleeding time may improve as gestation progresses.
- Postpartum hemorrhage may be a serious problem. The concentration of factor VIII appears to determine the risk of hemorrhage.
- Bleeding during pregnancy is rare because levels of factor VIII and vWF increase during pregnancy. However, shortly after delivery, they decline. If the factor VIII level is less than 50%, treatment during labor and delivery should be initiated. Hemorrhage can also occur several days postpartum.

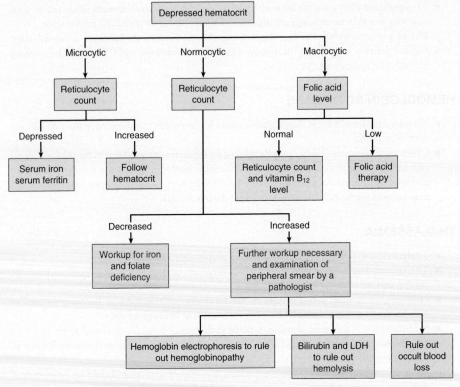

Fig. 44.1   Evaluation of anemia. LDH, lactate dehydrogenase.

- Antihemophiliac factor (Humate-P) is employed in women who do not respond to desmopressin or for those with vWD types other than 1A.
- Bleeding during pregnancy is rare in women with vWD.
- In an emergent situation, if the type of vWD is not known with certainty, factor VIII/vWF concentrate should be administered.

CHAPTER 45

Thromboembolic Disorders in Pregnancy

Christian M. Pettker ■ Charles J. Lockwood

KEY POINTS

- VTE is a leading cause of mortality and serious morbidity in pregnant women, with a prevalence of 1 per 1000 to 1 per 2000 pregnancies; the greatest risk of fatal PE occurs following CDs.
- Inherited and acquired thrombophilias account for most VTEs in pregnancy.
- VUS is the most common diagnostic modality used in the evaluation of patients with suspected DVT, with an overall sensitivity and specificity of 90% to 100% for proximal vein thromboses.
- In stable patients with suspected PE and leg signs or symptoms, VUS should be performed because it may avoid the risks of radiation exposure and may detect a DVT, the cause of the PE.
- Stable patients with suspected PE should have a chest radiograph to determine the diagnostic test to be used. A nondiagnostic chest radiograph should therefore prompt performance of a V/Q scan. A patient with abnormal chest radiography should be evaluated with spiral CT pulmonary angiography.
- Heparin remains the mainstay of therapy for VTE, with its most serious but rare complication being immunoglobulin-mediated heparin-induced thrombocytopenia type 2, which usually occurs 5 to 14 days following initiation of therapy and paradoxically increases the risk of thrombosis.
- Thromboprophylaxis is warranted in high- and moderate-risk groups based on a history of VTE and the presence of thrombophilia and should be selected according to overall risk for recurrence.
- Protamine sulfate can entirely reverse the anticoagulant effect of unfractionated heparain and can partially (80%) reverse the effect of LMWH.
- Graduated elastic compression stockings and pneumatic compression devices appear to reduce the likelihood of VTE in pregnancy and, at a minimum, should be used in all high-risk patients and should be strongly considered for all patients undergoing CD.

Epidemiology and Incidence

- Occurring in approximately in 1 in 1500 pregnancies, venous thromboembolism (VTE) is a relatively uncommon disorder but is a leading cause of mortality and serious morbidity in pregnant women.[1-8] This rate represents a nearly tenfold increase compared with nonpregnant women of comparable childbearing age.

Genetics

- Factor V Leiden is the most common mutation and accounts for over 40% of inherited thrombophilias in most studies.

Pathophysiology of Thrombosis in Pregnancy

- A doubling occurs in circulating concentrations of fibrinogen, and 20% to 1000% increases are seen in factors VII, VIII, IX, X, and XII, all of which peak at term in preparation for delivery.[9] Concomitantly, there is a 40% to 60% decrease in the levels of free protein S, conferring an overall resistance to activated protein C.[9,10]
- Coagulation factors generally return to baseline at 6 to 12 weeks.
- Venous stasis in the lower extremities results from compression of the inferior vena cava and pelvic veins by the enlarging uterus.[11,12]
- The incidence of thrombosis is far greater in the left leg than in the right.[1,13]

ANTIPHOSPHOLIPID SYNDROME

- Antiphospholipid syndrome is responsible for approximately 14% of thromboembolic events in pregnancy.[14,15]
- Providers should use caution when ordering and interpreting tests in the absence of antiphospholipid syndrome–qualifying clinical criteria.

INHERITED THROMBOPHILIAS

- All patients who present with VTE in pregnancy or postpartum should be considered for an appropriate workup for inherited thrombophilias.

RISK FACTORS AND ASSOCIATIONS

- Virchow triad—vascular stasis, hypercoagulability, and vascular trauma—describes the three classic antecedents to thrombosis, and many of the physiologic changes of pregnancy contribute to these criteria.
- Admission to the hospital in pregnancy may be associated with a 17-fold increased risk for VTE compared with a nonhospitalized cohort, with this risk remaining high (sixfold) for the 28 days after admission.[16]

Risk-Scoring System

- Three factors—symptoms in the left leg, a leg circumference discrepancy of 2 cm or more, or first-trimester presentation—were highly predictive of deep vein thrombosis (DVT).

Imaging

- The most common diagnostic modality used in the evaluation of patients with suspected DVT is venous ultrasonography (VUS) with or without color Doppler.
- The most accurate ultrasonic criterion for diagnosing venous thrombosis is noncompressibility of the venous lumen in a transverse plane under gentle probe pressure using duplex and color flow Doppler imaging.[17]

D-Dimer Assays

- Normal pregnancy causes a physiologic increase in D-dimer, with levels that exceed the threshold for normal in 78% and 100% of patients in the second and third trimesters, respectively.[18]

Ventilation-Perfusion Scanning

- Given that most young, healthy women have little underlying lung pulmonary pathology, the diagnostic efficacy of V/Q scanning in pregnancy is substantially higher than that in older, nonpregnant patients.

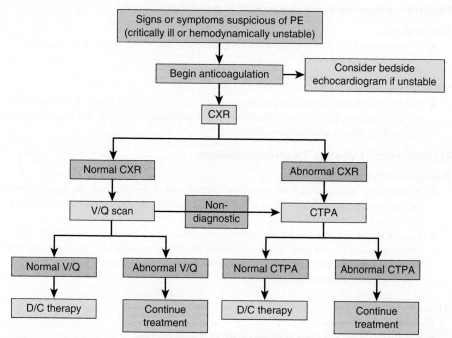

Fig. 45.1 Diagnostic algorithm for suspected pulmonary embolism (PE) in a critically ill or hemodynamically unstable patient. CTPA, computed tomographic pulmonary angiography; CXR, chest radiograph; D/C, discontinue; V/Q, ventilation-perfusion.

Spiral Computed Tomographic Pulmonary Angiography

■ CT pulmonary angiography performs less well in pregnant compared with nonpregnant cohorts.

Ventilation-Perfusion Scanning Versus Computed Tomographic Pulmonary Angiography

■ V/Q scanning is the modality of choice for pregnant patients with suspected pulmonary embolism (PE) and a normal chest radiograph.

D-Dimer Assays

■ There is no role for D-dimer testing in the workup of pregnant patients with suspected PE.

Lower Extremity Evaluation

■ Most PEs (90%) arise from lower extremity DVTs, and among patients with the diagnosis of PE, half will be found to harbor a lower extremity DVT; this includes up to 20% of PE patients without signs or symptoms of lower extremity DVT.[19–21]

Workup of Patients With Suspected Pulmonary Embolus

■ Chest radiography should definitely be performed when VUS is negative or when no lower extremity signs or symptoms are apparent. Although the chest radiograph is not typically used in the actual diagnosis, it allows for proper selection of the next diagnostic test. V/Q scan is performed if the chest radiograph is normal.

■ In the critically ill patient, anticoagulation should be started—in the absence of contraindications—and a similar protocol is followed (Fig. 45.1).

Radiation Exposure From Diagnostic Procedures

Fetal Exposure
- A combination of chest radiograph, V/Q scan, and pulmonary angiography exposes the fetus to less than 0.5 rads.[6]

Maternal Exposure
- Radiation exposure to the maternal breast is also an important consideration when choosing tests because the increased glandularity and proliferative state of the pregnant breast presumably make it more radiosensitive.

Management of Venous Thromboembolism

Perioperative Prevention
- Perioperative administration of low-dose unfractionated heparin may be appropriate in patients undergoing CD with clear risk factors such as obesity, malignancy, immobility, or a high-risk chronic medical disease.
- Because stockings and pneumatic compression devices pose no hemorrhagic risk and do little harm, they should be strongly considered for thromboprophylaxis in all patients with risk factors, such as those patients who are hospitalized or immobilized, including pregnant or postoperative cesarean patients.

Therapy
Unfractionated Heparin
- Heparin-induced thrombocytopenia occurs in 3% of patients.
- Protamine sulfate reverses the effect of intravenously administered unfractionated heparin.

Low-Molecular-Weight Heparin
- Regional anesthesia is contraindicated within 18 to 24 hours of therapeutic low-molecular-weight heparin (LMWH) administration.

Coumarin
- Warfarin is a pregnancy category X medication because fetal exposure can cause nasal and midface hypoplasia, microphthalmia, mental retardation, and other ocular, skeletal, and central nervous system malformations.

Treatment of Acute Deep Venous Thrombosis or Pulmonary Embolus
- Therapeutic doses of the LMWH enoxaparin may start at 1 mg/kg subcutaneously twice daily.

Prophylactic Anticoagulation Recommendations for Low-, Moderate-, and High-Risk Groups
- The postpartum period represents a time of elevated risk, particularly in patients with risk factors.
- The various thrombophilias can be classified into high- and low-risk types, and anticoagulation recommendations for each type will be different depending on whether the patient has a personal history of VTE.
- Patients with recurrent VTE who have tested negative for the known inherited thrombophilias likely have an underlying pathology (e.g., an undiagnosed genetic malformation in a step in the coagulation cascade) and should be cared for cautiously.
- Typical prophylactic doses of the LMWH enoxaparin may start at 40 mg subcutaneously daily.

References for this chapter are available at ExpertConsult.com.

CHAPTER 46

Collagen Vascular Diseases in Pregnancy

Jeanette R. Carpenter ■ D. Ware Branch

KEY POINTS

- SLE is the most common serious autoimmune disease that affects women of reproductive age.
- SLE disease activity at the onset of pregnancy is the most important determinant of the course of the disease in pregnancy.
- Women with SLE should be counseled to postpone pregnancy until a sustained remission for at least 6 months has been achieved.
- For women with lupus nephritis, moderate renal insufficiency (serum creatinine 1.5 to 2 mg/dL) is a relative contraindication to pregnancy, and advanced renal insufficiency (creatinine >2 mg/dL) should be considered an absolute contraindication to pregnancy.
- Women with SLE who become pregnant on hydroxychloroquine should generally continue this medication because it may decrease the risk of disease flares.
- The diagnosis of APS is incumbent upon either arterial or venous thrombosis or obstetric morbidity and repeatedly positive testing for lupus anticoagulant and/or medium to high titers of anticardiolipin or aβ2-GP-I IgG or IgM antibodies.
- All women with APS and prior thrombosis should receive full anticoagulation during pregnancy and postpartum.
- Pregnant women with an APS diagnosis based upon recurrent early miscarriage without prior thrombosis should receive either low-dose aspirin alone or combined with a prophylactic dose of heparin.
- Pregnant women with an APS diagnosis based upon fetal death, early preeclampsia, or placental insufficiency and without prior thrombosis should generally receive low-dose aspirin combined with prophylactic heparin.
- Most women with rheumatoid arthritis will experience an improvement in symptoms during pregnancy, but the risk for postpartum relapse is high.
- Women with systemic sclerosis generally have favorable pregnancy outcomes but should be carefully assessed for visceral organ (i.e., renal, cardiac, or pulmonary) involvement.

Systemic Lupus Erythematosus

EPIDEMIOLOGY AND ETIOLOGY

■ Systemic lupus erythematosus (SLE) is a chronic inflammatory and autoimmune disorder that can affect multiple organ systems, including the skin, joints, kidneys, central nervous system, heart, lungs, and liver.

- SLE is more prevalent among women than men, and most women who are affected by the disease manifest it at some point during their reproductive years.
- Significant racial differences are apparent in disease prevalence: black women have a prevalence of 405 per 100,000 compared with a prevalence of 164 per 100,000 among white women.

CLINICAL MANIFESTATIONS

- The clinical course of SLE is characterized by periods of disease "flares" interspersed with periods of remission. The most common presenting symptoms of SLE include arthralgias, fatigue, malaise, weight change, Raynaud phenomenon, fever, photosensitive rash, and alopecia.
- Most patients also have skin manifestations at some point in the course of the disease, and the classic presentation is a malar "butterfly" rash that worsens with sun exposure.

DIAGNOSIS

- A patient must have at least 4 of the 11 clinical and laboratory criteria, either serially or simultaneously. It should be emphasized, however, that some women with features of SLE might not meet the strict diagnostic criteria but can still be at risk for pregnancy complications. These women may benefit from increased surveillance and even treatment.
- Because nearly all individuals with SLE will have a positive antinuclear antibody (ANA) titer, this is a reasonable initial screening test for women with suggestive symptoms. If the ANA test is negative, a diagnosis of SLE is highly unlikely.
- Anti–double-stranded DNA and anti-Smith antibodies are more highly specific for SLE, albeit less sensitive.
- Patients with either SLE or Sjögren syndrome may also have anti-Ro/SSA and anti-La/SSB antibodies, which are particularly relevant to the obstetric patient because of the association with neonatal lupus erythematosus (NLE) and congenital heart block (CHB).

LUPUS FLARE IN PREGNANCY

- The best predictor of the course of SLE during gestation is the state of disease activity at the onset of pregnancy.
- Women with SLE should be counseled to delay pregnancy until their disease has been in remission for at least 6 months.
- Flares in pregnancy most commonly manifest as fatigue, joint pain, rash, and proteinuria. Assessing anti–double-stranded DNA titers and complement (C3 and C4) levels may provide additional evidence of disease flares in women with clinical symptoms.

LUPUS NEPHRITIS IN PREGNANCY

- Renal manifestations are present in approximately half of all patients with SLE.
- Women with lupus nephritis (LN), particularly active disease, are at especially increased risk for adverse pregnancy outcomes that include hypertensive disorders of pregnancy, disease flares, low-birthweight infants, and indicated preterm delivery.
- As a general rule, a serum creatinine of 1.4 to 1.9 mg/dL (estimated glomerular filtration rate ~30 to 59 mL/min/1.73 m^2) is a relative contraindication to pregnancy given the substantial risk of midterm pregnancy complications that might require preterm delivery. Most experts consider a serum creatinine of 2.0 mg/dL or greater (estimated glomerular filtration rate ~15 to 29 mL/min/1.73 m^2) to be an absolute contraindication to pregnancy, again

because of the substantial risk of pregnancy complications requiring extreme preterm birth (PTB) and the threat to long-term renal function.

- Women with LN often have increasing proteinuria across gestation, related in part to increased glomerular filtration.
- Women with severe LN are often treated with mycophenolate mofetil (MMF), a significant teratogen that is contraindicated in pregnancy.

PREGNANCY COMPLICATIONS

- Women with SLE do not appear to be less fertile than women without SLE, but they are at increased risk for multiple adverse pregnancy outcomes that include pregnancy loss, PTB, preeclampsia, and intrauterine growth restriction (IUGR).
- The overall fetal death rate among these women is 4%, and the neonatal death rate is 1%.[1]
- Although the rate of IUGR among pregnancies complicated by SLE has been reported to be as high as 40%, modern treatments and improved pregnancy surveillance have probably decreased this rate.
- Women with SLE have an approximately threefold increased risk for PTB.
- Hypertensive disorders (gestational hypertension or preeclampsia) occur in 10% to 30% of pregnancies with SLE.
- Daily low-dose aspirin (typically 81 mg in the United States) beginning early in pregnancy is recommended for women with SLE, particularly those with renal manifestations, because evidence suggests this may modestly decrease the risk of developing preeclampsia.[2]

NEONATAL LUPUS ERYTHEMATOSUS

- Neonatal lupus erythematosus is an acquired autoimmune condition related to the transplacental transfer of anti-Ro/SSA and anti-La/SSB antibodies.
- Among all pregnant women with SLE, the risk of NLE is less than 5%.
- The most serious manifestation of NLE is complete heart block. It is most frequently diagnosed at a routine prenatal visit when a fixed fetal bradycardia of 50 to 80 beats/min is detected. CHB is most commonly diagnosed between 16 and 24 weeks' gestation, and it is rarely diagnosed in the third trimester.
- Although many clinicians routinely test pregnant women with SLE for anti-Ro/SSA and anti-La/SSB antibodies, this practice is not without controversy given that CHB is infrequent, antenatal treatment to alter outcome is of uncertain efficacy, and a positive test result may cause unnecessary maternal anxiety.
- Complete CHB is irreversible and is associated with an overall perinatal mortality rate of at least 20% (5% stillborn). The majority of survivors require a pacemaker.

MANAGEMENT OF PREGNANCIES COMPLICATED BY SYSTEMIC LUPUS ERYTHEMATOSUS

- Ideally, women with SLE would present for a preconception visit such that disease remission could be ensured, medications reviewed, and counseling performed.
- Key components include the assessment of disease activity and renal manifestations, surveillance for preeclampsia, surveillance of fetal growth, and antenatal testing. Comanagement with a rheumatologist is particularly important for women with severe manifestations or active disease.

- Even with early detection of cardiac conduction abnormalities or new-onset CHB, no credible evidence suggests that medical interventions alter outcomes.

DRUG USED TO TREAT SYSTEMIC LUPUS ERYTHEMATOSUS AND PREGNANCY CONSIDERATIONS

Hydroxychloroquine

- Past concerns regarding hydroxychloroquine being associated with fetal ocular toxicity and ototoxicity (FDA category C) have not been confirmed by studies published within the past 15 years.
- Hydroxychloroquine is compatible with breastfeeding.

Glucocorticoids

- SLE flares in pregnancy are most commonly treated with glucocorticoids. Nonfluorinated steroids, such as prednisone and methylprednisolone (both FDA category C) are preferred in pregnancy.
- Prolonged use of glucocorticoids is associated with an increased risk for maternal bone loss, gestational diabetes, hypertension and preeclampsia, and adrenal suppression.
- Prednisone is compatible with breastfeeding, although for women who take more than 20 mg/day, it may be prudent to delay feeding for 4 hours after the dose.

Nonsteroidal Antiinflammatory Drugs

- Third-trimester nonsteroidal antiinflammatory drug (NSAID) use may cause premature closure of the fetal ductus arteriosus, particularly after 30 weeks' gestation, and oligohydramnios. For these reasons, NSAIDs are FDA category C before 30 weeks and category D thereafter.
- NSAIDs are compatible with breastfeeding.

Azathioprine

- Azathioprine, often in combination with glucocorticoids, is the preferred treatment for severe or active SLE in pregnancy. Most experts consider azathioprine to be compatible with breastfeeding, although long-term follow-up of exposed infants is limited.

Cyclosporine A

- Data obtained primarily from organ transplant patients indicate a very low risk of teratogenicity, but the risk for PTB and small-for-gestational-age infants may be increased.[3]
- Women on cyclosporine are generally discouraged from breastfeeding, although data are limited regarding adverse outcomes.

Cyclophosphamide

- This drug is teratogenic and should not be used at all in the first trimester.
- Cyclophosphamide is not compatible with breastfeeding.

Mycophenolate Mofetil

- MMF is absolutely contraindicated in pregnancy due its abortifacient and teratogenic properties.
- No data are available regarding MMF use and breastfeeding, and it is considered contraindicated.

Antiphospholipid Syndrome

- Antiphospholipid syndrome (APS) is an autoimmune condition associated with venous and arterial thrombosis, and adverse pregnancy outcomes that include recurrent early miscarriage, fetal death, early preeclampsia, and placental insufficiency. Diagnosis of APS is confirmed by persistently positive aPLs.
- The diagnosis of APS is confirmed by the detection of one or more of three antiphospholipid antibodies (aPLs): lupus anticoagulant, anticardiolipin antibodies, and anti–β2-glycoprotein I (aβ2-GP-I) antibodies.
- In the absence of a history of thrombosis or pregnancy morbidity, the risks associated with an incidentally identified positive test for aPL among otherwise healthy women are not well understood, and these women should not be diagnosed with APS.

DIAGNOSIS

- As defined by the international criteria, at least one clinical criterion and positive aPL are required for the diagnosis of definite APS (see Box 46.1).[4]
- It should also be emphasized that lupus anticoagulant is a better predictor of pregnancy morbidity or thrombosis than anticardiolipin antibodies or aβ2-GP-I antibodies.

Catastrophic Antiphospholipid Syndrome

- Catastrophic antiphospholipid syndrome can occur in pregnancy and should be considered in the differential diagnosis that includes hemolytic-uremic syndrome and thrombotic thrombocytopenic purpura. According to international criteria, the diagnosis of catastrophic antiphospholipid syndrome is based on thromboses in three or more organs in less than a week, microthrombosis in at least one organ, and persistent aPL positivity.

Treatment During Pregnancy

- Management of APS during pregnancy is aimed at minimizing or eliminating the risks of thrombosis, miscarriage, fetal death, preeclampsia, placental insufficiency, and iatrogenic PTB. With currently recommended management strategies, the likelihood of a successful pregnancy (delivery of a viable infant) in a woman diagnosed with APS exceeds 70%.
- The combination of a heparin agent and low-dose aspirin is the current recommended treatment for APS in pregnancy.
- Heparin is usually begun in the early first trimester after demonstrating either an appropriately rising serum human chorionic gonadotropin or the presence of a live embryo on ultrasonography.
- A Cochrane systematic review concluded that although the quality of available studies was not high, "combined unfractionated heparin (UFH) and aspirin may reduce pregnancy loss by 54%" in women with APS based on recurrent early miscarriage.[5]
- A recent ACOG practice bulletin states that for women with APS without a preceding thrombotic event, either clinical surveillance or prophylactic heparin may be used in the antepartum period but that "prophylactic doses of heparin and low-dose aspirin during pregnancy...should be considered."[6]
- Postpartum thromboprophylaxis with unfractionated heparin, low-molecular-weight heparin, or warfarin (international normalized ratio, 2 to 3) should be strongly considered in all women with APS and is absolutely indicated in women with prior thrombosis.
- Both heparin and warfarin are safe for breastfeeding mothers.

BOX 46.1 ■ Revised Classification Criteria for the Antiphospholipid Antibody Syndrome*

Clinical Criteria

Vascular Thrombosis†

1. One or more clinical episodes of arterial, venous, or small-vessel thrombosis in any tissue or organ *and*
2. Thrombosis confirmed by objective, validated criteria (i.e., unequivocal findings of appropriate imaging studies or histopathology) *and*
3. For histopathologic confirmation, thrombosis should be present without significant evidence of inflammation in the vessel wall

Pregnancy Morbidity

1. One or more unexplained deaths of a morphologically normal fetus at or beyond the 10th week of gestation, with normal fetal morphology documented by ultrasound or by direct examination of the fetus *or*
2. One or more premature births of a morphologically normal neonate at or before the 34th week of gestation because of eclampsia or severe preeclampsia or placental insufficiency‡ *or*
3. Three or more unexplained consecutive spontaneous abortions before the 10th week of gestation with maternal anatomic or hormonal abnormalities and paternal and maternal chromosomal causes excluded

Laboratory Criteria

1. Lupus anticoagulant present in plasma on two or more occasions at least 12 weeks apart, detected according to the guidelines of the International Society on Thrombosis and Hemostasis
2. Anticardiolipin antibody of IgG and/or IgM isotype in blood present in medium or high titer (i.e., >40 GPL or MPL or >99th percentile) on at least two occasions at least 12 weeks apart, measured by standardized ELISA
3. Anti–β2-glycoprotein I antibody of IgG and/or IgM isotype in serum or plasma (in titer >99th percentile) present in medium or high titer on at least two occasions at least 12 weeks apart, measured by standardized ELISA

---

*Must meet at least one clinical and one laboratory criterion for diagnosis of "definite" APS.
†Superficial venous thrombosis is not included in the clinical criteria.
‡Features of placental insufficiency may include (1) abnormal or nonreassuring fetal surveillance, such as a nonreactive nonstress test; (2) abnormal Doppler flow in the umbilical artery (e.g., absent end-diastolic flow); (3) oligohydramnios; or (4) infant birthweight below the 10th percentile for gestational age.
ELISA, *enzyme-linked immunosorbent assay;* GPL, *IgG phospholipid units;* Ig, *immunoglobulin;* MPL, *IgM phospholipid units.*
Modified from Miyakis S, Lockshin MD, Atsumi T, et al. International consensus statement on an update of the classification criteria for definite antiphospholipid syndrome (APS). J Thromb Haemost. 2006;4:295-306.

Rheumatoid Arthritis

- Rheumatoid arthritis (RA) is an autoimmune disease characterized by chronic, symmetric inflammatory arthritis of the synovial joints. RA affects 1% to 2% of U.S. adults; as with SLE, RA is more common among females than males.
- The onset of RA is often insidious, with the gradual development of symmetric peripheral polyarthritis and morning stiffness. Involvement of the metacarpophalangeal and proximal interphalangeal joints is characteristic, and significant deformity of these joints may become apparent as the disease progresses.

DIAGNOSIS

- "Definite" RA is based on confirmed synovitis in at least one joint, absence of another cause for the synovitis, and a score of at least 6 out of 10 on a standardized assessment in 4 clinical domains: (1) degree of joint involvement, (2) serologic testing, (3) response from acute-phase reactants, and (4) duration of symptoms.
- 70% to 80% of patients with RA test positive for rheumatoid factor (RF) antibodies.
- However, RF antibodies are somewhat nonspecific because 5% to 10% of the general, healthy population will test positive for RF.

PREGNANCY CONSIDERATIONS

- The majority of women, perhaps as many as 80% to 90%, experience some improvement in their RA symptoms during pregnancy, although only approximately 50% have more than moderate improvement.
- Most women who experience an improvement in symptoms during pregnancy will relapse postpartum, typically in the first 3 months. It does not appear that pregnancy has any significant effects on the long-term course of RA.
- RA disease activity does not appear to significantly impact pregnancy outcomes.

MANAGEMENT OF PREGNANCIES COMPLICATED BY RHEUMATOID ARTHRITIS

- Mild to moderate joint pain can usually be managed with acetaminophen or low-dose glucocorticoids.
- No alterations to routine prenatal care are necessary for women with mild, uncomplicated RA.
- Because the risk of postpartum disease exacerbation is high, it is important to assess symptoms at postpartum visits and to arrange appropriate follow-up with rheumatology.

ANTIRHEUMATIC DRUGS

Sulfasalazine

- Sulfasalazine is compatible with breastfeeding.

Tumor Necrosis Factor-α Inhibitors

- Although human data are somewhat limited, tumor necrosis factor inhibitors are considered to be compatible with pregnancy.
- The choice to breastfeed while taking tumor necrosis factor inhibitors should be made after a thorough discussion of potential risks and benefits.

Biologic Agents

- These drugs may be used to treat autoimmune disease not sufficiently controlled with traditional therapies, but data regarding the use of these medications in pregnancy are extremely limited.
- It is prudent to avoid their use unless the woman is refractory to other therapies and the severity of disease warrants continuation.
- Patients who choose to breastfeed should do so only after a thorough discussion of potential risks and benefits.

Methotrexate

- Methotrexate (MTX) is an abortifacient in early pregnancy and a potent teratogen.
- All reproductive-aged women taking MTX should be warned of its teratogenic risks and advised to remain on effective contraception.
- MTX is found in low levels in breast milk and is considered contraindicated in breastfeeding.

Leflunomide

- Leflunomide is teratogenic in humans and is absolutely contraindicated in pregnancy.
- No data are available regarding leflunomide and breastfeeding, and it is considered contraindicated.

Systemic Sclerosis

- Systemic sclerosis (SSc), or systemic scleroderma, is a heterogeneous autoimmune disorder characterized by small-vessel vasculopathy, the presence of characteristic autoantibodies, and fibroblast dysfunction that leads to increased extracellular matrix deposition and progressive fibrosis of the skin and visceral tissues.
- SSc is infrequently encountered in pregnancy because the peak age of onset is in the fifth decade.
- The most frequent visceral symptoms of SSc are heartburn and dysphagia related to esophageal dysmotility.

DIAGNOSIS

- The presence of skin thickening of the fingers extending proximal to the metacarpophalangeal joints is sufficient for the diagnosis of SSc.
- Most patients with SSc have a positive ANA.

PREGNANCY CONSIDERATIONS

- If SSc is clinically stable at the onset of pregnancy and the woman is without obvious renal, cardiac, or pulmonary disease, maternal outcomes are generally good.
- PTB is more common among women with SSc, particularly those with diffuse disease. The risks for preeclampsia and IUGR are threefold higher among women with SSc when compared with the general population

MANAGEMENT OF PREGNANCIES COMPLICATED BY SYSTEMIC SCLEROSIS

- Preconceptional counseling is critical for women with SSc. Women should be evaluated for pulmonary hypertension, which is a contraindication to pregnancy.
- SSc renal crisis carries such a high risk of morbidity and mortality that the use of an angiotensin-converting enzyme inhibitor in pregnancy may be justified in this specific circumstance.
- Particular attention should be paid to those women with diffuse disease, and an increase in the frequency of prenatal visits to every 1 to 2 weeks is prudent.
- Among those with diffuse and severe disease, a multidisciplinary approach with rheumatology, anesthesiology, and even nephrology, cardiology, or pulmonology (depending on the specific organs involved) is recommended.

Sjögren Syndrome

- Sjögren syndrome (SS) is a chronic autoimmune disorder characterized by decreased lacrimal and salivary gland function, which leads to dry eyes and dry mouth.
- Pregnancy outcomes among women with SS are similar to those without the disease. However, women with SS may be positive for anti-Ro/SSA antibodies, with the accompanying risks for NLE and CHB.

References for this chapter are available at ExpertConsult.com.

CHAPTER 47

Hepatic Disorders During Pregnancy

Mitchell S. Cappell

KEY POINTS

- The differential of hepatobiliary conditions is extensive in pregnancy and includes pregnancy-related disorders in addition to disorders unrelated to pregnancy. Indeed, several clinical syndromes are unique to pregnancy, such as intrahepatic cholestasis of pregnancy and AFLP.
- Pregnancy affects the normative values of serum parameters of liver function and pancreatic injury. During pregnancy, the serum level of albumin declines, and the serum levels of amylase, alkaline phosphatase, bile acids, cholesterol, and triglycerides rise. Yet these serum parameters are still clinically important measures of liver function and pancreatic injury during pregnancy, provided the changes in normative values are appreciated.
- Many causes of significant to severe liver dysfunction during pregnancy—including preeclampsia, eclampsia, HELLP syndrome, and AFLP—are rapidly relieved and completely reversed by delivery of the infant. Delivery is generally the definitive therapy for these disorders.
- Pregnancy aggravates preexisting portal hypertension and increases the risk of variceal hemorrhage. As in nonpregnant patients, endoscopic banding and sclerotherapy appear to be first-line therapies for esophageal variceal bleeding in pregnant patients.
- Pregnancy greatly aggravates acute hepatitis E infection, hepatocellular adenomas, acute intermittent porphyria, and herpes simplex hepatitis.
- Neonates born to mothers who have acute or chronic hepatitis B are at high risk of vertical transmission of infection during delivery. Such infants should be passively immunized with hepatitis B hyperimmune globulin and actively immunized with hepatitis B vaccine at birth to prevent this infection.

Overview

- Hepatic, biliary, and pancreatic disorders are relatively uncommon but are not rare during pregnancy. For example, during pregnancy about 3% of women develop serum liver function test abnormalities,[1] and about 1 in 500 develop potentially life-threatening hepatic diseases that endanger fetal viability.[2,3]
- The interests of both the mother and the fetus must be considered in therapeutic decisions. Usually these interests do not conflict, because generally, what is good for the mother is good for the fetus.

Differential Diagnosis of Hepatobiliary Symptoms and Conditions During Pregnancy

MATERNAL JAUNDICE

- As in the general population, acute viral hepatitis is the most common cause of jaundice during pregnancy.[2,3] The differential diagnosis of jaundice during the first and second trimesters of pregnancy also includes drug hepatotoxicity and gallstone disease such as acute cholecystitis, choledocholithiasis, ascending cholangitis, or gallstone pancreatitis.

RIGHT UPPER QUADRANT ABDOMINAL PAIN

- Biliary colic
- Acute cholecystitis
- Acute pancreatitis
- Laboratory evaluation of significant abdominal pain routinely includes a complete blood count, serum electrolytes, and liver function tests as well as a leukocyte differential, coagulation profile, and serum lipase determination.
- Right upper quadrant pain and abnormal liver function tests in the setting of new-onset hypertension should strongly suggest preeclampsia with hepatic involvement.

NAUSEA AND VOMITING

- Hyperemesis gravidarum is a serious and potentially life-threatening form of nausea and vomiting of pregnancy associated with loss of more than 5% of the pregravid weight.
- The differential diagnosis of nausea and vomiting during pregnancy also includes hepatic and pancreatobiliary diseases such as pancreatitis, viral hepatitis, symptomatic cholelithiasis, acute cholecystitis, acute fatty liver of pregnancy (AFLP), and occasionally intrahepatic cholestasis of pregnancy.

PRURITUS

- Important clues that pruritus may be due to the intrahepatic cholestasis of pregnancy include pruritus that begins during the third trimester of pregnancy with no history of chronic liver disease, absence of abdominal pain, pruritus that affects mostly the hands and feet, and only mild to moderately elevated serum transaminase and bilirubin levels.

Abdominal Imaging During Pregnancy

- Fetal safety during diagnostic imaging is a concern for pregnant patients. Ultrasonography is considered safe and is the preferred abdominal imaging modality during pregnancy.[4]
- No reported harmful effects result from MRI during pregnancy,
- Gadolinium has not been associated with adverse fetal outcomes in a number of individual case reports or in limited case series.
- Diagnostic studies with high radiation exposure, such as abdominal CT, typically expose the fetus to less than 1 rad and should therefore be considered when indicated.[5]

THERAPEUTIC ENDOSCOPIC RETROGRADE CHOLANGIOPANCREATOGRAPHY

- Choledocholithiasis usually requires urgent therapy because of potentially life-threatening ascending cholangitis or gallstone pancreatitis. Symptomatic choledocholithiasis is best managed by therapeutic endoscopic retrograde cholangiopancreatography (ERCP).
- ERCP is justifiable during pregnancy for appropriate indications and contemplated therapeutic intervention.
- Therapeutic ERCP can be performed during pregnancy to help avoid complex biliary surgery or to postpone cholecystectomy until after parturition.

ENDOSCOPIC VARICEAL SCLEROTHERAPY OR BANDING

- Pregnancy appears to increase the risk of variceal bleeding from portal hypertension because of the gestational increase in plasma volume.[6] Endoscopic ligation (banding) or sclerotherapy are particularly attractive therapies for variceal bleeding during pregnancy because the alternative of transjugular intrahepatic portosystemic shunt requires radiation, and the surgical alternatives can cause fetal loss.

TEAM APPROACH AND INFORMED CONSENT

- Complex hepatic problems during pregnancy are best handled at a tertiary hospital with the requisite experience and expertise.

Pancreatobiliary Disease

ACUTE PANCREATITIS

- Acute pancreatitis occurs in about 1 per 3000 pregnancies, most commonly during the third trimester.[7,8] Gallstones cause about 70% of cases because alcoholism is relatively uncommon during pregnancy.[9,10]
- Pregnancy does not significantly alter the clinical presentation of acute pancreatitis.[9,10] Epigastric pain is the most common symptom.
- Acute pancreatitis is diagnosed by finding typical abnormalities in two of the following three parameters: (1) clinical presentation, (2) laboratory tests, or (3) radiologic examinations. Typical symptoms of pancreatitis include epigastric or right upper quadrant pain and nausea and vomiting. Serum lipase is a reliable marker of acute pancreatitis during pregnancy.
- Acute pancreatitis during pregnancy is often mild and usually responds to medical therapy that includes IV fluid administration, gastric acid suppression, analgesia, sometimes nasogastric suction, and discontinuation of oral intake.
- Laparoscopic cholecystectomy can be utilized during pregnancy and is best performed during the second trimester after organogenesis has occurred and before the growing gravid uterus interferes with visualization of the laparoscopic field.

CHOLELITHIASIS AND CHOLECYSTITIS

- Most gallstones are asymptomatic during pregnancy,[13] although symptoms of gallstone disease during pregnancy are the same as those in other patients.[12,13]

- More severe complications of cholelithiasis include cholecystitis, choledocholithiasis, jaundice, ascending cholangitis, hepatic abscess, and gallstone pancreatitis. Pregnancy does not increase the frequency or severity of these complications.[13] Acute cholecystitis is a chemical inflammation usually caused by cystic duct obstruction by a gallstone.
- The third most common nonobstetric surgical emergency during pregnancy with an incidence of about 4 cases per 10,000 pregnancies.[10]
- Ultrasound is very helpful in diagnosing acute cholecystitis during pregnancy.
- Most cases of biliary colic and some cases of very mild acute cholecystitis can be managed conservatively with close observation, expectant management, and deferral of surgery to the immediate postpartum period.[11,15] However, most patients with recurrent biliary colic or acute cholecystitis undergo cholecystectomy.[12,14,16]
- Cholecystectomy is best performed during the second trimester; cholecystectomy during the first trimester is occasionally associated with fetal loss, and cholecystectomy during the third trimester may be associated with premature labor.[14,16]

Common Liver Diseases Incidental to Pregnancy

CHRONIC HEPATITIS B

- Maternal chronic hepatitis B infection may be transmitted to the neonate, usually during delivery.[17] The risk of vertical transmission is about 90% in mothers who are positive for the hepatitis B e antigen, but it is about 25% in mothers who are hepatitis B e antigen negative.
- Infants born to mothers with acute or chronic hepatitis B infection should be passively immunized with hepatitis B hyperimmune globulin and should be actively immunized with hepatitis B vaccine immediately after birth.

CHRONIC HEPATITIS C

- Women with chronic hepatitis C may exhibit transient normalization of their serum aminotransferase levels associated with an increase in the serum viral load during pregnancy, possibly because of mildly attenuated immunity.[18]
- The risk of vertical transmission of hepatitis C from a chronically infected mother with viremia to the neonate is about 5%.[19]

BUDD-CHIARI SYNDROME

- Budd-Chiari syndrome refers to hepatic vein thrombosis or occlusion that increases the hepatic sinusoidal pressure, and it can lead to portal hypertension or hepatic necrosis.[20]
- This syndrome is diagnosed by pulsed Doppler ultrasound, hepatic venography, or magnetic resonance angiography.[21–23]
- Definitive therapy is liver transplantation.

PREGNANCY AFTER LIVER TRANSPLANTATION

- Immunosuppressive therapy should be maintained during pregnancy after liver transplantation.

INTRAHEPATIC CHOLESTASIS OF PREGNANCY

- The incidence of intrahepatic cholestasis of pregnancy ranges from about 2 per 10,000 in the United States to about 20 per 10,000 in Europe.[24] The cardinal symptom is pruritus due to cholestasis and accumulated bile salts in the dermis.
- Ursodeoxycholic acid is the generally recommended therapy.[25]
- Vitamin K deficiency that results from mild steatorrhea, associated with the cholestasis itself or the cholestyramine therapy for the cholestasis, increases the risk of postpartum hemorrhage. The prothrombin time may be monitored during pregnancy, especially near parturition, and vitamin K can be administered as necessary.

ACUTE FATTY LIVER OF PREGNANCY

- AFLP is a rare but severe disease characterized by hepatic microvesicular steatosis associated with mitochondrial dysfunction.
- Characteristic laboratory findings in severely affected patients include a prolonged prothrombin time, hypofibrinogenemia, and increased serum levels of fibrin split products from disseminated intravascular coagulation and/or hepatic decompensation. Other laboratory abnormalities include increased serum levels of ammonia, uric acid, blood urea nitrogen, and creatinine.[20,27,28]
- AFLP differs from severe acute viral hepatitis in that the serum aminotransferase levels in AFLP rarely exceed 1000 U/L, the viral serologic tests are negative, and hepatic pathologic analysis reveals much less inflammatory infiltration and hepatocytic necrosis.[20,26–28] AFLP may be difficult to distinguish from HELLP syndrome (hemolysis, elevated liver enzymes, and low platelet count) and preeclampsia or eclampsia with disseminated intravascular coagulation.
- Fortunately, the definitive treatment for all these disorders is prompt delivery after maternal stabilization.
- AFLP rarely recurs in subsequent pregnancies.[27]

References for this chapter are available at ExpertConsult.com.

CHAPTER 48

Gastrointestinal Disorders During Pregnancy

Mitchell S. Cappell

KEY POINTS

- The differential diagnosis of GI symptoms and signs such as abdominal pain is particularly extensive during pregnancy. Aside from GI and other intraabdominal disorders incidental to pregnancy, the differential includes obstetric, gynecologic, and GI disorders related to pregnancy.
- Pregnancy can affect the clinical presentation, frequency, or severity of GI diseases. For example, GERD markedly increases in frequency, and peptic ulcer disease decreases in frequency or may become inactive during pregnancy.
- Abdominal ultrasound is the safest and most commonly used abdominal imaging modality to evaluate GI conditions during pregnancy. Other common abdominal imaging modalities, particularly computed tomography, raise serious concerns about fetal safety.
- EGD and flexible sigmoidoscopy can be performed when strongly indicated during pregnancy, such as for significant acute upper and lower GI bleeding, respectively.
- Most GI drugs appear to be relatively safe for the fetus (FDA categories B and C) and can be used with caution when clearly indicated during pregnancy, especially during the second and third trimesters after organogenesis has occurred. Drugs to be avoided during pregnancy include methotrexate (category X), some chemotherapeutic agents, and a few antibiotics.

Differential Diagnosis and Evaluation of Gastrointestinal Symptoms During Pregnancy

ABDOMINAL PAIN

- The differential diagnosis of abdominal pain during pregnancy is extensive in that it includes obstetric conditions in addition to the usual gastrointestinal (GI) and other intraabdominal conditions in the general population.[1]
- The abdominal pain is typically localized to the abdominal quadrant in which the afflicted organ is located, as illustrated for pain in the right lower quadrant in Box 48.1.
- When the diagnosis is uncertain, close and vigilant monitoring by a surgical team with frequent abdominal examination and regular laboratory tests can often clarify the diagnosis. The character, severity, localization, or instigating factors of abdominal pain often change with time. For example, acute appendicitis typically changes from a dull, poorly localized, moderate pain to an intense and focal pain as the inflammation extends from the appendiceal wall to the surrounding peritoneum. The differential diagnosis of severe abdominal pain is described in Table 48.1.

BOX 48.1 ■ Differential Diagnosis of Right Lower Quadrant Abdominal Pain

Gastrointestinal Disorders
  Appendicitis
  Crohn disease
  Ruptured Meckel diverticulum
  Intestinal intussusception
  Cecal perforation
  Colon cancer
  Ischemic colitis
  Irritable bowel syndrome

Renal Diseases
  Nephrolithiasis
  Cystitis
  Pyelonephritis

Obstetric and Gynecologic Diseases
  Ruptured ectopic pregnancy
  Ovarian tumors
  Ovarian cyst rupture
  Ovarian torsion
  Endometriosis
  Uterine leiomyomas

Other
  Trochanteric bursitis

TABLE 48.1 ■ Common Causes of Acute, Severe Abdominal Pain During Pregnancy: Pain Characteristics and Diagnostic Tests

Condition	Location	Character	Radiation	Diagnostic Tests
Ruptured ectopic pregnancy	Lower abdomen or pelvis	Localized, severe	None	Serum β-hCG, abdominal ultrasound
Pelvic inflammatory disease	Lower abdomen or pelvis	Gradual in onset, localized	Flanks and thighs	Abdominal ultrasound
Appendicitis	First periumbilical, later RLQ (RUQ in late pregnancy)	Gradual in onset, becomes focal	Back or flank	Abdominal ultrasound in appropriate clinical setting
Acute cholecystitis	RUQ	Focal	Right scapula, shoulder, or back	Abdominal ultrasound, serum liver function tests
Pancreatitis	Epigastric	Localized, boring	Middle of back	Serum lipase and amylase, abdominal ultrasound

Continued

TABLE 48.1 ■ Common Causes of Acute, Severe Abdominal Pain During Pregnancy: Pain Characteristics and Diagnostic Tests—cont'd

Condition	Location	Character	Radiation	Diagnostic Tests
Perforated peptic ulcer	Epigastric or RUQ	Burning, boring	Right back	Abdominal ultrasound, laparotomy
Urolithiasis	Abdomen or flanks	Varies from intermittent and aching to severe and unremitting	Groin	Urinalysis, abdominal ultrasound, and occasionally fluoroscopy with contrast urography

hCG, human chorionic gonadotropin; *RLQ,* right lower quadrant; *RUQ,* right upper quadrant.

SELECTED GASTROINTESTINAL SYMPTOMS

Hematemesis

- The most common causes of GI hemorrhage during pregnancy are gastroesophageal reflux disease (GERD), gastritis, Mallory-Weiss tears, and ulcers.[2,3]
- The hematocrit is an even less reliable indicator of bleeding severity during pregnancy because of the conflicting effects of intravascular fluid accumulation and increased erythrocyte mass during normal pregnancy.

Constipation

- Constipation is very common in pregnant women and affects up to one-fourth of this population.[4]
- Laxatives to be avoided during pregnancy include castor oil, because it may initiate premature uterine contractions, and hypertonic saline laxatives such as phospho soda, because they promote sodium and water retention, which is inadvisable during pregnancy; in addition, they may cause renal failure in patients who are dehydrated or have preexisting renal insufficiency.[5,6]

Red Blood Per Rectum

- Hemorrhoids are the most common cause of rectal bleeding during pregnancy.

Diagnostic Testing During Pregnancy

RADIOLOGIC IMAGING

- Ultrasonography is considered safe during pregnancy and is the preferred imaging modality for abdominal pain during pregnancy.[7]

ENDOSCOPY DURING PREGNANCY

- Sigmoidoscopy seems to be relatively safe during pregnancy.
- Data are currently limited on colonoscopy during pregnancy.

TABLE 48.2 ■ **General Principles to Improve the Risk/Benefit Ratio of Gastrointestinal Endoscopy During Pregnancy**

Principle	Example
Perform endoscopy only for strong indications	Colonoscopy for suspected colon cancer
Avoid endoscopy or defer it until delivery for weak or elective indications	Colonoscopy for routine colon cancer screening
Use the safest drugs (Food and Drug Administration category B preferable or at most category C) in the lowest possible dosages for sedation and analgesia	Propofol (category B) or fentanyl (category C) but not diazepam (category D) because of possible, albeit unlikely, association with congenital cleft palate
Consult an anesthesiologist regarding drug safety during pregnancy	Monitored anesthesia care with anesthesiologist present during endoscopy
It is preferable to perform endoscopy in the second trimester, if possible, to avoid potential teratogenicity during fetal organogenesis in the first trimester and to avoid premature labor or adverse effects on the neonate after delivery in the third trimester	If possible, defer endoscopy during the first trimester until the second trimester, and defer endoscopy during the third trimester until after delivery
Minimize procedure time	Performed by an experienced, expert endoscopist
Obstetric support should be available for a pregnancy-related procedure complication	Performed in an in-hospital endoscopy suite rather than a physician's office or ambulatory surgical center

Modified from Cappell MS. Endoscopy in pregnancy: risks versus benefits. Nature Clin Pract Gastroenterol Hepatol. 2005;2(9):376-377; Cappell MS. The fetal safety and clinical efficacy of gastrointestinal endoscopy during pregnancy. Gastroenterol Clin North Am. 2003;32:123-79; Cappell MS. Sedation and analgesia for gastrointestinal endoscopy during pregnancy. Gastrointest Endosc Clin North Am. 2006;16(1):1-31; and American Society for Gastrointestinal Endoscopy. ASGE guideline: guidelines for endoscopy in pregnant and lactating women. Gastrointest Endosc. 2005;61(3):357-362.

- Esophagogastroduodenoscopy (EGD) is recommended during pregnancy for hemodynamically significant upperGI bleeding. It is relatively safe for the fetus and the mother.
- General measures to increase the risk/benefit ratio of endoscopy during pregnancy are listed in Table 48.2.[8–11]

Nausea and Vomiting of Pregnancy and Hyperemesis Gravidarum

- Hyperemesis gravidarum is a severe, pathologic form of nausea and vomiting of pregnancy (NVP) characterized by a greater than 5% loss of prepregnancy weight and otherwise unexplained ketonuria.
- NVP and hyperemesis gravidarum are diagnoses of exclusion arrived at only after excluding other conditions by appropriate tests.
- Patients with mild nausea during pregnancy typically require counseling and reassurance without pharmacologic therapy.
- Vitamin B_6 (pyridoxine), a component of Bendectin, has been used by itself to treat mild-to-moderate NVP with some success.[12]

Gastroesophageal Reflux and Peptic Ulcer Disease

- The incidence of pyrosis approaches 80% during pregnancy.[1] The incidence of GERD is likewise high during pregnancy[13] and may relate to a hypotonic lower esophageal sphincter and delayed GI transit attributed to gestational hormones, especially progesterone, and gastric compression by the gravid uterus.

- Nausea, emesis, dyspepsia, and anorexia are so frequent during pregnancy that peptic ulcer disease (PUD) cannot be diagnosed solely by symptomatology during pregnancy.[14]
- Pregnant patients with GERD or PUD should avoid caffeine, alcohol, smoking cigarettes, and nonsteroidal antiinflammatory drug use, although acetaminophen is safe and the cyclooxygenase 2 inhibitors are less gastrotoxic than the nonselective nonsteroidal antiinflammatory drugs.[15] Patients with GERD should elevate the head of their bed and avoid wearing tight belts. They should avoid recumbency after eating and discontinue oral intake 3 hours before bedtime.
- Antacids are generally safe for the fetus, although those that contain sodium bicarbonate should be used with caution throughout pregnancy because such antacids may cause fluid overload or metabolic alkalosis.[16]
- Proton pump inhibitors were initially reserved for refractory, severe, or complicated GERD or PUD during pregnancy but have recently been increasingly used for moderate disease because of accumulating evidence of relative fetal safety.
- Drug therapy for *Helicobacter pylori* eradication should be deferred until after parturition and lactation because of concern about the fetal safety of antibiotics, such as clarithromycin and metronidazole.[17]
- Surgery for GERD is best performed either before or after pregnancy.[18,19]

Acute Appendicitis

- Acute appendicitis is the most common nonobstetric surgical emergency during pregnancy with an incidence of about 1 per 1000 pregnancies.[20,21] Appendiceal obstruction, usually from an appendicolith, is the primary etiologic event, although stasis and other factors are also implicated. As the appendiceal lumen distends secondary to appendiceal obstruction, the patient initially experiences poorly localized periumbilical pain. Severe luminal distention, mural inflammation and edema, and bacterial translocation produce somatic pain that becomes severe and well localized at the McBurney point, which is located in the right lower quadrant one-third of the way from the anterior superior iliac spine to the umbilicus. Displacement of the appendix by the gravid uterus during late pregnancy may cause the point of maximal abdominal pain and tenderness to migrate superiorly and laterally from the McBurney point, but this migration typically extends only a few centimeters away from the McBurney point during late pregnancy.[1]
- Sonography is the initial imaging test of choice during pregnancy.
- Appendicitis cannot be excluded if the appendix is not visualized on ultrasound.
- MRI is the appropriate next test in the pregnant patient if the abdominal ultrasound is inconclusive.
- Up to one-quarter of pregnant women with appendicitis develop an appendiceal perforation.[1] This high rate is attributed to delayed diagnosis during pregnancy.
- Appendicitis during pregnancy mandates prompt appendectomy after IV hydration and correction of electrolyte abnormalities.
- Laparoscopy should be considered during the first two trimesters or even later by experienced operators for nonperforated appendicitis or when the diagnosis is uncertain.[22]

Intestinal Obstruction

- Acute intestinal obstruction is the second most common nonobstetric abdominal emergency with an incidence of 1 per 2500 pregnancies.[23–25]
- Intestinal obstruction classically presents with a symptomatic triad of abdominal pain, emesis, and obstipation.[23,24]

- The approach to intestinal obstruction is the same in pregnancy as in the general population except that decisions are more urgently required because both the fetus and the mother are at risk.
- Surgery is recommended for unremitting and complete intestinal obstruction, whereas medical management is recommended for intermittent or partial obstruction.[23]

Intestinal Pseudoobstruction

- Intestinal pseudoobstruction, adynamic ileus, is characterized by severe abdominal distention detected on physical examination and diffuse intestinal dilatation noted on abdominal roentgenogram.
- Intestinal pseudoobstruction is a well-described but uncommon complication of cesarean or vaginal delivery.[26,27] Patients with pseudoobstruction have nausea, emesis, obstipation, and diffuse abdominal pain that typically evolves over several days.[26]
- Treatment includes nasogastric aspiration, parenteral fluid administration, repletion of electrolytes, and rectal tube decompression. The pseudoobstruction usually spontaneously resolves.[26]

Inflammatory Bowel Disease

- The inflammatory bowel diseases (IBDs), ulcerative colitis (UC) and Crohn disease (CD), are immunologically mediated disorders that peak in incidence during a woman's reproductive life. In women younger than 40 years of age, the incidence of UC is 40 to 100 per 100,000, and the incidence of CD is 5 to 10 per 100,000.[1] UC is a colonic mucosal disease manifested by bloody diarrhea, crampy abdominal pain, and pyrexia. CD can involve any part of the GI tract but most commonly involves the terminal ileum or colon. It is characterized by diarrhea, abdominal pain, anorexia, pyrexia, and malnutrition. Patients with CD may have fistulae and anorectal disease. Extraintestinal manifestations of IBD include arthritis, uveitis, sclerosing cholangitis, and cutaneous lesions.
- Patients with inactive or mild disease before conception tend to have the same disease activity during pregnancy. Active disease at conception increases the likelihood of active disease during pregnancy and of a poor pregnancy outcome that includes spontaneous abortion, miscarriage, stillbirth, or premature delivery.[28,29]
- The beneficial effects of IBD therapy on the mother and fetus must be weighed against the potential of fetal toxicity and teratogenicity (Table 48.3; see Chapter 8).
- Active disease poses greater risk to the fetus than most therapies.[30]
- Sulfasalazine and 5-aminosalicylates are safe and should be used when required during pregnancy.[28,31]
- The FDA categorizes azathioprine and 6-mercaptopurine as class D drugs during pregnancy, but many gastroenterologists continue these medications during pregnancy if required to maintain remission.[28,32]

Hemorrhoids

- Hemorrhoids are common in adults and are particularly common during pregnancy, especially during the third trimester or immediately postpartum, with an estimated incidence of 25% during pregnancy.[33]
- Hemorrhoids characteristically produce a clinical triad of bright red blood per rectum that resembles the color of arterial blood; blood coating, rather than blood admixed with stool; and postdefecatory bleeding, most commonly noted on the toilet paper.[34]

Irritable Bowel Syndrome

- Irritable bowel syndrome (IBS) is diagnosed, according to the Rome III criteria, by the presence of both abdominal pain and disordered defecation for at least 6 months with at

TABLE 48.3 ▦ Pharmacologic Therapy for Inflammatory Bowel Disease During Pregnancy

Drug	FDA Category During Pregnancy	Recommendation During Pregnancy
Sulfasalazine	B	Relatively safe, but concern exists about sulfa moiety causing neonatal jaundice
Mesalamine	B	Mesalamine is relatively safe
Infliximab (anti-TNF)	B	Not teratogenic in mice exposed to an analogous antibody, but clinical data are insufficient
Adalimumab (anti-TNF)	B	Believed to be relatively safe drug during pregnancy based on animal data, little clinical data; drug manufacturer is placing patients receiving this drug during pregnancy on a national registry
Certolizumab (anti-TNF)	B	Animal studies have not revealed fetal toxicity, and clinical data are sparse
Loperamide	B	Loperamide is relatively safe
Metronidazole	B	Avoid during first trimester (carcinogenic in rodents)
Corticosteroids	C	Relatively safe, concern regarding fetal adrenal function and maternal hyperglycemia; monitor the neonates of mothers who received substantial doses of corticosteroids during pregnancy
Ciprofloxacin	C	Use with caution, small studies show no significant risk during pregnancy
Diphenoxylate	C	Avoid; a possible teratogen
Cyclosporine	C	Cyclosporine is embryotoxic and fetotoxic at very high doses in rats and rabbits
6-Mercaptopurine	D	Avoid starting after conception, might cause IUGR
Azathioprine	D	Avoid starting after conception, might cause IUGR, teratogenic in laboratory animals
Methotrexate	X	Methotrexate is a contraindicated teratogen and abortifacient

FDA, Food and Drug Administration; *IUGR,* intrauterine growth restriction; *TNF,* tumor necrosis factor.

least two of the following: (1) pain relief by a bowel movement, (2) onset of pain related to a change in stool frequency, and (3) onset of pain related to a change in stool appearance.[35] Endoscopic, radiologic, and histologic intestinal studies reveal no evident organic disease. Young women typically have diarrhea-predominant IBS but sometimes have primarily constipation or alternating diarrhea and constipation. Abdominal bloating and distention are common symptoms.

- IBS is believed to be generally mild during pregnancy,[36] and gestational hormones—particularly progesterone—may exacerbate the symptoms of IBS.[37]
- Symptoms of IBS are best treated during pregnancy by dietary modification or behavioral therapy.

References for this chapter are available at ExpertConsult.com.

CHAPTER 49

Neurologic Disorders in Pregnancy

Elizabeth E. Gerard ■ Philip Samuels

KEY POINTS

- Epilepsy affects approximately 1% of the general population and is the most frequent neurologic complication of pregnancy.
- Prepregnancy counseling is imperative in the patient with epilepsy.
- Valproic acid has been associated with a significantly increased risk of major congenital malformations and adverse cognitive outcomes, including lower IQs and an increased risk of autism, when compared with other AEDs and with the general population.
- AEDs known to have a low risk of structural teratogenesis—such as lamotrigine, levetiracetam, or carbamazepine—should be tried as first-line agents in women with epilepsy over AEDs that have been less well studied or valproic acid.
- Ultimately, the AED that best controls the patient's seizures should be used during pregnancy. Efforts to reach the minimum therapeutic dose should be attempted well in advance of pregnancy.
- Because of the changes in plasma volume, drug distribution, and metabolism that occur during pregnancy, anticonvulsant levels should be checked prior to conception and monthly during pregnancy. Dose adjustments to maintain prepregnancy levels are an important part of seizure control for many AEDs, especially lamotrigine.
- Women using AEDs should take folic acid 0.4 mg to 4 mg daily prior to and throughout pregnancy. They should also be offered a specialized ultrasound for careful assessment of major congenital malformations.
- Pregnancy does not hasten the onset or progression of MS. DMAs used to decrease the rate of relapses and disability in MS are typically not recommended during pregnancy because MS relapses tend to be less frequent. A washout period is recommended for many DMAs.
- For some patients, certain DMAs—such as glatiramer acetate and interferon-β—can be used in pregnancy.
- Breastfeeding in MS is controversial. Exclusive breastfeeding may reduce the risk of MS relapses, but treatment with DMAs is typically not recommended for women who are breastfeeding.
- Any new headache or new headache type that presents in pregnancy requires workup for an underlying potentially deleterious cause.
- Nonpharmacologic treatments are considered first-line therapies for migraine in pregnancy, which typically improves without treatment.
- Carpal tunnel syndrome is common in pregnancy and usually responds to conservative splinting, glucocorticoid injection, or both. Surgery can be safely undertaken if indicated during pregnancy.

Epilepsy and Seizures

- Epilepsy affects approximately 1% of the general population and is the most frequent major neurologic complication encountered in pregnancy.
- A diagnosis of epilepsy is made in the setting of two unprovoked seizures or one seizure in a patient with clinical features that make a second seizure likely, such as findings on brain MRI or electroencephalogram that are consistent with a diagnosis of epilepsy or a family history of epilepsy.
- Focal epilepsy is the most common type of epilepsy in adult patients. It may occur secondary to an acquired abnormality such as a tumor, vascular malformation, brain injury, or infectious or autoimmune disorder that affects the brain.
- The mainstay of epilepsy therapy, especially in women of childbearing age, is to try to find the one antiepileptic drug (AED) that best controls a patient's seizures at the minimum therapeutic dose or level. In certain cases, polytherapy may be preferable to monotherapy.
- Lamotrigine and levetiracetam are now the most commonly prescribed AEDs for women of childbearing age.
- Most women with epilepsy will need to remain on AEDs during their childbearing years and throughout pregnancy.
- Uncontrolled seizures increase the risk of maternal injury and death and potentially expose the infant to transient anoxia. Women with epilepsy were 10 times more likely to die during pregnancy or during the postpartum period.
- The majority of pregnant women with seizure disorders can have a successful pregnancy with minimal risk to mother and fetus with the support of their obstetrician and neurologist.

TERATOGENIC EFFECTS OF ANTIEPILEPTIC DRUGS

- Women with epilepsy on AEDs are at increased risk for major congenital malformations (Table 49.1). The risk of major malformations has been shown to be dose related for several AEDs.
- Valproate carries a risk of major congenital malformations (neural tube defects, cardiac anomalies, hypospadias, oral clefts) significantly greater than that of other AEDs and baseline population rates, and adverse cognitive and behavioral developmental outcomes.
- Rates of major malformations with lamotrigine exposure have been consistently low and range from 2% to 4.6%, across eight prospective registries, and developmental scores of infants prenatally exposed to lamotrigine did not differ from those of controls.
- Rates of specific malformations with phenytoin exposure are 0.4% for cardiac malformations, 0% for neural tube defects, 0.2% for oral clefts, and 0.5% for hypospadias.
- Phenobarbital is rarely used as a first-line AED in developed countries given its adverse cognitive and metabolic side effects and the availability of alternative medications with fewer adverse effects.
- Toprimate is associated with a tenfold increased risk of oral clefts or an absolute risk of 1.4%, which resulted in the U.S. Food and Drug Administration reclassification of topiramate from class C to class D for pregnancy.

EFFECTS OF PREGNANCY ON ANTICONVULSANT MEDICATIONS

- AED metabolism varies greatly by individual; each patient has her own therapeutic drug level at which seizures are best controlled. This is typically within the standard window but may be above or below it. It is important to establish this drug level prior to pregnancy whenever

TABLE 49.1 ■ Rate of Major Congenital Malformations With Individual Antiepileptic Drugs When Used as Monotherapy

Registry	Study	Rate of Major Congenital Malformations With Individual Antiepileptic Drugs as Monotherapy*								
		CBZ	GBP	LTG	LEV	OXC	PHB	PHT	TPM	VPA
Australian Pregnancy Registry	Vajda, 2014	5.5% (346)	0% (14)	4.6% (307)	2.4% (82)	5.9% (17)	0% (4)	2.4% (41)	2.4% (42)	13.8% (253)
Danish Registry	Molgaard, 2011		1.7% (59)	3.7% (1019)	0% (58)	2.8% (393)			4.6% (108)	
EURAP	Tomson, 2011	5.6% (1402)		2.9% (1280)	1.6% (126)	3.3% (184)	7.4% (217)	5.8% (103)	6.8% (73)	9.7% (1010)
Finland National Birth Registry	Artama, 2005	2.7% (805)								10.7% (263)
GSK Lamotrigine Registry	Cunnington, 2011			2.2% (1558)						
North American AED Pregnancy Registry	Hernandez, 2012	3.0% (1033)	0.7% (145)	2.0% (1562)	2.4% (450)	2.2% (182)	5.5% (199)	2.9% (416)	4.2% (359)	9.3% (323)
Norwegian Medical Birth Registry	Veiby, 2014	2.9% (685)	0% (18)	3.4% (833)	1.7% (118)	1.8% (57)	7.4% (27)		4.2% (48)	6.3% (333)
Swedish Medical Birth Registry	Tomson, 2012	2.7% (1430)	0% (18)	2.9% (1100)	0% (61)	3.7% (27)	14% (7)	6.7% (119)	7.7% (52)	4.7% (619)
U.K./Ireland pregnancy registry	Campbell, 2014 Mawhinney, 2013 Morrow, 2006 Hunt, 2008	2.6% (1657)	3.2% (32)	2.3% (2098)	0.7% (304)			3.7% (82)	9% (203)	6.7% (1290)

Data from Gerard E. Pack AM. Pregnancy registries: what do they mean to clinical practice? Curr Neurol Neurosci Rep. 2008;8(4):325-332.
*Numbers in parentheses indicate number of pregnancies enrolled.
AED, antiepileptic drug; CBZ, carbamazepine; GBP, gabapentin; LEV, levetiracetam; LTG, lamotrigine; OXC, oxcarbazepine; PHB, phenobarbital; PHT, phenytoin; TPM, topiramate; VPA, valproic acid.

possible, because levels of anticonvulsant medications can change dramatically during pregnancy, and in many cases, decreasing AED levels have been associated with loss of seizure control.

- Many factors—including altered protein binding, delayed gastric emptying, nausea and vomiting, changes in plasma volume, changes in the volume of distribution, and even folic acid supplementation—can affect the levels of anticonvulsant medications. Additionally, changes in AED metabolism can be dramatically altered by the pregnant state.
- Over the course of a pregnancy, lamotrigine clearance increases by over 200% in the majority of women with epilepsy. Lamotrigine doses need to be increased substantially during pregnancy to maintain prepregnancy levels and seizure control.
- Checking AED drug levels monthly is recommended for all AEDs.

PREGNANCY AND SEIZURE FREQUENCY

- For the majority of women with epilepsy (54% to 80%), seizure frequency will remain similar to their baseline seizure frequency.
- Seizure freedom for 9 months prior to pregnancy is associated with an 84% to 92% chance of remaining seizure-free during pregnancy.

OBSTETRIC AND NEONATAL OUTCOMES

- Women with epilepsy may be at increased risk for obstetric complications such as a small-for-gestational-age infant. Bleeding complications at delivery may also be increased, although again studies have been conflicting on this point.
- Epilepsy and AED use are typically not indications for cesarean delivery (CD).

PRECONCEPTION COUNSELING FOR WOMEN WITH EPILEPSY

- Lamotrigine and levetiracetam are quickly becoming the most commonly prescribed drugs for women of childbearing age with epilepsy.
- Baseline AED levels should be established prior to pregnancy in order to set a target for dose adjustment during pregnancy.
- Changing AEDs once a woman is already pregnant is usually not recommended.
- If the patient has had no seizures during the past 2 to 4 years, an attempt may be made to withdraw her from anticonvulsant medications.
- Supplementation with folate (0.4 to 1 mg) in all women of childbearing age taking AEDs should be recommended.
- Vitamin D deficiency is also common in women with epilepsy and 25-hydroxyvitamin D levels should be checked and optimized prior to pregnancy.

Antepartum Management

- At 18 to 22 weeks, the patient should undergo a detailed anatomic ultrasound to determine whether congenital malformations are present.
- Antepartum fetal evaluation is not necessary in all mothers with seizure disorders, but it should be considered for patients who have active seizures in the third trimester.

Vitamin K Supplementation

- A more recent study of 662 women with epilepsy taking enzyme-inducing antiepileptic drugs did not find any increased risk of bleeding in the neonate if the infant received 1 mg of vitamin K intramuscularly at birth.

LABOR AND DELIVERY

- Although epidemiologically there may be an increased risk of induction of labor and cesarean delivery in women with epilepsy, these interventions should not be recommended to women with epilepsy without specific additional obstetric, medical, or neurologic indications.

NEW ONSET OF SEIZURES IN PREGNANCY AND IN THE PUERPERIUM

- If the seizures occur in the third trimester, they are eclampsia until proven otherwise and should be treated as such until the physician can perform a proper evaluation.
- If the patient develops seizures for the first time at an earlier gestational age, she should be evaluated and started on the proper medication.
- For new-onset epilepsy, levetiracetam is often used first because it can be started quickly and does not carry a high risk of rash. It is typically not practical to start lamotrigine when epilepsy presents in pregnancy.

BREASTFEEDING AND THE POSTPARTUM PERIOD

- If the patient's medication dosages were increased during pregnancy, they will need to be decreased over the 3 weeks after delivery to levels at or slightly higher than that of the pre-pregnancy period.
- Whereas AEDs taken by the mother are present in breast milk to varying degrees, few data suggest neonatal harm from exposure through breast milk.

Multiple Sclerosis

- Multiple sclerosis (MS) is a chronic autoimmune demyelinating disease that affects women more often than men. The onset of symptoms usually occurs between the ages of 20 and 40 years; thus it commonly affects women of childbearing age.
- The most common form of the disease, relapsing remitting MS, is characterized by periodic exacerbations with complete or partial remissions.
- The risk of MS relapses is reduced during gestation but may increase transiently in the postpartum period.
- MS does not seem to have any significant effect on the course of pregnancy or fetal outcomes and no association between MS and preterm birth or neonatal birth weight.

DISEASE-MODIFYING AGENTS AND PREGNANCY

- The mainstay of treatment for acute MS relapses is corticosteroids or, rarely, other immunomodulatory treatments. These therapies are utilized to reduce relapse rates; decrease MRI progression, one marker of MS disease activity; and lessen cumulative disability in patients with MS. They are not used to treat acute MS relapses.
- Given that few data are available on the safety of disease-modifying agents (DMAs) in pregnancy and the fact that MS attacks are usually less frequent in pregnancy, most experts recommend stopping DMAs prior to conception.
- Of the first-line therapies, experts agree that interferon-β and glatiramer acetate can be continued up to the time that contraception is stopped. Glatiramer acetate is the DMA of choice if one must be used during pregnancy, although the patient's history of response to this drug must also be considered.

- Mitoxantrone is a second-line agent for the treatment of MS, and cyclophosphamide is occasionally used for severe cases. Both treatments can cause amenorrhea in one-third of patients, and cyclophosphamide is associated with ovarian toxicity.

PREPREGNANCY COUNSELING FOR PATIENTS WITH MULTIPLE SCLEROSIS

- Patients should be reassured that the vast majority of women with MS can have healthy pregnancies and that MS in the mother does not pose an adverse risk to the fetus.
- The risk of developing MS in a child with a single parent with MS is 2% to 2.5%.

MANAGEMENT OF MULTIPLE SCLEROSIS DURING PREGNANCY

- No specific changes in routine obstetric care are recommended for women with MS.
- CD is usually not indicated in women with MS.

BREASTFEEDING AND THE POSTPARTUM PERIOD

- Breastfeeding in women with MS is a controversial and actively debated. The PRIMS study found that breastfeeding had no effect on the rate of MS relapses in the first 3 months postpartum.
- Most experts state that DMAs should not be resumed while a woman is breastfeeding. This recommendation is based on a lack of evidence about the safety of these drugs in breastfeeding rather than evidence of harm.

MIGRAINE

- Migraine symptoms tend to improve during pregnancy, although dietary factors may precipitate migraine attacks.
- Recent studies have demonstrated that sumatriptan can be used during pregnancy including the first trimester. In a large Norwegian database, no increase in congenital anomalies or other adverse pregnancy outcomes was reported. No significant difference in prematurity or low birthweight has been observed.
- Ergotamine should be avoided during pregnancy.

HEADACHE IN PREGNANCY

- Headaches during pregnancy can be a symptom of underlying intracranial pathology.
- Symptoms that should prompt further evaluation include abrupt onset of symptoms, persistent headache, and positional component. Any associated focal neurologic signs or vision changes should also prompt additional investigation unless they are a typical part of a patient's migraine aura.
- Patients with primary headache disorders (migraine and tension-type headaches) can get secondary headaches, so any change in pattern or new symptoms should also be considered evidence of a possible underlying problem.

Idiopathic Intracranial Hypertension (Pseudotumor Cerebri)

- More than 90% of patients with idiopathic intracranial hypertension (IIH) have headaches, and 40% have horizontal diplopia. Papilledema is a characteristic feature of the condition and is present in the majority of cases. If left untreated, IIH can progress to permanent visual loss.

- Pregnancy outcome appears to be unaffected by IIH, and no increase in fetal wastage or congenital anomalies are reported.
- The main objectives of treatment for IIH are relief of pain and preservation of vision.
- IIH is not usually an indication for CD. Both epidural and spinal anesthesia, when expertly administered, can be safely used in patients with IIH.

Cerebral Vein Thrombosis

- Patients typically present with a subacute, progressive, unremitting headache that may be worse when lying down.
- MRI and magnetic resonance venogram of the brain are the diagnostic tests of choice.
- Women who have had a cerebral vein thrombosis during pregnancy should avoid hormonal contraception, and women with a history of clotting while on hormonal contraception should use prophylactic anticoagulation during pregnancy.

Subarachnoid Hemorrhage

- Subarachnoid hemorrhage usually manifests with a sudden "thunderclap" headache that is often associated with vomiting, stiff neck, and fluctuations of consciousness.

Reversible Cerebral Vasoconstriction

- Reversible cerebral vasoconstriction syndrome can present with a similar "thunderclap" headache. It may also present with focal neurologic deficits, seizures, and fluctuating levels of consciousness.

Stroke

- Preeclampsia and eclampsia are risk factors for both ischemic and hemorrhagic strokes.

ISCHEMIC STROKE

- Ischemic stroke typically presents with acute focal neurologic symptoms.
- Although tissue plasminogen activator can be considered for pregnant women with arterial occlusion, it should probably be avoided in patients with preeclampsia/eclampsia given the increased risk of intracranial hemorrhage in these cases.

HEMORRHAGIC STROKE AND VASCULAR MALFORMATIONS

- A woman with a known arteriovenous malformation (AVM) should consider treatment prior to conceiving, and when an AVM is discovered during pregnancy, risks of treatment should be weighed against the risk of hemorrhage.
- If the patient has undergone corrective surgery for an aneurysm or an AVM, she should be allowed to deliver vaginally.

Carpal Tunnel Syndrome

- The median nerve and flexor tendons pass through this carpal tunnel, which has little room for expansion. If the wrist is extremely flexed or extended, the volume of the carpal tunnel is reduced. In pregnancy, weight gain and edema can produce a carpal tunnel syndrome that results from compression of the median nerve.
- Commonly, the syndrome consists of pain, numbness, and tingling in the distribution of the median nerve in the hand and wrist. This includes the thumb, index finger, long finger, and radial side of the ring finger on the palmar aspect.

- The syndrome appeared to be more common in primigravidae with generalized edema.
- Supportive and conservative therapies are usually adequate for the treatment of carpal tunnel syndrome. Splints placed on the dorsum of the hand, which keep the wrist in a neutral position and maximize the capacity of the carpal tunnel, often provide dramatic relief.
- It is important to warn patients that carpal tunnel syndrome can persist for several years postpartum and can recur in future pregnancies.

CHAPTER 50

Malignant Diseases and Pregnancy

Ritu Salani ■ Larry J. Copeland

KEY POINTS

- Because many of the common complaints of pregnancy are also early symptoms of metastatic cancer, pregnant women with cancer are at risk for delays in diagnosis and therapeutic intervention.
- The safest time for most cancer therapies in pregnancy is in the second and third trimesters, thereby avoiding induction of teratogenic risks or miscarriage in the first trimester. For most malignancies diagnosed during the second trimester, chemotherapy should be undertaken as indicated because fetal risk is generally lower than the risk of delaying treatment or proceeding with preterm delivery.
- Antimetabolites and alkylating agents present the greatest hazard to the developing fetus.
- Diagnostic delays for breast cancer in pregnancy are often attributed to physician reluctance to properly evaluate breast complaints or abnormal findings in pregnancy.
- Treatment for Hodgkin disease may compromise the reproductive potential, and combined treatment with irradiation and chemotherapy are associated with the highest risk of ovarian failure.
- When corrected for tumor thickness, pregnancy does not appear to be an independent prognostic variable for survival in case of melanoma.
- After stratifying for stage and age, patients with pregnancy-associated cervical carcinoma have survival rates similar to those of the nonpregnant patient.
- Because most malignant ovarian tumors found in pregnancy are either germ cell tumors or low-grade, early-stage epithelial tumors, the therapeutic plan will usually permit continuation of the pregnancy and preservation of fertility.
- Although rare, most colorectal carcinomas in pregnancy are detectable on rectal examination, underscoring the need for a rectal examination at the patient's first prenatal visit.
- Phantom β-hCG should be ruled out in patients suspected of having gestational trophoblastic disease when not documented by other clear clinical evidence (histology, imaging, and clinical history), especially when β-hCG titers are low.

Introduction

■ Cancer in pregnancy complicates the management of both the cancer and the pregnancy. Diagnostic and therapeutic interventions must carefully address the associated risks to both the patient and the fetus.

- Although cancer is the second most common cause of death for women in their reproductive years, only about 1 in 1000 pregnancies is complicated by cancer.[1]
- Delays in diagnosis of cancer during pregnancy are common for various reasons: (1) many of the presenting symptoms of cancer are often attributed to the pregnancy; (2) many of the physiologic and anatomic alterations of pregnancy can compromise physical examination; (3) serum tumor markers such as β-human chorionic gonadotropin (β-hCG), alpha-fetoprotein, and cancer antigen 125 are increased during pregnancy; and (4) the ability to optimally perform either imaging studies or invasive diagnostic procedures may be altered during pregnancy.
- Because the gestational age is significant when evaluating the risks of treatments, it is important to determine gestational age accurately.
- A successful outcome is dependent on a cooperative multidisciplinary approach.

Cancer Therapy During Pregnancy

GENERAL EFFECTS OF CHEMOTHERAPY DURING PREGNANCY AND LACTATION

- Because pregnancy alters physiology, there is potential for altered pharmacokinetics associated with chemotherapy. Orally administered medications are subjected to altered gastrointestinal motility and the 50% expansion in plasma volume, producing a longer drug half-life. The increase in plasma proteins and fall in albumin may also alter drug availability, and amniotic fluid may act as a pharmacologic third space, potentially increasing toxicity due to delayed metabolism and excretion.
- If continuation of the pregnancy is desired, chemotherapy is not advised in the first trimester because of an increased rate of major malformations that ranges from 10% to 17% with single-agent therapy and up to 25% with combination chemotherapy.
- The risk of teratogenicity during the second and third trimesters is significantly reduced and is likely no different from that for pregnant women who are not exposed to chemotherapy,[2] although neonatal myelosuppression and hearing loss have been reported (see Chapter 5). However, administration in the second and third trimester can be associated with intrauterine growth restriction, stillbirth, and low birthweight.[3,4] Maternal effects, such as chemotherapy-induced nausea and vomiting, may also affect fetal growth and birthweight.[5]
- Because most antineoplastic agents can be found in breast milk, breastfeeding is contraindicated (see Chapter 5).[2]

SPECIFIC EFFECTS OF CHEMOTHERAPY AGENTS DURING PREGNANCY AND LACTATION

Antimetabolites

- In the first trimester, methotrexate has been associated with skeletal and central nervous system defects. Though no anomalies were reported in the second and third trimester, methotrexate was associated with low birthweight and neonatal myelosuppresion.[6]

Alkylating Agents

- Cyclophosphamide and chlorambucil have demonstrated some teratogenic potential when administered in the first trimester, including renal agenesis, ocular abnormalities, and cleft palate.[5] In the second and third trimester, alkylating agents have been shown to be acceptably safe.[6,7]

Antitumor Antibiotics

- Even when administered in early pregnancy, antitumor antibiotics such as doxorubicin, idarubicin, bleomycin, and daunorubicin appear to demonstrate a low risk of teratogenicity.

Vinca Alkaloids

- Although potent teratogens in animals, vincristine and vinblastine do not appear to be as teratogenic in humans.[5]

Platinum Agents

- Platinum agents have been used with relatively acceptable risks. Reports of normal outcomes have been reported; however, there are cases of intrauterine growth restriction as well.

Targeted Therapies

- Trastuzumab, rituximab, and imatinib have been used only inadvertently in pregnancy and required more data on safety before used.

Radiation Therapy

- Ionizing radiation is a known teratogen, and the developing embryo is particularly sensitive to its effects. Doses higher than 0.20 gray are considered teratogenic.
- Radiation therapy should be postponed until the postpartum period, and consideration should be given to suitable alternative therapies such as surgery or chemotherapy. If delay of therapy is not possible, termination of the pregnancy may be required.

Surgery and Anesthesia

- If flexibility in timing exists, abdominal or pelvic surgery is best performed in the second trimester to limit the risk of first-trimester spontaneous abortion or preterm labor.
- There is no evidence that there are significant risks of anesthesia independent of coexisting disease.[8]

Pregnancy Following Cancer Treatment

- A number of women with early cervical cancer have received fertility preservation surgery with radical trachelectomy and regional lymphadenectomy and the preliminary fertility and pregnancy outcomes have been favorable.
- In women with estrogen receptor–positive breast cancer, there is no evidence that subsequent pregnancy adversely affects survival.
- It has been recommended that after a cancer diagnosis, pregnancy should be delayed for at least 2 years, during which recurrence risk is highest.

Cancer During Pregnancy

BREAST CANCER

- Recent publications are consistent with a frequency of breast cancer concurrent with pregnancy of 1 per 3000 to 10,000 live births, but this incidence is increasing with advancing maternal age at first birth.[9]

Diagnosis and Staging

- Breast abnormalities should be evaluated in the same manner as in a nonpregnant patient.
- The lengths of delays in diagnosis of breast cancer in pregnancy are commonly 3 to 7 months or longer and may result in more advanced stages of diagnosis compared with the general population.[10,11]
- Bloody nipple discharge should be evaluated with mammography and ultrasound.[12]
- Breast ultrasound has a high sensitivity and specificity and can distinguish between solid and cystic masses, which makes it the preferred imaging modality for pregnant women.
- For breast masses, a core needle biopsy is the preferred method for histologic diagnosis.[10]
- Before proceeding with treatment, staging should be undertaken.
- The contralateral breast must be carefully assessed. Laboratory tests should include baseline liver function tests and serum tumor markers, carcinoembryonic antigen, and also cancer antigen 15-3, which appears to be a useful tumor marker for monitoring breast cancer in pregnancy.[13]

Treatment

- Therapy must be individualized in accordance with present knowledge and with the specific desires of the patient, gestational age, and tumor stage and biology.
- At all times, maternal treatment should adhere to standard recommendations.
- At the time of diagnosis, it is important to have a baseline assessment of fetal growth/development by ultrasound as well as routine fetal monitoring throughout the pregnancy/treatment.[14]

Local Therapy
- Consideration should be given to the delay of irradiation until after delivery.

Pregnancy Termination
- Survival outcomes are similar if the patient has a spontaneous pregnancy loss, choses to terminate, or continues with the pregnancy.[5,15]

Chemotherapy
- Women who present with either metastatic breast carcinoma or rapidly progressive inflammatory carcinoma should avoid any delays in therapy.
- If there is a clinical indication for adjuvant chemotherapy other than inflammatory carcinoma, the delay of instituting chemotherapy and awaiting fetal pulmonary maturity should be considered in select third-trimester situations.

Prognosis

- Outcomes in stage I and II disease are favorable, and survival rates approach 86% to 100%. However, the presence and extent of nodal involvement is especially predictive of prognosis in both nonpregnant and pregnant patients.[5]
- Probably because of the associated delays in diagnosis, pregnancy appears to increase the frequency of nodal disease, with 53% to 71% of patients exhibiting nodal involvement at diagnosis.[16,17]

Subsequent Pregnancy
- It is generally advised that women with node-negative disease wait 2 to 3 years, and this interval should be extended to 5 years for patients with positive nodes.

Lactation and Breast Reconstruction

- Lactation is possible in a small percentage of patients after breast-conserving therapy for early-stage breast cancer.[18]
- Because data are limited, it may be best to address reconstruction in the postpartum period.

HEMATOLOGIC MALIGNANCIES

Hodgkin Lymphoma

- Hodgkin lymphoma (HL) is the second most commonly diagnosed cancer in women aged 15 to 29 years, and it presents at a mean age of 32 years.
- The routine evaluation for HL during pregnancy includes a single anterior/posterior view chest radiograph, liver function tests, serum creatinine clearance, complete blood cell count, erythrocyte sedimentation rate, and lymph node and bone marrow biopsy.
- Most investigators agree that treatment should not be withheld during pregnancy except in early-stage disease, particularly if the diagnosis is made in late gestation. Termination of pregnancy should therefore not be routinely advised.[19,20]
- General recommendations, therefore, include delaying therapy until at least the second trimester due to the increased first-trimester fetal risk. After the first trimester, therapy should not be delayed for patients with symptomatic, subdiaphragmatic, or progressive HL. Radiotherapy to the supradiaphragmatic regions may be performed with abdominal shielding after the first trimester.
- Following therapy for HL, it has been suggested that pregnancy planning should take into consideration that about 80% of recurrences manifest within 2 years.
- More recent series have shown the pregnancy rate among reproductive-age HL survivors to be similar to that of the normal female population.

Non-Hodgkin Lymphoma

- In general, non-Hodgkin lymphoma is more likely to complicate pregnancy because more patients have an aggressive histology and advanced-stage disease.
- With the exception of aggressive histologic types, the management of lymphoma may be deferred in the first trimester due to the typical, indolent nature of disease.

ACUTE LEUKEMIA

- Acute leukemia represents about 90% of leukemias that coexist with pregnancy. Acute myeloid leukemia accounts for about 60% and acute lymphoblastic leukemia for about 30% of cases. More than three-fourths of the cases are diagnosed after the first trimester.[19,21] The prognosis for acute leukemia in pregnancy is guarded.[21]
- Acute leukemia requires immediate treatment regardless of gestational age because delay may result in poorer maternal outcomes. However, numerous reports have documented successful pregnancies in patients with acute leukemia who were aggressively treated with leukapheresis and combination chemotherapy in the second and third trimesters.[19]
- Though reports have shown no serious long-term effects of in utero exposure to chemotherapy, it is important to counsel patients that acute leukemia and its therapy are associated with a high rates of spontaneous abortions, stillbirths, preterm deliveries, and fetal growth restriction.
- If the mother is exposed to cytotoxic drugs within 1 month of delivery, the newborn should be monitored closely for evidence of granulocytopenia or thrombocytopenia.

CHRONIC LEUKEMIA

- Chronic myelocytic leukemia tends to be indolent, and normal hematopoiesis is only mildly affected in the early stages of disease. Therefore delay of aggressive treatment is more feasible than with acute leukemia.

MELANOMA

- The incidence of malignant melanoma is increasing in the childbearing years, with reported ranges from 1% to 3.3% in pregnant or lactating women. It accounts for 8% of malignancies diagnosed in gestation.[1,7,22]
- After correcting for tumor thickness, survival rates are similar, and there is no increase in poor prognostic location of lesions in the pregnant patient and comparable survival outcomes to nonpregnant cohorts.[22,23]
- The methods used to describe the depth of invasion for melanoma are depicted in Fig. 50.1. Wide surgical excision with appropriate margins remains the most effective modality for the treatment of melanoma.
- Given the aggressive nature of the current therapies available for metastatic disease, it is appropriate to consider termination when managing advanced disease presenting in the first trimester.
- It is generally recommended that patients wait 2 to 3 years before attempting another pregnancy, especially with nodal disease.[24]

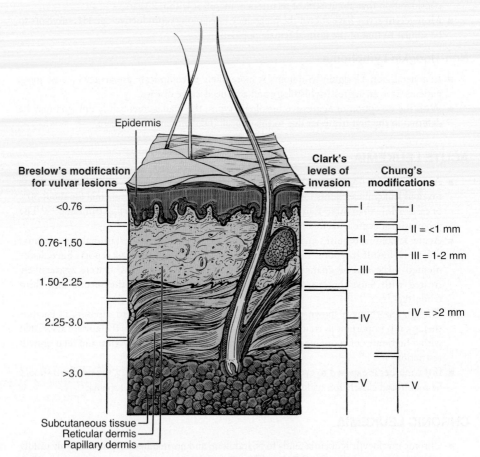

Fig. 50.1 Schematic comparison of the different levels of invasion for melanoma. (*From Gordon AN. Vulvar tumors. In Copeland LJ [ed]:* Textbook of Gynecology, *ed 2. Philadelphia: WB Saunders; 2000:1202.*)

CERVICAL CANCER

- Cervical cancer is the most common gynecologic malignancy associated with pregnancy. It occurs in approximately 1 to 2 per 2000 to 10,000 pregnancies, and approximately 3% (1 in 34 cases) of all invasive cervical cancers occur during pregnancy.[1,7,9]
- False-negative cervical cytology is at increased risk in pregnancy owing to excess mucus and bleeding from cervical eversion. Therefore it is necessary to obtain a biopsy to ensure that tissue friability or a lesion is not secondary to tumor.
- Although endocervical curettage is not recommended during pregnancy, lesions that involve the lower endocervical canal can often be directly visualized and biopsied. Whereas the pregnant cervix is hypervascular, serious hemorrhage from an outpatient biopsy is uncommon, and the risk of bleeding is offset by the risk of missing an early invasive cancer.
- Therapeutic conization for intraepithelial squamous lesions is contraindicated during pregnancy. Diagnostic cone biopsy in pregnancy is reserved for patients whose colposcopic-directed biopsy has shown superficial invasion (suspected microinvasion) or in other situations in which an invasive lesion is suspected but cannot be confirmed by biopsy.
- The diagnosis of cervical cancer is commonly made postpartum rather than during pregnancy. Furthermore, although stage IB disease is the most common stage found, all stages are represented in significant numbers.

Microinvasion

- In patients with a microinvasive squamous carcinoma with negative margins on cone biopsy, consideration can be given to conservative management until delivery.

Invasive, Early-Stage Disease

- Because the definitive treatment of invasive cervical cancer is not compatible with continuation of pregnancy, the clinical question that must be addressed is when to proceed with delivery so that therapy can be completed.
- Treatment options will be influenced by gestational age, tumor stage and metastatic evaluation, and maternal desires and expectations regarding the pregnancy.

Invasive, Locally Advanced Disease

- The patient with a first-trimester pregnancy can usually be treated in the standard fashion with initiation of chemotherapy and external radiation therapy to the pelvis or an extended field, as dictated by standard treatment guidelines. Most of these patients proceed to miscarry within 2 to 5 weeks of initiating the radiation.

Invasive, Distant Metastasis

- Metastatic disease to extrapelvic sites carries a poor prognosis. Although a select few patients with aortic node metastasis may receive curative therapy, it is unlikely for the patient with pulmonary metastasis, bone metastasis, or supraclavicular lymph node metastasis to be cured.
- Personal patient choices and ethical considerations are the major factors guiding treatment in these situations.

Method of Delivery

- Whether vaginal delivery promotes systemic dissemination of tumor cells is unknown, although the general opinion is that survival rates are not influenced by the mode of delivery.
- The episiotomy should be carefully followed in a cervical cancer patient who delivers vaginally.

Survival

- Although some authors have suggested that the survival of patients with cervical cancer associated with pregnancy is compromised, most reports indicate that the prognosis is not altered.[25]

OVARIAN CANCER

- Although adnexal masses are often observed in pregnancy, only 2% to 5% are malignant ovarian tumors.[26] Overall, ovarian cancer occurs in approximately 1 in 10,000 to 1 in 56,000 pregnancies.[9,26]
- Whereas the three major categories of ovarian tumors (i.e., epithelial), including borderline tumors, germ cell, and sex-cord stromal, occur during pregnancy, the majority are diagnosed in early stages and result in favorable outcomes.[26]
- The majority of epithelial ovarian tumors that complicate pregnancy are grade 1, or low malignant potential, or early stage; not uncommonly, these tumors are both low grade and stage I.
- Skilled sonographic examination or MRI (Fig. 50.2) is essential to determining the potential for malignancy based on size and imaging characteristics.
- Prompt surgical exploration is also performed for the mass associated with ascites or when metastatic disease is evident.
- When a malignant ovarian tumor is encountered at laparotomy, surgical intervention should be similar to that for the nonpregnant patient.
- Virilizing ovarian tumors during pregnancy are most commonly secondary to thecalutein cysts, and their evaluation and management should be conservative.

Postoperative Adjuvant Therapy

- Patients with advanced epithelial tumors should receive combination chemotherapy. The standard therapy is the combination of a platinum agent and paclitaxel, and tolerability of this regimen in pregnancy has been demonstrated.[27]

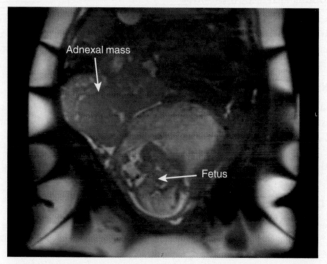

Fig. 50.2 Magnetic resonance imaging of an ovarian malignancy diagnosed during pregnancy.

VULVAR AND VAGINAL CANCER

- Because vulvar and vaginal cancers usually occur after age 40 years, the diagnosis of either disease concurrent with pregnancy is rare.

ENDOMETRIAL CANCER

- With a thorough evaluation excluding metastatic disease and extensive counseling, these patients may be candidates for conservative treatment with hormonal manipulation, repeat endometrial evaluation, and modifications of risk factors in order to preserve fertility.

GASTROINTESTINAL CANCERS

Upper Gastrointestinal Cancers

- Stomach and hepatic cancer are rarely diagnosed in women during the reproductive years.
- During pregnancy, persistent severe upper gastrointestinal symptoms are best evaluated by gastroduodenoscopy rather than radiologic studies.
- In patients with unresectable hepatomas, therapeutic abortion can be considered to decrease the risk of subsequent rupture and bleeding.

Colon and Rectal Cancer

- The incidence of colon cancer during pregnancy is about 1 in 13,000 live-born deliveries.[28]
- The majority of colorectal carcinomas during pregnancy are rectal and palpable on rectal examination, in contrast to more proximal lesions found in the nonpregnant patient.[28]
- Management of colon cancer is determined by gestational age at diagnosis and tumor stage. During the first half of pregnancy, colon resection with anastomosis is indicated for colon or appendiceal cancers.[29] In late pregnancy, a diverting colostomy may be necessary to relieve a colonic obstruction and allow the development of fetal maturity before instituting definitive therapy.

URINARY TRACT CANCERS

- Bladder and renal cancers are extremely rare during pregnancy.
- Diagnosis of renal cell carcinoma is typically made by a combination of symptoms, including the presence of a palpable mass, flank pain, refractory urinary tract symptoms, or hematuria.
- Bladder cancer common symptoms are painless hematuria, abdominal pain, and it can be diagnosed on routine obstetric ultrasound examination.

Central Nervous System Tumors

- The spectrum of central nervous system tumors found in pregnant patients is similar to those found in nonpregnant patients.[30]
- Whereas high-grade glial tumors should undergo prompt diagnosis and treatment, low-grade glial tumors such as astrocytomas and oligodendrogliomas do not usually require immediate intervention.

Neonatal Outcomes

- The impact of cancer and its therapy on the fetus/neonate needs to be considered. Consultation with maternal-fetal medicine and the neonatology team as soon as possible is recommended.

- Around 50% will be admitted to the neonatal intensive care unit with prematurity as the most common indication.[3] Neonates who were exposed to chemotherapy for acute lymphoblastic leukemia or near the time of delivery may experience hematologic toxicity.

Fetal-Placental Metastasis

- Metastatic spread of a maternal primary tumor to the placenta or fetus is rare. In general, the biologically aggressive spectrum of malignancies seem to carry the highest risk for fetal metastases.
- Malignant melanoma is the most frequently reported tumor metastatic to the placenta, and it also has a high rate of fetal metastases.[31,32]

Fertility Preservation

- The risk of infertility may be a direct result of the disease, surgery, chemotherapy agents and dose, radiation, and age.
- Though based on limited studies and selection bias, the use of fertility preservation techniques in appropriately selected patients has not been shown to have inferior oncologic outcomes when compared to standard therapy.
- Surgical options for fertility preservation include radical trachelectomy and ovarian transposition for cervical cancer and retention of the contralateral ovary and uterus in ovarian cancer.

Gestational Trophoblastic Disease and Pregnancy-Related Issues

HYDATIDIFORM MOLE (COMPLETE MOLE)

- The incidence of hydatidiform mole has great geographic variability. In the United States, it occurs in approximately 1 in 1000 to 1 in 1500 pregnancies. Approximately 95% of complete hydatidiform moles have a 46, XX paternal homologous chromosomal pattern.
- The safest technique for evacuating a hydatidiform mole is with the suction aspiration technique. Oxytocin should not be initiated until the patient is in the operating room and evacuation is imminent in order to minimize the risk of embolization of trophoblastic tissue.
- For the patient with a complete molar pregnancy, the risk of requiring chemotherapy for persistent gestational trophoblastic disease (GTD) is approximately 20%.

INVASIVE MOLE (CHORIOADENOMA DESTRUENS)

- Because invasion of the myometrium by molar tissue is clinically occult, it is difficult to assess the true incidence, and it is estimated to be between 5% and 10%.
- The clinical hallmark of an invasive mole is hemorrhage, which can be severe, and either vaginal or intraperitoneal.

PARTIAL HYDATIDIFORM MOLE

- Most partial moles have a triploid (paternally inherited, diandric, triploidies) karyotype, and the next most common are tetraploidies.
- The management of a patient with sonographic findings suggestive of a diagnosis of a partial mole is particularly challenging if the karyotype analysis of the fetus is diploid, especially if the diagnosis is made in the second or third trimester.
- Approximately 2% to 6% of patients develop persistent GTD after a partial molar pregnancy.[33]

PLACENTAL SITE TROPHOBLASTIC TUMOR

- Less than 1% of all patients with GTD have placental site trophoblastic tumor.
- This tumor usually presents with abnormal vaginal bleeding following a term pregnancy. The β-hCG level may not reliably reflect disease progression.

CHORIOCARCINOMA

- Choriocarcinoma develops in approximately 1 in every 40,000 term pregnancies, and this clinical presentation represents about one-fourth of all cases of choriocarcinoma. The other cases follow molar disease or an abortion (spontaneous, therapeutic, or ectopic).
- Choriocarcinoma is notorious for masquerading as other diseases. This is secondary to hemorrhagic metastases producing symptoms such as hematuria, hemoptysis, hematemesis, hematochezia, stroke, or vaginal bleeding. It is also important to rule out phantom β-hCG production if the clinical scenario warrants, such as situations with low titers and no histologic or convincing imaging evidence of GTD.

References for this chapter are available at ExpertConsult.com.

CHAPTER 51

Skin Disease and Pregnancy

Annie R. Wang ■ George Kroumpouzos

KEY POINTS

- With the physiologic skin changes of pregnancy, no risks are incurred for the mother or fetus. The changes should be expected to resolve postpartum.
- Preexisting melanocytic nevi may show mild changes in pregnancy, but no increased risk for malignant transformation exists.
- Preexisting skin disorders are more likely to worsen than improve in pregnancy; atopic dermatitis (eczema) is the most common dermatosis in pregnancy.
- Prognosis of melanoma is not adversely affected by pregnancy.
- Pruritus occurs in up to 3% to 14% of pregnancies. A constellation of clinical and laboratory findings is crucial to establishing etiology.
- Impetigo herpetiformis (pustular psoriasis of pregnancy) is often associated with reduced calcium or vitamin D. Serious maternal and fetal risks are associated with this disease.
- PG typically flares at delivery, and treatment is with oral steroids. Mild fetal risks—such as small-for-gestational-age infants, preterm delivery, and neonatal PG—have been associated with this disease.
- PEP commonly starts in the abdominal striae and spares the periumbilical area. It is associated with multiple gestation pregnancy, but no maternal or fetal risks are apparent.
- PP and PFP carry no maternal or fetal risks.

Physiologic Skin Changes Induced by Pregnancy

- Although they may prompt cosmetic complaints, such physiologic changes are not associated with risks to the mother or fetus and can be expected to resolve or improve postpartum (Box 51.1).
- Mild forms of localized or generalized hyperpigmentation occur to some extent in up to 90% of pregnant women.
- Melasma usually resolves postpartum but may recur in subsequent pregnancies or with the use of oral contraceptives (Fig. 51.1).
- The pyogenic granuloma of pregnancy, known as *granuloma gravidarum* or *pregnancy epulis,* is a benign proliferation of capillaries that usually occurs in the gingiva.
- *Striae gravidarum,* also called *striae distensae* or "stretch marks," develop in up to 90% of white women between the sixth and seventh months of gestation.
- Increased eccrine function has been reported during pregnancy and may account for the increased prevalence of miliaria, hyperhidrosis, and dyshidrosis. Conversely, apocrine activity may decrease.
- Postpartum hair shedding (*telogen effluvium*) may be noted as a greater proportion of hairs enter the telogen phase.

BOX 51.1 ■ Physiologic Skin Changes in Pregnancy

Pigmentary

Common

Hyperpigmentation
Melasma

Uncommon

Jaundice
Pseudoacanthotic changes
Dermal melanocytosis
Hyperkeratosis of the nipple
Vulvar melanosis

Hair Cycle and Growth

Hirsutism
Postpartum telogen effluvium
Postpartum male-pattern alopecia
Diffuse hair thinning (late pregnancy)

Nail

Subungual hyperkeratosis
Distal onycholysis
Transverse grooving
Brittleness and softening

Glandular

Increased eccrine function
Increased sebaceous function
Decreased apocrine function

Connective Tissue

Striae
Skin tags (*molluscum fibrosum gravidarum*)

Vascular

Spider telangiectasias
Pyogenic granuloma (*granuloma gravidarum*)
Palmar erythema
Nonpitting edema
Severe labial edema
Varicosities
Vasomotor instability
Gingival hyperemia
Hemorrhoids

Mucous Membrane

Gingivitis
Chadwick sign
Goodell sign

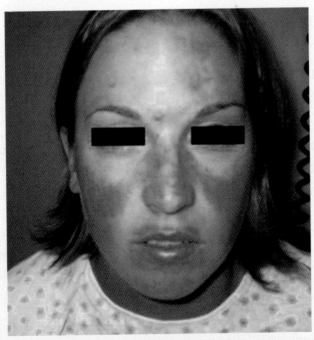

Fig. 51.1   Centrofacial type of melasma involving the cheeks, nose, upper lip, and forehead.

Preexisting Skin Diseases and Tumors Affected by Pregnancy

- Pregnancy can aggravate or, less often, improve many skin conditions and primary skin tumors.

ATOPIC ECZEMA AND DERMATITIS

- Treatment for gestational exacerbations of atopic dermatitis (AD) is primarily symptomatic. A moisturizer and low-potency to mid-potentcy topical steroid is the first-line treatment.

ACNE VULGARIS

- In one study, pregnancy affected acne in approximately 70% of women, with 41% reporting improvement and 29% reporting a worsening with pregnancy.

OTHER INFLAMMATORY SKIN DISEASES

- Women with existing chronic psoriasis can be counseled that between 40% and 63% of women have symptomatic improvement, compared with only 14% of women who have symptomatic deterioration.

AUTOIMMUNE PROGESTERONE DERMATITIS

- Autoimmune progesterone dermatitis is caused by hypersensitivity to progesterone through autoimmune or nonimmune mechanisms.

IMPETIGO HERPETIFORMIS

- Impetigo herpetiformis is a rare variant of generalized pustular psoriasis that develops primarily during pregnancy, often in association with hypocalcemia or low serum levels of vitamin D (Fig. 51.2).
- Whereas maternal prognosis is excellent with early diagnosis, aggressive treatment, and supportive care, an increased risk of perinatal mortality may persist despite maternal treatment.

Cutaneous Manifestations of Autoimmune Disorders

BULLOUS DISORDERS

- Pemphigus vulgaris, vegetans, or foliaceus may develop or worsen during pregnancy.

SKIN TUMORS

- Melanocytic nevi may develop, enlarge, or darken during pregnancy, but these changes are less dramatic than previously thought.

MALIGNANT MELANOMA

- Several epidemiologic studies to evaluate the effect of pregnancy status at diagnosis suggest that the 5-year survival rate is not affected after controlling for confounding factors.

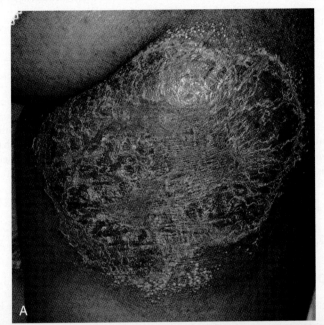

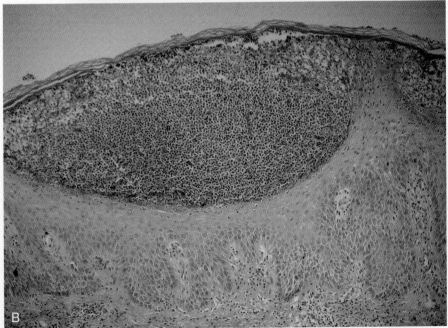

Fig. 51.2 **A,** Impetigo herpetiformis: discrete, grouped, sterile pustules at the periphery of an erythematous crusted plaque. **B,** Histopathology of impetigo herpetiformis shows the characteristic Kogoj spongiform pustule, formed of neutrophils in the uppermost portion of the spinous layer (hematoxylin-eosin stain). (*Courtesy Aleksandr Itkin, MD.*)

- Wide local excision of the primary melanoma should be performed in stages I through III, and conservative excision should be undertaken in stage IV.
- Sentinel lymph node biopsy is the most powerful prognostic factor in clinically localized melanoma.
- Melanoma is the most common type of malignancy to metastasize to the placenta and fetus, and it represents 31% of such metastases.

Pruritus in Pregnancy

- Itching is the most common dermatologic symptom in pregnancy. Mild prurutis is common and occurs most frequently over the abdomen. However, a broad differential diagnosis needs to be considered; the constellation of clinical and laboratory findings will help establish a diagnosis and guide management decisions.

Specific Dermatoses of Pregnancy

- Specific dermatoses of pregnancy refer only to those skin diseases that result directly from the state of gestation or the products of conception (Table 51.1).

PEMPHIGOID (HERPES) GESTATIONIS

- Pemphigoid gestationis (PG) is a rare autoimmune skin disease that affects between 1 in 7000 and 1 in 50,000 pregnancies.
- PG usually presents in the second or third trimester of pregnancy with extremely pruritic urticarial lesions that typically begin on the abdomen and trunk and commonly involve the umbilicus (Fig. 51.3, *A*).
- Although the differential diagnosis of PG includes drug eruption, erythema multiforme, and allergic contact dermatitis, the most common diagnosis to exclude is the far more common polymorphic eruption of pregnancy (PEP) (see below). PEP can manifest with urticarial and/or vesicular lesions almost indistinguishable from those of PG, although PEP classically begins in the abdominal striae and spares the umbilicus.
- Oral corticosteroids remain the cornerstone of treatment in PG.
- An association with small-for-gestational-age infants and preterm delivery has been reported.
- Approximately 5% to 10% of neonates will manifest bullous skin lesions (neonatal PG) secondary to passive transplacental transfer of PG antibody.

POLYMORPHIC ERUPTION OF PREGNANCY

- PEP, also known as *pruritic urticarial papules and plaques of pregnancy*, is the most common specific dermatosis of pregnancy and affects between 1 in 130 and 1 in 300 pregnancies.
- Lesions typically begin in the abdominal striae and spare the periumbilical region in up to two-thirds of cases (Fig. 51.4, *A*).
- A meta-analysis revealed a tenfold higher prevalence of multiple gestation in pregnancies affected by PEP.
- PEP is not associated with adverse maternal or fetal outcomes.

ATOPIC ERUPTION OF PREGNANCY

- Atopic eruption of pregnancy (AEP) is a clinical entity that encompasses prurigo of pregnancy (PP), pruritic folliculitis of pregnancy (PFP), and AD; this includes *new* AD, defined as AD that develops for the first time in gestation.

TABLE 51.1 ■ Overview of Specific Dermatoses of Pregnancy

	U.S. Rates	Clinical Data	Lesion Morphology and Distribution	Important Laboratory Findings	Fetal Risks
Pemphigoid gestationis (PG)	1:50,000	Second or third trimester or postpartum Flare at delivery (75%) Resolution postpartum with a good chance of recurrence in future pregnancies	Abdominal urticarial lesions progress into a generalized bullous eruption.	Skin immunofluorescence shows linear deposition of C3 along basement membrane.	Neonatal PG SGA infants Preterm delivery
Polymorphic eruption of pregnancy (PEP)	1:130 to 1:300	Third trimester or postpartum Primigravidae Resolution postpartum Association with multiple gestation No recurrence in future pregnancies	Polymorphous eruption starts in the abdominal striae and shows periumbilical sparing.	None	None
Atopic eruption of pregnancy (AEP)	>50% of pruritic dermatoses	First or second trimester Resolution postpartum with possible recurrence in future pregnancies	Flexural surfaces, neck, chest, trunk	Serum IgE elevations (20% to 70%)	None
Prurigo of pregnancy (PP)	1:300 to 1:450	Second or third trimester Resolution postpartum with recurrence in future pregnancies	Grouped excoriated papules over the extensor extremities and occasionally the abdomen	None	None
Pruritic folliculitis of pregnancy (PFP)	>30 cases	Second or third trimester Resolution postpartum with possible recurrence in future pregnancies	Follicular papules and pustules	Biopsy: sterile folliculitis	None

Modified from Kroumpouzos, G, Cohen LM. Specific dermatoses of pregnancy: an evidence-based systematic review. *Am J Obstet Gynecol.* 2003;188:1082–1092. Ig, immunoglobulin; SGA, small for gestational age.

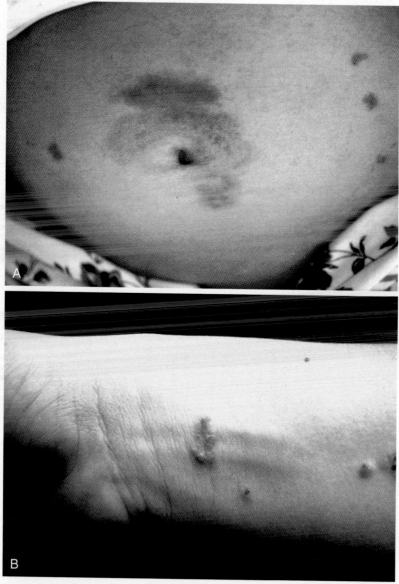

Fig. 51.3   A, Pruritic abdominal urticarial plaques develop in the early phase of pemphigoid (herpes) gestationis and typically involve the umbilicus. **B,** Characteristic tense vesicles on an erythematous base on the forearm in a patient with PG. (*From Kroumpouzos G: Skin disease. In James DK, Steer PJ, Weiner CP, Gonik B, Crowther CA, Robson SC:* High-Risk Pregnancy: Management Options, *4th ed, Philadelphia: Elsevier Saunders; 2011, p. 929.*)

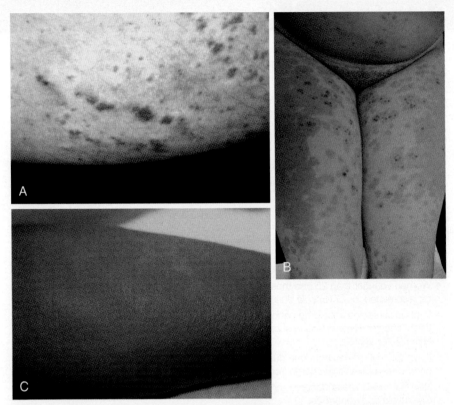

Fig. 51.4   A, Pruritic urticarial papules and plaques of pregnancy (PUPPP) include urticarial lesions that typically start in the abdominal striae. **B,** Vesicular lesions superimposed on urticarial plaques and targetoid lesions reminiscent of erythema multiforme or pemphigoid (herpes) gestationis. **C,** Widespread PUPPP may resemble a toxic erythema or atopic dermatitis. (*Courtesy Helen Raynham, MD.*)

- The earlier onset, prior to the third trimester, may help distinguish AEP from other pregnancy dermatoses such as pemphigoid gestationis and PEP.

PRURIGO OF PREGNANCY

- PP affects between 1 in 300 and 1 in 450 pregnancies. It manifests itself with grouped excoriated or crusted pruritic papules over the extensor surfaces of the extremities and occasionally on the trunk and elsewhere (see Table 51.1).
- PP has not been associated with increased maternal risk.
- It has been proposed that PP and intrahepatic cholestasis of pregnancy are closely related conditions, distinguished only by the absence of primary lesions in intrahepatic cholestasis of pregnancy.

PRURITIC FOLLICULITIS OF PREGNANCY

- PFP is a rare specific dermatosis of pregnancy.
- PFP presents with pruritic follicular erythematous papules and pustules that affect primarily the trunk.
- PFP resolves postpartum and has not been associated with substantial risks for the fetus.

CHAPTER 52

Maternal and Perinatal Infection: *Chlamydia,* Gonorrhea, and Syphilis in Pregnancy

Jessica L. Nyholm ■ Kirk D. Ramin ■ Daniel V. Landers

KEY POINTS

- All pregnant women younger than 25 years or those at increased risk should be screened for *Chlamydia* and gonorrhea during pregnancy.
- Women younger than 25 and those at high risk for sexually transmitted infections should be rescreened for *Chlamydia* during the third trimester.
- Syphilis screening should be performed at the first prenatal visit as well as early in the third trimester. Repeat testing should be performed at the time of delivery in patients at high risk for syphilis.
- If syphilis testing was not done during pregnancy, it should be performed postpartum prior to the patient's discharge from the hospital.
- NAATs of urine, the endocervix, or the vagina is the preferred screening test for both *Chlamydia* and gonorrhea.
- Screening for syphilis can be performed using either a treponemal or nontreponemal test.
- Penicillin is the antimicrobial of choice in treating syphilis among pregnant women and for reducing the incidence of congenital syphilis.
- Pregnant women with a penicillin allergy and syphilis infection should undergo penicillin desensitization with subsequent penicillin therapy.

Chlamydia

EPIDEMIOLOGY

- The two most valuable sources of incidence and prevalence data on sexually transmitted pathogens are provided by the Centers for Disease Control and Prevention (CDC) and the World Health Organization (WHO).
- Overall, the WHO 2008 global estimate places the incidence at 105.7 million new cases of *Chlamydia* infection, 106.1 million new cases of gonorrhea, and 10.6 million new cases of syphilis among people aged 15 to 49 years.
- Genital tract chlamydial infections are generally ascribed to *Chlamydia trachomatis* and account for the most prevalent reported infectious disease in the United States.
- These infections present unique problems for public health control programs because 50% to 70% of these infections are clinically silent in women.

- Most reported infections occur in the 15- to 24-year-old age group.
- The endorsement of a nationwide broad-based screening program by both the CDC and Institute of Medicine.

PATHOGENESIS

- Only *C. trachomatis* and *C. pneumoniae* claim primates as their endogenous hosts.
- Chlamydiae are obligate intracellular bacteria that grow in eukaryotic epithelial cells, and they have a unique growth cycle, distinct from all other pathogens.
- Because chlamydiae depend on their host cell for the generation of adenosine triphosphate, they require viable cells for survival.[1]
- Major outer membrane protein is a major target for protective host immune responses, such as neutralizing antibodies and possibly protective T-cell responses.[2,3]
- Chronic immune activation plays a role in propagating clinical disease.[4]
- Aberrations in humoral immunity also appear to modulate clinical disease.

DIAGNOSIS

- Because curative antibiotic therapies for chlamydial infections are available and inexpensive, early diagnosis is an essential component of management and prevention.
- Chlamydial culture has been replaced by nucleic acid amplification tests (NAATs).
- NAATs can be utilized to test for *C. trachomatis* in endocervical swabs from women, urethral swabs from men, first-catch urine from both men and women, and vaginal swabs from women.[5] The ability of NAATs to detect *C. trachomatis* without a pelvic examination is a key advantage of NAATs, and this ability facilitates screening men and women in nontraditional screening venues.
- Other antigen-detection methods—such as enzyme immunoassay, direct fluorescence assay, nucleic acid hybridization/probe tests, and nucleic acid genetic transformation tests—are also available but are generally not recommended for routine testing for genital tract specimens.

TREATMENT

- In pregnancy, the CDC recommends azithromycin in a single 1-g oral dose (Box 52.1).
- Doxycycline, ofloxacin, and levofloxacin are part of the treatment options in a nonpregnant patient; however, they are contraindicated in pregnancy and should not be used in this population.
- A repeat chlamydial test should be performed 3 to 4 weeks after treatment is completed.
- Women under the age of 25 and patients at high risk for *Chlamydia* infection should be retested in the third trimester of pregnancy.

Gonorrhea

EPIDEMIOLOGY

- The single greatest determinant of gonorrhea incidence since 1975 has so far been age: annual reported cases are highest in adolescents aged 15 to 19 years (459.2 per 100,000) and in young adults aged 20 to 24 years (541.6 per 100,000).[6]

PATHOGENESIS

- *Neisseria gonorrhoeae* is a gram-negative diplococcus for which humans are the only natural host.
- Rather, gonococci persist in the host by virtue of their ability to alter the host environment.

> **BOX 52.1 ■ Recommended Treatment Regimens* for *Chlamydia trachomatis* Infections in Pregnancy†**
>
> **Recommended Regimen†**
>
> Azithromycin, 1 g orally in a single dose
>
> **Alternative Regimens**
>
> Amoxicillin 500 mg orally 3 times a day for 7 days *or*
> Erythromycin base, 500 mg orally 4 times a day for 7 days *or*
> Erythromycin base, 250 mg orally 4 times a day for 14 days *or*
> Erythromycin ethylsuccinate, 800 mg orally 4 times a day for 7 days *or*
> Erythromycin ethylsuccinate, 400 mg orally 4 times a day for 14 days
>
> ---
>
> **The Centers for Disease Control and Prevention recommends treating individuals with a positive* Chlamydia*-sensitive nucleic acid amplification test. Although tetracycline and doxycycline have the greatest activity against* C. trachomatis, *these drugs should not be used in pregnancy because of their effects on bone and on dental enamel of the developing fetus (see Chapter 8). Owing to gastrointestinal side effects with erythromycin, azithromycin is the drug of choice in pregnancy.*
> *†Sex partners within the preceding 60 days of diagnosis or the most recent sex partner, if that has been longer than 60 days, should be evaluated and treated also.*
> *Modified from Workowski KA, Bolan GA; Centers for Disease Control and Prevention. Sexually transmitted diseases treatment guidelines, 2015. MMWR Morb Mortal Wkly Rep. 2015;64(RR-03):1-137.*

DIAGNOSIS

- The gold standard for diagnosis of gonorrhea infection was previously isolation of the organism by culture.
- Antimicrobial therapy should be initiated following an initial presumptive test result, but additional tests must be performed to confirm the identity of an isolate as *N. gonorrhoeae*.
- Indications for culture for *N. gonorrhoeae* include testing in suspected cases of treatment failure, monitoring antibiotic resistance, and testing in cases of suspected extragenital infection and exposure due to sexual abuse.
- The current recommended test for routine screening for *N. gonorrhoeae* is NAATs.
- NAATs can be utilized to test for *N. gonorrhoeae* in endocervical swabs from women, urethral swabs from men, first-catch urine from both men and women, and vaginal swabs from women.[5] The ability of NAATs to detect *N. gonorrhoeae* without a pelvic examination is a key advantage of NAATs, and this ability facilitates screening men and women in nontraditional screening venues.
- Given the performance of NAATs, supplemental testing of NAAT-positive specimens is no longer recommended by the CDC.

TREATMENT

- Because of the risk for coinfectivity with *N. gonorrhoeae* and *C. trachomatis,* the CDC recommends empirically treating patients with positive gonorrhea test results for both gonorrhea and *Chlamydia.*[5]
- In 2007, the Gonococcal Isolate Surveillance Project found 27% of *N. gonorrhoeae* infections were resistant to penicillin, tetracycline, ciprofloxacin, or a combination of these antibiotics. In 2009, the CDC Working Group for Cephalosporin-Resistant Gonorrhea Outbreak Response Plan was convened to address the growing resistance to these antibiotics by *N. gonorrhoeae.*[7] In their *Morbidity and Mortality Weekly Report* from May of 2011,

the CDC reviewed five cases of urethral gonorrhea with high mean inhibitory capacities (9.1%) of azithromycin, which represented 10% of those treated for *N. gonorrhoeae* in San Diego County from August to October of 2009.[8] In this monograph, the CDC reinforced the 2010 STD Treatment Guidelines that recommend dual therapy with 250 mg ceftriaxone and 1 g of azithromycin orally for uncomplicated urogenital, rectal, and pharyngeal gonorrhea. The CDC does not recommend azithromycin as monotherapy in the treatment of gonorrhea due to the concern over development of resistance and reported treatment failures. Spectinomycin can be used to treat uncomplicated urogenital infections with good success; however, it is expensive and not produced in the United States.

Syphilis

EPIDEMIOLOGY

- Historically, syphilis has long been recognized as a chronic systemic infectious process secondary to infection with the spirochete *Treponema pallidum*.

PATHOGENESIS

- Syphilis is a chronic disease caused by the spirochete *T. pallidum*.
- Following mucosal invasion, an incubation period of about 1 week to 3 months ensues until the chancre appears to herald the primary infection. The chancre arises at the point of entry by the spirochetes and is a broad-based, typically nontender ulcerated lesion that gives a characteristic "woody" or "rubbery" feel on palpation. It is seldom secondarily infected, and it resolves without medical treatment in 3 to 6 weeks. The organism then hematogenously spreads through the body during the period in which the immune system has responded, usually about 4 to 10 weeks.[9] Secondary syphilis is characterized by a generalized maculopapular eruption, constitutional symptoms, major organ involvement, and lymphadenopathy. Like the other major organ systems, the central nervous system is invaded in about 40% of individuals during this hematogenous phase.[10,11] Secondary syphilis resolves over 2 to 6 weeks as the patient enters the latent phase of the disease.[9] The latent phase is divided into *early latent* (<1 year) and *late latent* (>1 year) disease, during which no symptoms or signs of clinical disease are noted. If left untreated, progression to tertiary disease with cardiovascular system, central nervous system, and musculoskeletal system involvement occurs. The organism has an affinity for the arterioles, and the inflammatory response that follows results in obliterative endarteritis and subsequent end-organ destruction.[12]

DIAGNOSIS

- The ability to diagnose infection with *T. pallidum* has been problematic for two primary reasons. The first is the failure of the organism, as of yet, to be cultured on an artificial medium. The second lies in the long-recognized tendency of the clinical manifestations to mimic a variety of other diseases.
- If primary syphilis is suspected, examination of the serous exudates from the chancre under darkfield microscopy can definitively diagnose the condition by identification of the flexuous-bodied (spiral) organism.
- Because most individuals infected with *T. pallidum* are in the asymptomatic latent phase of the disease, serologic testing is the primary means of diagnosis.
- For most individuals, the treponemal tests remain positive lifelong.[13]
- The following recommendations for diagnosing syphilis in HIV-infected individuals have been made by the CDC.[14]

BOX 52.2 ■ Recommended Treatment Regimens* for *Treponema pallidum* Infections

Primary, Secondary, Early Latent Disease
Benzathine penicillin G, 2.4 million U IM as a single dose

Late Latent and Latent Disease of Unknown Duration
Benzathine penicillin G, 2.4 miU IM weekly for 3 doses (7.2 miU total)

Tertiary Disease

Neurosyphilis
Aqueous crystalline penicillin G, 18 to 24 miU/day IV (3 to 4 miU every 4 hours or continuous infusion) for 10 to 14 days *or*
Procaine penicillin G, 2.4 miU IM once daily with probenecid 500 mg PO 4 times a day for 10 to 14 days if compliance can be ensured

Without Neurosyphilis
Benzathine penicillin G, 2.4 miU IM weekly for 3 weeks (7.2 miU total)

Penicillin Allergy (Documented)

In Pregnancy
Desensitization and penicillin therapy as above

---

*The CDC recommends penicillin as the treatment of choice in individuals with syphilis.
IM, intramuscularly; *IV,* intravenously; *miU,* million units; *PO,* per os.
Modified from Workowski KA, Bolan GA; Centers for Disease Control and Prevention (CDC). Sexually transmitted diseases treatment guidelines, 2015. MMWR Morb Mortal Wkly Rep. 2015;64(RR-03):1-137.

TREATMENT

- Penicillin has been effective in the treatment of disease and in the prevention of disease progression in both nonpregnant and pregnant women, and it has also been used in the prevention and treatment of congenital syphilis (Box 52.2).[15,16]
- The initial evaluation of patients with a penicillin allergy should begin with skin testing with both major and minor determinants.[15] Those with a reported penicillin allergy and negative skin testing may receive penicillin therapy. However, patients who have had a positive skin test should undergo penicillin desensitization with subsequent administration of penicillin therapy.[15,17]

Congenital Syphilis

- Congenital syphilis infection results from transplacental migration of the organism to the fetus. Congenital disease can occur at any stage of maternal infection and at any gestational age.[18]
- Transplacental infection must be close to 100% during the early stages of maternal disease because of the known hematogenous spread, with rates of transmission falling to 10% as bacteremia abates with the subsequent mounting of the maternal immunologic response during late latent disease.[19–21]
- The risk for adverse pregnancy outcome in pregnant women with syphilis that was untreated is approximately 52%.[22] The specific risks include a higher risk for miscarriage or stillbirth (21%), neonatal death (9.3%), premature birth or low birthweight (5.8%), and clinical evidence of congenital infection (15%) when compared with the risks in women without syphilis.[22]

- Nonimmune fetal hydrops, polyhydramnios, and intrauterine fetal demise have long been associated with congenital syphilis.
- Hollier and colleagues[23] prospectively identified and followed 24 women with untreated syphilis to better define the pathophysiology of fetal disease.
- Maternal stage of disease—primary, secondary, and early latent—correlated with fetal infection rates of 50%, 67%, and 83%, respectively. Ultrasound examination was abnormal in 16 of the 24 fetuses (67%).
- This study demonstrates the utility of ultrasound examination in the diagnosis and management of the syphilis-infected gravida and her unborn child. This is supported by the CDC, which recommends sonographic evaluation of the fetus for evidence of congenital infection if syphilis is diagnosed after 20 weeks' gestation.
- In an effort to reduce the incidence of congenital syphilis, the CDC recommends screening all pregnant women at the time of their first prenatal visit and again early in the third trimester. In addition, women should be screened at delivery if not previously screened, or if they are at high risk.[15]
- It was estimated by the WHO that approximately one-third of women who received prenatal care were not tested for syphilis.[24]
- Almost 90% of stillbirths attributed to congenital syphilis occur among women who are never treated or who are treated inappropriately.[25]

⊘ *References for this chapter are available at* ExpertConsult.com.

CHAPTER 53

Maternal and Perinatal Infection in Pregnancy: Viral

Helene B. Bernstein

KEY POINTS

- Rubella immunization and HBV and HIV infection screening is standard. HIV screening should be performed via an "opt out" approach, and in high prevalence areas, repeat screening in the third trimester should be considered. Varicella screening may be considered in women without a history of infection. Routine CMV screening is not recommended secondary to high seroprevalence.

- The ACOG and the CDC recommend seasonal influenza vaccination (October through May) for all pregnant women with intramuscular inactivated vaccine. Hepatitis A virus and HBV vaccination are also safe in pregnancy and should be offered based on risk and susceptibility. Live attenuated vaccines for rubeola, rubella, and varicella infection should be deferred until after pregnancy.

- Rapid intrapartum HIV testing should be accessible to women without documented HIV status because most perinatally infected infants are born to women unaware of their HIV status.

- The standard of care for HIV infection is cART with at least three drugs from at least two classes of antiretrovirals. Early, sustained control of viral replication is associated with decreased HIV transmission. Fully suppressive preconception therapy is recommended, and cART should be started as early in pregnancy as possible for women entering pregnancy not already on cART.

- Pregnant women suspected to be infected with influenza should receive treatment immediately, without delay for diagnostic confirmation.

- Fetal parvovirus infection may result in fetal anemia and hydrops. Women with documented infection should be screened with serial ultrasounds. Middle cerebral artery Doppler studies may also be used.

- Rubeola (measles) is one of the most infectious viruses, and 75% to 90% of exposed, susceptible contacts become infected. Measles infection can cause subacute sclerosing panencephalitis, a progressive, uniformly fatal neurologic disease. Infection may originate in individuals born outside the United States, but gaps in vaccination permit the spread of outbreaks in the United States.

- CMV transmission is highest during the third trimester with a 30% to 40% fetal transmission risk. Serious sequelae are most common following first-trimester infection, whereby 24% of infected fetuses have sensorineural hearing loss and 32% have other central nervous system sequelae.

- Susceptible varicella-exposed women should receive VZIG to reduce the risk of infection and transmission. The addition of prophylactic acyclovir may further reduce maternal infection risk.

Viral Infections

- Viruses are obligate intracellular parasites that utilize the host cell's structural and functional components while exhibiting remarkably diverse strategies for gene expression and replication.
- Infection is typically initiated by the virus binding to a specific host cell receptor. For productive infection to occur, viruses must enter cells, replicate their genome, and release infectious virions.
- The host immune response to viral infection encompasses both local and systemic effects via activation of immune cells, the induction of an adaptive immune response, and the release of cytokines, chemokines, and antibodies.

Human Immunodeficiency Virus

- Human immunodeficiency virus (HIV) is a member of the Retroviridae family, characterized by spherical, enveloped viruses. Retroviruses are unique because the viral genome is transcribed into DNA via the viral enzyme reverse transcriptase, followed by integration into the host cell genome via the viral enzyme integrase. HIV also has the capacity to become latent within quiescent infected cells, which has made eradication of the virus thus far impossible.
- HIV predominantly infects CD4+ cells, including T cells, monocytes, and macrophages.
- Following exposure and primary infection, 50% to 70% of individuals infected with HIV develop the acute retroviral syndrome.

EPIDEMIOLOGY

- Most HIV-infected individuals reside outside the United States. Global HIV burden is estimated at 37 million individuals; moreover, women account for more than half of all people living with HIV. In contrast, approximately 50,000 Americans are diagnosed with HIV infection annually; women account for 20% of new HIV infections and 23% of existing infections. Women typically acquire HIV infection by heterosexual contact, and about 65% of new infections occur in black Americans.

DIAGNOSIS

- Current recommendations are to screen with an HIV-1/2 antigen/antibody combination immunoassay, or "combo assay," with confirmation of infection with an HIV-1/HIV-2 antibody differentiation immunoassay and HIV-1 nucleic acid test (Fig. 53.1).

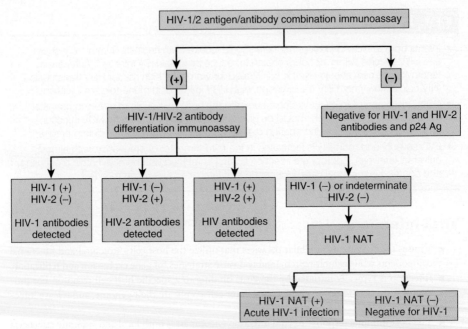

Fig. 53.1 Diagnosis of human immunodeficiency virus (HIV) infection. Ag, antigen; HIV, human immunodeficiency virus; NAT, nucleic acid test; +, reactive test result; –, nonreactive test result.

- Both the American College of Obstetrics and Gynecology (ACOG) and Centers for Disease Control and Prevention (CDC) recommend an "opt out" approach to ensure routine HIV screening for all pregnant women, ideally performed at the first prenatal visit.
- Clinicians should be aware of local legal requirements in regard to confidentiality and disclosure of HIV-related health information.

TREATMENT OBJECTIVES

- Treatment objectives for *all* infected individuals are to maximally and durably suppress viral load.
- When caring for HIV-infected pregnant women, two separate but related goals emerge: (1) treatment of maternal infection and (2) chemoprophylaxis to reduce the risk of perinatal HIV transmission.

MANAGEMENT DURING PREGNANCY

- Plasma HIV RNA (viral load) is determined using reverse transcriptase–polymerase chain reaction technology.
- Combination care with at least three drugs from at least two classes of antiretroviral drugs (ARVs) is standard care for HIV infection in the United States (Table 53.1).
- Commonly used drug classes include nucleoside/nucleotide reverse transcriptase inhibitors (NRTIs), nonnucleoside reverse transcriptase inhibitors (NNRTIs), and protease inhibitors (Table 53.2).

TABLE 53.1 ■ Treatment Recommendations for Antiretroviral-Naive Pregnant Women

Preferred Backbones and Regimens

	FDCs	Comment
Two-NRTI Backbones		
TDF/FTC or TDF/3TC	Truvada 200 mg FTC+ 300 mg TDF tablet	The recommended NRTI backbone for nonpregnant adults; can be administered once daily. TDF has potential renal toxicity and should be used with caution in patients with renal insufficiency.
ABC/3TC	Epzicom 300 mg 3TC + 600 mg ABC tablet	Can be administered once daily; ABC is associated with HSRs and should not be used in HLA-B*5701–positive patients; it may be less efficacious than TDF/FTC in patients with HIV RNA level >100,000.
ZDV/3TC	Combivir 150 mg 3TC + 200 mg ZDV tablet	Backbone with the most experience in pregnancy, disadvantages include twice-daily administration and increased toxicity; not a preferred backbone in nonpregnant adults.
PI Regimens		
ATV/r + two-NRTI backbone		Once-daily administration of ATV/r; no longer preferred in nonpregnant adults secondary to increased toxicity-related discontinuation compared with DRV- and RAL-based regimens.
DRV/r + two-NRTI backbone		Twice-daily administration of DRV/r in pregnancy; preferred PI in nonpregnant adults, increasing experience with use in pregnancy.
NNRTI Regimen		
EFV + two-NRTI backbone	Atripla 200 mg FTC + 300 mg TDF + 600 mg EFV tablet	Atripla enables once-daily administration of a single tablet regimen; concern due to observed birth defects in primates, although human risk is unconfirmed; postpartum contraception must be ensured; preferred regimen in women who require coadministration of drugs with significant PI interactions.
INSTI Regimen		
RAL + two-NRTI backbone		Twice-daily administration of RAL; preferred NRTI regimen in nonpregnant adults, increasing experience and established PK in pregnancy. Rapid viral load reduction; however, twice-daily dosing required.
Alternative Regimens		
RPV/TDF/FTC		Available in coformulated single-pill, once-daily regimen with PK pregnancy data. However, relatively little clinical experience in pregnancy and not recommended for pretreatment HIV RNA >100,000 or CD4 count <200 cells/mm³.
LPV/r + two-NRTI backbone		Twice-daily administration; once-daily LPV/r is not recommended for use in pregnant women; not a preferred PI in adults secondary to higher rates of GI side effects, hyperlipidemia, and insulin resistance.
No Longer Recommended		
SQV/r + two-NRTI backbone		Not recommended based on potential toxicity and dosing disadvantages. Baseline ECG recommended before initiation secondary to potential PR and QT prolongation; contraindicated with preexisting cardiac conduction system disease; large pill burden.

Continued

TABLE 53.1 ■ **Treatment Recommendations for Antiretroviral-Naive Pregnant Women—cont'd**

Preferred Backbones and Regimens

FDCs	Comment
NVP + two-NRTI backbone	No longer recommended secondary to higher adverse event potential, complex lead-in dosing and low resistance barrier. NVP is administered twice daily; caution should be used when initiating ART in women with CD4 count >250 cells/mm³. Use NVP and ABC together with caution; both can cause HSRs within the first few weeks after initiation.

From Panel on Treatment of HIV-Infected Pregnant Women and Prevention of Perinatal Transmission. Recommendations for Use of Antiretroviral Drugs in Pregnant HIV-1-Infected Women for Maternal Health and Interventions to Reduce Perinatal HIV Transmission in the United States. Available at http://aidsinfo.nih.gov/contentfiles/lvguidelines/PerinatalGL.pdf.

3TC, lamivudine; ABC, abacavir; ART, antiretroviral therapy; ATV/r, atazanavir/ritonavir; DRV/r, darunavir/ritonavir; ECG, electrocardiogram; EFV, efavirenz; FDC, fixed-dose combination; FTC, emtricitabine; GI, gastrointestinal; HIV, human immunodeficiency virus; HLA, human leukocyte antigen; HSR, hypersensitivity reaction; INSTI, integrase strand transfer inhibitor; LPV/r, lopinavir/ritonavir; NNRTI, nonnucleotide reverse transcriptase inhibitor; NRTI, nucleotide/nucleoside reverse transcriptase inhibitor; NVP, nevirapine; PI, protease inhibitor; PK, pharmacokinetic; RAL, raltegravir; SQV, saquinavir; TDF, tenofovir disoproxil fumarate; ZDV, zidovudine.

TABLE 53.2 ■ **Stages of HIV Infection**

CDC Stage	CD4+ T-Lymphocyte Count and Percentages
Stage 1 (HIV infection)	CD4+ T-lymphocyte count ≥500 cells/μL or ≥ 29%
Stage 2 (HIV infection)	CD4+ T-lymphocyte count 200 to 499 cells/μL or 14% to 29%
Stage 3 (AIDS)	CD4+ T-lymphocyte count <200 cells/μL or <14%

AIDS, acquired immune deficiency syndrome; CDC, Centers for Disease Control and Prevention; HIV, human immunodeficiency virus.

- Efavirenz (EFV) remains the preferred NNRTI in pregnancy. Current perinatal HIV treatment guidelines support initiation of EFV after the first 8 weeks of pregnancy.
- All NRTIs bind to mitochondrial γ-DNA polymerase, potentially causing dysfunction that manifests as clinically significant myopathy, cardiomyopathy, neuropathy, lactic acidosis, or fatty liver—which resembles hemolysis, elevated liver enzymes, low platelets (HELLP) syndrome.
- With longer duration of antenatal ARV prophylaxis, starting prior to 28 weeks' gestation, each additional week of therapy corresponds to a 10% reduced risk of HIV transmission after adjusting for viral load, mode of delivery, and sex of the infant.
- All HIV-infected women should be screened for hepatitis B virus (HBV) and hepatitis C virus (HCV) unless they are known to be infected.
- Patients with a CD4 count below 200 cells/mm³ should also receive prophylaxis against opportunistic infections.
- Patients on stable antiretroviral therapy (ART) regimens and with suppressed viremia can have viral loads checked each trimester.

Factors That Influence Transmission

- Most perinatal HIV transmission occurs within the intrapartum period; thus effective combined ART (cART) or scheduled cesarean delivery (CD) in patients without viral suppression substantially reduces transmission.
- Early and sustained control of viral replication is associated with decreased HIV transmission, which supports cART initiation as early in pregnancy as possible for all women not treated preconceptionally.
- ART is recommended for all women, independent of viral load suppression.
- Most perinatal HIV transmission in the United States occurs in women who are not known to be HIV infected prior to the birth of their child.
- Evidence to date suggests no increased risk of HIV transmission in women with fully suppressed viral loads undergoing invasive prenatal testing.

INTRAPARTUM MANAGEMENT OF HUMAN IMMUNODEFICIENCY VIRUS

- Intrapartum IV zidovudine (ZDV) is no longer recommended for HIV-infected women who receive a combination ARV with sustained viral suppression (HIV RNA consistently ≤1000 copies/mL during late pregnancy) and no medication adherence concerns.
- The newest perinatal HIV treatment guidelines suggest intrapartum ZDV administration consistent with the elective CD recommendations.
- During labor, every effort should be made to avoid instrumentation that increases the neonate's exposure to infected maternal blood and secretions.
- Scheduled CD at 38 weeks' gestation, confirmed by early ultrasonography, is recommended for women with HIV RNA levels greater than 1000 copies/mL and for women with unknown HIV RNA levels near the time of delivery.
- Given that prolonged spontaneous rupture of membranes does not appreciably increase HIV transmission risk in term patients, we do not recommend elective CD because it is unlikely to reduce perinatal HIV transmission risk in patients being actively managed using oxytocin for augmentation or induction.
- For HIV-infected women who do not receive ART before labor, IV ZDV should be given during labor.
- Rapid HIV testing should be performed for all laboring women without documented HIV status during pregnancy.

POSTPARTUM CARE OF WOMEN WITH HUMAN IMMUNODEFICIENCY VIRUS

- Guidelines for managing HIV infection in adults recommend cART for all infected individuals.
- Because the benefits of breastfeeding in the United States do not outweigh the risk of HIV transmission, breastfeeding is not recommended for HIV-infected women in the United States.

HUMAN IMMUNODEFICIENCY VIRUS–DISCORDANT COUPLES

- Recommendations are to review and encourage safe sexual practices, including consistent use of barrier contraception, preexposure prophylaxis (PrEP), and a plan for HIV screening.
- Preexposure prophylaxis is the use of ARV medications by HIV-uninfected individuals to maintain blood and genital drug levels sufficient to prevent HIV acquisition.

Influenza

- The World Health Organization and U.S. Public Health Service recommend strains to be included in the annual vaccine based on recent prevalence.
- Influenza is spread by respiratory droplets, is highly contagious, and occurs as an epidemic typically during the winter months.
- Pregnant women suspected to be infected with influenza should be treated immediately, independent of vaccination status, without waiting for diagnostic confirmation (Table 53.3).
- To prevent maternal influenza infection and associated perinatal morbidity and mortality, both the ACOG and the CDC recommend annual vaccination of all pregnant women during influenza season (October to May) using the intramuscular inactivated vaccine.
- The intranasal vaccine contains live virus and should *not* be used during pregnancy.

Parvovirus

- The most common presentation of B19 parvovirus infection is erythema infectiosum, which is characterized by a facial rash consistent with a slapped-cheek appearance and a reticulated or lacelike rash on the trunk and extremities (Fig. 53.2).
- Fetal infection occurs following approximately 33% of maternal infections and can be asymptomatic or characterized by aplastic anemia of varying severity (Table 53.4). Severe anemia can lead to high-output congestive heart failure and nonimmune hydrops.
- Serial ultrasounds to evaluate the fetus for hydrops should be performed for 8 to 10 weeks after maternal illness.

Measles

- Rubeola (measles) is one of the most infectious viruses, spread primarily via respiratory droplets; with exposure, 75% to 90% of susceptible contacts become infected.
- The diagnosis of measles is usually made based on clinical presentation (Table 53.5).

TABLE 53.3 ■ Antiviral Medication Dosing Recommendations for Influenza

Antiviral Agent	Activity	Action	Use	Dosage	Duration	Contraindications
Oseltamivir (Tamiflu)	Influenza A and B	NA inhibitor	Treatment	75 mg BID	5 days	None
			Prophylaxis	75 mg QD	7 days	
Zanamivir (Relenza)	Influenza A and B	NA inhibitor	Treatment	10 mg BID inhaled	5 days	Underlying respiratory disease
			Prophylaxis	10 mg QD inhaled	7 days	
Peramivir (Rapivab)	Influenza A and B	NA inhibitor	Treatment	600 mg IV infusion over 15 to 30 min		Category C, limited experience in pregnancy, use only if clearly needed

BID, twice per day; *NA,* neuraminidase; *QD,* once per day.

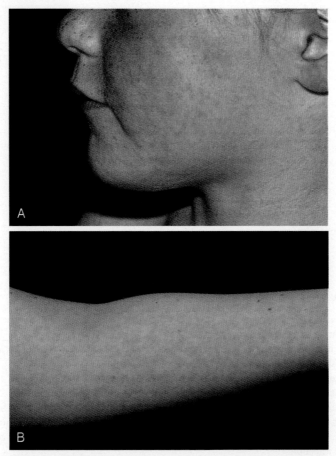

Fig. 53.2 A, Characteristic "slapped cheek" rash of erythema infectiosum. B, Note lacelike rash on upper extremity. (*From Ferri F, et al.* Ferri's Fast Facts in Dermatology. *Philadelphia: Saunders; 2011.*)

TABLE 53.4 ■ Association Between Gestational Age at Time of Exposure and Risk of Fetal Parvovirus Infection

Time of Exposure (Weeks of Gestation)	Frequency of Severely Affected Fetuses
1-12	19%
13-20	15%
>20	6%

- The largest, most recently reported study of measles in pregnancy revealed that pregnant women were twice as likely to require hospitalization (60%), three times as likely to acquire pneumonia (26%), and six times as likely to die of complications (3%) compared with nonpregnant adults.
- The risk of spontaneous abortion and preterm delivery following measles infection during pregnancy is 20% to 60%.
- The most effective way to prevent measles infection in pregnancy is to ensure vaccination prior to pregnancy using a two-dose series, usually a component of the trivalent measles, mumps, and rubella vaccine.

TABLE 53.5 ■ **Differential Diagnosis of Measles**

	Conjunctivitis	Rhinitis	Sore Throat	Exanthem	Leukocytosis	Specific Laboratory Tests
Measles	++	++	−	+	−	+
Rubella	−	±	±	−	−	+
Exanthem subitum	−	±	−	−	−	+
Enterovirus infection	−	±	±	−	−	+
Adenovirus infection	+	+	+	−	−	+
Scarlet fever	±	±	++	−	+	+
Infectious mononucleosis	−	−	++	±	±	+
Drug rash	−	−	−	−	−	−

RUBELLA

- Rubella serology is typically performed at the initial prenatal visit to identify women with inadequate levels of antibody.
- When maternal infection occurs within the first 12 weeks of pregnancy and is accompanied by a rash, over 80% of fetuses become infected with rubella.
- Congenital rubella infection is associated with miscarriage and stillbirth and can have significant deleterious effects on the fetus.
- The most common manifestation of congenital rubella is growth restriction. Sensorineural hearing loss is the most common single defect and affects up to 90% of congenitally infected infants. The rate of hearing loss is inversely related to the gestational age of congenital rubella infection.
- No cases of congenital rubella syndrome have been reported in approximately 1000 infants born following inadvertent vaccination during pregnancy.

Cytomegalovirus Infection

- Day-care workers are at high risk for infection.
- Congenital cytomegalovirus (CMV) is the leading cause of hearing loss in children.
- Antepartum CMV detection does not predict the severity of congenital CMV infection, and 80% to 90% of children with congenital CMV infection have no neurologic sequelae.
- Intrauterine CMV transmission is highest in the third trimester with an overall 30% to 40% risk of fetal transmission. Serious sequelae occur most frequently following first-trimester infection: 24% of infected fetuses have sensorineural hearing loss and 32% have other central nervous system sequelae.
- 15% of subclinical congenital CMV infection is associated with hearing loss.
- Routine CMV screening during pregnancy is not recommended secondary to high seroprevalence.
- Pregnant women should be counseled regarding preventive measures: careful handling of potentially infected articles such as diapers, clothing, and toys; avoidance of sharing food and utensils; and frequent hand washing.

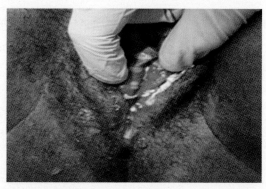

Fig. 53.3 Ulcerated lesions characteristic of herpes simplex infection. (*From Ferri F, et al.* Ferri's Fast Facts in Dermatology. *Philadelphia: Saunders; 2011.*)

- Avoiding maternal CMV infection is the only effective prevention for congenital CMV infection.
- Ultrasound can be useful in identifying a congenitally infected infant with likely impairment.

Herpesvirus

- Herpes simplex virus (HSV)-1 infection is normally manifested by herpes simplex labialis (cold sores), whereas HSV-2 infection customarily involves the genitals and includes the vulva, vagina, and/or cervix (Fig. 53.3).
- One-third of HSV-infected individuals have no recurrences, one-third have approximately three recurrences per year, and another third have more than three recurrences per year (Table 53.6).
- Definitive diagnosis of active HSV infection is made by viral culture or by nucleic acid detection of HSV, which is faster and more sensitive.
- Maternal primary infection with HSV prior to labor does not usually impact the fetus.
- Women with more than two HSV recurrences per year should be offered prophylaxis to decrease the frequency and severity of recurrences (Table 53.7).
- Intrapartum HSV exposure is associated with neonatal infection, which complicates approximately 1 in 3500 deliveries in the United States and is associated with significant neonatal morbidity and mortality.
- Primary maternal HSV infection, not recurrent infection, accounts for the vast majority of neonatal HSV infections.

Varicella

- Patients should be carefully observed for the development of varicella pneumonia, which occurs in almost 20% of infections during pregnancy.
- Oral acyclovir (800 mg by mouth 5 times per day) or valacyclovir (1 g by mouth 3 times a day) are safe in pregnancy and should be given to all infected women because they decrease illness duration if instituted within 24 hours of rash emergence.
- If maternal varicella occurs within 5 days before and 2 days after delivery, varicella zoster immune globulin (VZIG) should be given to the newborn to prevent neonatal varicella.

TABLE 53.6 ■ Comparison of Primary Versus Recurrent Herpes Simplex Virus Infection

Stage of Illness	Primary (Days)	Recurrent (Days)
Incubation period and/or prodrome	2-10	1-2
Vesicle, pustule	6	2
Wet ulcer	6	3
Dry crust	8	7
Total	22-30	13-14

TABLE 53.7 ■ Herpes Simplex Virus Treatment

Drug	Primary Infection	Recurrent Infection	Prophylaxis
Acyclovir	400 mg TID for 7 to 10 days	800 mg BID for 5 days or 800 mg TID for 2 days	400 mg BID
Valacyclovir	1 g BID for 7 to 10 days	500 mg BID for 3 days or 1 g QD for 5 days	500 to 1000 mg QD
Famciclovir	250 mg TID for 7 to 10 days	500 mg followed by 250 mg BID for 2 days or 1 g BID for 1 day	250 mg BID

BID, twice daily; *TID,* three times a day; *QD,* once per day.

- Prevention includes ascertaining varicella zoster virus (VZV) status prior to pregnancy in women without a clinical history of infection and offering live attenuated VZV vaccine (Varivax, Merck) to susceptible women prior to conception.
- This live vaccine is contraindicated during gestation. Pregnancy should be deferred for 3 months following vaccination, although there is no evidence of congenital VZV infection following vaccination during pregnancy.
- With confirmed VZV susceptibility or the inability to obtain serology within 96 hours of exposure, the preferred prophylaxis is high-titer VZIG.

Hepatitis

HEPATITIS A

- Perinatal transmission has not been documented; however, infants delivered to an acutely infected mother should receive hepatitis A virus immune globulin to prevent horizontal transmission following delivery.

HEPATITIS B

- In the United States, 5 to 15 per 1000 pregnant women have chronic HBV infection, whereas 1 to 2 per 1000 have acute HBV infection.
- HBV is transmitted parenterally via sexual transmission and perinatal exposure. Without intervention, infants born to hepatitis B surface antigen (HBsAg)-positive mothers have a 90% risk of perinatal HBV infection.

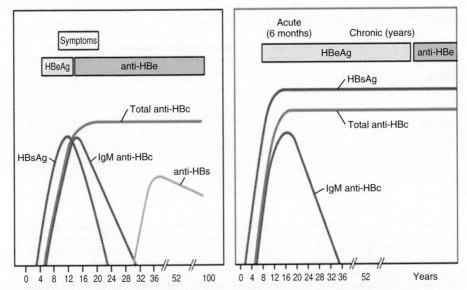

Fig. 53.4 Typical course of hepatitis B virus (HBV). *Left,* Typical course of acute HBV. *Right,* Chronic HBV. HBc, hepatitis B core; HBe, early hepatitis B; HBsAg, hepatitis B surface antigen; IgM, immunoglobulin M. (*From Koziel MJ, Thio CL. Hepatitis B virus and hepatitis delta virus. In Mandell GL, Bennett JE, Dolin R, eds. Mandell, Douglas, and Bennett's Principles and Practice of Infectious Disease, 7th ed., Philadelphia: Elsevier; 2010.*)

- Most newly infected adults (85% to 90%) clear their infection, whereas the remaining 10% to 15% become chronically infected (Fig. 53.4; Table 53.8). Chronic HBV infection has a 15% to 30% risk of liver cirrhosis and a substantially increased probability of hepatocellular carcinoma.
- HBV infection is prevented by a recombinant vaccination that is safe in pregnancy and should be offered to patients with significant risk factors, including those with a history of sexually transmitted diseases, health care workers, and those with infected household or sexual contacts.
- HBV-infected women can breastfeed because perinatal transmission is not increased in these patients.
- In the United States, all newborns are vaccinated against HBV.

HEPATITIS C

- 50% of HCV infections become chronic, which makes it the most common chronic blood-borne pathogen in the United States.
- Universal screening is not recommended, but individuals with risk factors should be tested once (Box 53.1), and annual testing is recommended for persons injecting drugs or with ongoing HCV exposure risk factors.
- Perinatal HCV transmission occurs in 3% to 10% of patients with detectable HCV RNA, whereas transmission in the absence of detectable viremia is rare.
- Given the potential for curative therapy, patients diagnosed with active HCV infection should be referred to a practitioner prepared to provide comprehensive ongoing management of their HCV disease.

TABLE 53.8 ■ Interpretation of Hepatitis B Serologic Tests

Test	Acute Infection	Immunity via Infection	Immunity Via Vaccination	Chronic Infection	Inactive Phase (Carrier)
HBsAg	+	−	−	+	+
Anti-HBs	−	+	+	−	−
HBeAg	+	−	−	+/−	
Anti-HBe	−	+/−	−	+/−	+
Anti-HBc*	+	+	−	+	+
IgM anti-HBc	+	−	−	−	−
HBV DNA†	+	−	−	+	+ (Low)
ALT	Elevated	Normal	Normal	Normal-elevated	Normal

From Koziel MJ, Thio CL. Hepatitis B virus and hepatitis delta virus. In Mandell GL, Bennett JE, Dolin R, eds. *Mandell, Douglas, and Bennett's Principles and Practice of Infectious Disease*, 7th ed., Philadelphia: Elsevier; 2010.
*Isolated anti-HBc IgG occurs during acute infection or can indicate remote prior infection (with loss of HBsAg or anti-HBs) or occult infection. HBV DNA assessment and hepatology consult is indicated.
†HBV DNA detection depends on assay sensitivity.
ALT, alanine aminotransferase; *HBc*, hepatitis B core; *HBe*, hepatitis B early antigen; *HBsAg*, hepatitis B surface antigen; *HBV*, hepatitis B virus; *IgM*, immunoglobulin M.

BOX 53.1 ■ Risk Factors for Hepatitis C Virus Infection

Definite Indications for Screening

　　Any history of intravenous drug use (even once)
　　HIV infection
　　Unexplained chronic liver disease including elevated aminotransferase levels
　　Hemodialysis
　　Blood transfusion or organ transplant prior to 1992
　　Receipt of clotting factor concentrates before 1987
　　Sexual contact with an individual infected with HIV, HBV, or HCV
　　History of incarceration
　　Intranasal illicit drug use
　　Individuals born to HCV-infected women
　　History of unregulated tattooing or body piercing
　　Health care worker with history of needle-stick injury
　　Persons born between 1945 and 1965

Consider Screening (Need Uncertain)

　　In vitro fertilization from anonymous donors
　　Known sexually transmitted disease or multiple partners
　　Steady sex partner of individual with history of injection drug use

---

HBV, hepatitis B virus; HCV, hepatitis C virus; HIV, human immunodeficiency virus.

HEPATITIS D

- Perinatal HBV prophylaxis also effectively prevents perinatal HDV transmission given the requirement for HBV coinfection.

HEPATITIS E

- Perinatal hepatitis E transmission is associated with significant perinatal morbidity and mortality.

Human Papillomavirus

- Trichloroacetic acid and/or cryotherapy are used to treat anogenital warts in pregnancy because podophyllin is contraindicated.

Ebola

- The critical element of clinical management is prompt patient isolation and implementation of recommended infection-control measures (standard contact and droplet precautions) using appropriate personal protective equipment when caring for any patient under investigation and patients with confirmed Ebola virus disease (EVD).
- We recommend advanced hemodynamic and fetal monitoring for pregnant women with suspected EVD, maintaining O_2 saturation above 95%, and utilizing vasopressors and ionotropic agents as needed to maintain cardiac output, blood pressure, and tissue perfusion.
- Pregnancy is thought to increase disease severity and mortality in the third trimester.
- Transmission via breastfeeding has been documented.

CHAPTER 54

Maternal and Perinatal Infection in Pregnancy: Bacterial

Patrick Duff ■ Meredith Birsner

Group B Streptococcal Infection

EPIDEMIOLOGY

- On average, about 20% to 25% of pregnant women in the United States harbor group B *Streptococcus* (GBS) in their lower genital tract and rectum. GBS is one of the most important causes of early-onset neonatal infection.
- About 80% to 85% of cases of neonatal GBS infection are early in onset and result almost exclusively from vertical transmission from a colonized mother.
- In preterm infants, the mortality rate from early-onset GBS infection may approach 25%. In term infants, the mortality rate is lower, averaging about 5%.[1]
- Major risk factors for early-onset infection include preterm labor, especially when complicated by preterm premature rupture of the membranes; intrapartum maternal fever (chorioamnionitis); prolonged rupture of membranes, defined as greater than 18 hours; previous delivery of an infected infant; young age; and black or Hispanic ethnicity.[2]

MATERNAL COMPLICATIONS

- Chorioamnionitis and postpartum endometritis
- Post-CD wound infection
- Lower urinary tract infections

DIAGNOSIS

- The gold standard for the diagnosis of GBS infection is bacteriologic culture.
- Specimens for culture should be obtained from the lower vagina, perineum, and perianal area using a simple cotton swab.

PREVENTION OF GROUP B STREPTOCOCCAL INFECTION

- The newest guidelines recommend universal cultures in all patients as the optimal method of prevention. Cultures should be performed at 35 to 37 weeks' gestation. All patients who test positive should receive intrapartum antibiotic prophylaxis with one of the regimens outlined in Fig. 54.1. Ideally, antibiotics should be administered at least 4 hours before delivery.
- Colonized patients scheduled for a planned cesarean delivery (CD) do not require intrapartum prophylaxis. Patients who tested positive for GBS in a previous pregnancy should not be assumed to be colonized and should be retested with each pregnancy.
- Patients who have GBS bacteriuria in pregnancy, even if treated, should be considered heavily colonized and should be targeted for intrapartum prophylaxis. Moreover, patients who had a previous infant with GBS infection also should be considered colonized and should be treated during labor.

Urinary Tract Infections

ACUTE URETHRITIS

- Acute urethritis, or acute urethral syndrome, is usually caused by one of three organisms: coliforms (principally *Escherichia coli*), *Neisseria gonorrhoeae*, and *Chlamydia trachomatis*.
- If gonococcal infection is suspected, the patient should be treated with intramuscular ceftriaxone (250 mg in a single dose) plus 1000 mg oral azithromycin.[3]
- If chlamydial infection is suspected or confirmed, the patient should be treated with azithromycin 1000 mg in a single dose.[2]

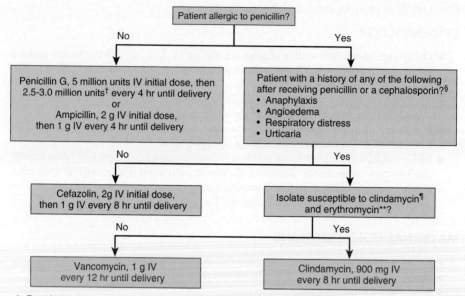

* Broader spectrum agents, including an agent active against GBS, might be necessary for treatment of chorioamnionitis.
† Doses ranging from 2.5 to 3.0 million units are acceptable for the doses administered every 4 hours following the initial dose. The choice of dose within that range should be guided by which formulations of penicillin G are readily available to reduce the need for pharmacies to specially prepare doses.
§ Penicillin-allergic patients with a history of anaphylaxis, angioedema, respiratory distress, or urticaria following administration of penicillin or a cephalosporin are considered to be at high risk for anaphylaxis and should not receive penicillin, ampicillin, or cefazolin for GBS intrapartum prophylaxis. For penicillin-allergic patients who do not have a history of those reactions, cefazolin is the preferred agent because pharmacologic data suggest it achieves effective intraamniotic concentrations. Vancomycin and clindamycin should be reserved for penicillin-allergic women at high risk for anaphylaxis.
¶ If laboratory facilities are adequate, clindamycin and erythromycin susceptibility testing should be performed on prenatal GBS isolates from penicillin-allergic women at high risk for anaphylaxis. If no susceptibility testing is performed, or the results are not available at the time of labor, vancomycin is the preferred agent for GBS intrapartum prophylaxis for penicillin-allergic women at high risk for anaphylaxis.
** Resistance to erythromycin is often but not always associated with clindamycin resistance. If an isolate is resistant to erythromycin, it might have inducible resistance to clindamycin, even if it appears susceptible to clindamycin. If a GBS isolate is susceptible to clindamycin, resistant to erythromycin, and testing for inducible clindamycin resistance has been performed and is negative (no inducible resistance), then clindamycin can be used for GBS intrapartum prophylaxis instead of vancomycin.

Fig. 54.1 Recommended regimens for intrapartum antibiotic prophylaxis for prevention of early-onset group B *Streptococcus* (GBS) disease. IV, intravenously.

ASYMPTOMATIC BACTERIURIA AND ACUTE CYSTITIS

- *E. coli* is responsible for at least 80% of cases of initial infections and about 70% of recurrent cases. *Klebsiella pneumoniae* and *Proteus* species also are important pathogens, particularly in patients who have a history of recurrent infection. Up to 10% of infections are caused by gram-positive organisms such as GBS, enterococci, and staphylococci.[4,5]
- All pregnant women should have a urine culture at their first prenatal appointment to detect preexisting asymptomatic bacteriuria.

- If the culture is positive—defined as greater than 10^5 colonies/mL urine from a midstream, clean-catch specimen—prompt treatment is necessary to prevent ascending infection. In the absence of effective treatment, about one-third of pregnant women with asymptomatic bacteriuria will develop acute pyelonephritis.
- Asymptomatic bacteriuria and acute cystitis characteristically respond well to short courses of oral antibiotics.
- A 3-day course of treatment appears to be comparable to a 7- to 10-day regimen for an initial infection.[4]
- In recent years, 20% to 30% of strains of *E. coli* and more than half the strains of *Klebsiella* have developed resistance to ampicillin.
- Nitrofurantoin monohydrate is more uniformly effective against the common uropathogens, except for *Proteus* species, than trimethoprim-sulfamethoxazole. Amoxicillin-clavulanic acid and trimethoprim-sulfamethoxazole usually are the best empiric agents for treatment of patients with suspected drug-resistant pathogens.
- Cultures during or immediately after treatment are indicated for patients who have a poor response to therapy or who have a history of recurrent infection.

ACUTE PYELONEPHRITIS

- The incidence of pyelonephritis in pregnancy is 1% to 2%.[5] Most cases develop as a consequence of undiagnosed or inadequately treated lower urinary tract infection.
- *E. coli* is again the principal pathogen.[5,6] *K. pneumoniae* and *Proteus* species also are important causes of infection, particularly in women with recurrent episodes of pyelonephritis.
- The usual clinical manifestations of acute pyelonephritis in pregnancy are fever, chills, flank pain and tenderness, urinary frequency or urgency, hematuria, and dysuria.
- Patients who appear to be moderately to severely ill or who show any signs of preterm labor should be hospitalized for IV antibiotic therapy.
- One reasonable choice for empiric IV antibiotic therapy is ceftriaxone 2 g every 24 hours.
- Once antibiotic therapy is initiated, about 75% of patients defervesce within 48 hours. By the end of 72 hours, almost 95% of patients are afebrile and asymptomatic.[5] The two most likely causes of treatment failure are a resistant microorganism and obstruction.
- Oral antibiotics should be prescribed to complete a total of 7 to 10 days of therapy.
- The most cost-effective way to reduce the frequency of recurrence is to administer a daily prophylactic dose of an antibiotic such as nitrofurantoin monohydrate 100 mg.

Upper Genital Tract Infections

CHORIOAMNIONITIS

Epidemiology

- Chorioamnionitis occurs in 1% to 5% of term pregnancies.[7] In patients with preterm delivery, the frequency of clinical or subclinical infection may approach 25%.[8]
- The principal pathogens are *Bacteroides* and *Prevotella* species, *E. coli*, anaerobic gram-positive cocci, GBS, and genital mycoplasmas.
- Several clinical risk factors for chorioamnionitis have been identified. The most important are young age, low socioeconomic status, nulliparity, extended duration of labor and ruptured membranes, multiple vaginal examinations, and preexisting infections of the lower genital tract.

Diagnosis

- In most situations, the diagnosis of chorioamnionitis can be established on the basis of the clinical findings of maternal fever and maternal and fetal tachycardia in the absence of other localizing signs of infection.

Management

- To prevent maternal and neonatal complications, parenteral antibiotic therapy should be initiated as soon as the diagnosis of chorioamnionitis is made, unless delivery is imminent.
- The most extensively tested IV antibiotic regimen for treatment of chorioamnionitis is the combination of ampicillin (2 g every 6 hours) or penicillin (5 million U every 6 hours) plus gentamicin.
- If a patient with chorioamnionitis requires CD, a drug with activity against anaerobic organisms should be added to the antibiotic regimen. Either clindamycin (900 mg) or metronidazole (500 mg) is an excellent choice for this purpose.

PUERPERAL ENDOMETRITIS
Epidemiology

- Similarly to chorioamnionitis, endometritis is a polymicrobial infection caused by microorganisms that are part of the normal vaginal flora.
- The principal risk factors for endometritis are CD, young age, low socioeconomic status, extended duration of labor and ruptured membranes, and multiple vaginal examinations. In addition, preexisting infection or colonization of the lower genital tract (gonorrhea, GBS, bacterial vaginosis) also predisposes to ascending infection.

Clinical Presentation and Diagnosis

- The initial differential diagnosis of puerperal fever should include endometritis, atelectasis, pneumonia, viral syndrome, pyelonephritis, and appendicitis.

Management

- Patients who have mild to moderately severe infections, particularly after vaginal delivery, can be treated with short IV courses of single agents such as the extended-spectrum cephalosporins and penicillins or carbapenem antibiotics such as imipenem-cilastatin, meropenem, and ertapenem.
- Once antibiotics are begun, approximately 90% of patients defervesce within 48 to 72 hours. When the patient has been afebrile and asymptomatic for 24 hours, parenteral antibiotics should be discontinued and the patient should be discharged. As a general rule, an extended course of oral antibiotics is not necessary after discharge.[9,10]
- Patients who fail to respond to the antibiotic therapy outlined earlier usually have one of two problems. The first is a resistant organism.
- The second major cause of treatment failure is a wound infection.
- Mortality is 30% to 50% when associated with sepsis, known as *streptococcal toxic shock syndrome.* Group A *Streptococcus* infections are invasive, and toxin production allows the organism to spread across tissue planes and cause necrosis while evading containment and abscess formation by the maternal immune system. Presentation is atypical and may involve extremes of temperature, unusual and vague pain, and pain in extremities. Endometrial biopsy may be a useful rapid diagnostic tool.

Prevention of Puerperal Endometritis

- We recommend that both low- and high-risk patients having CD receive antibiotics 30 to 60 minutes before the start of surgery. We recommend use of cefazolin, 1 g if body mass index is less than 30 m²/kg (or <80 kg) and 2 g if body mass index is greater than 30 m²/kg (or >80 kg), given as a rapid IV infusion.[11] We also recommend that, whenever possible, the placenta be removed by traction on the umbilical cord rather than by manual extraction.

Wound Infection

- The principal causative organisms are skin flora (*Staphylococcus aureus*, aerobic streptococci) and the pelvic flora (aerobic and anaerobic bacilli).[12]
- The diagnosis of wound infection should always be considered in patients who have a poor clinical response to antibiotic therapy for endometritis.
- Once the wound is opened, a careful inspection should be made to be certain that the fascial layer is intact. If it is disrupted, surgical intervention is necessary to reapproximate the fascia.
- *Necrotizing fasciitis* is an uncommon but extremely serious complication of abdominal wound infection.
- Necrotizing fasciitis should be suspected when the margins of the wound become discolored, cyanotic, and devoid of sensation.
- Necrotizing fasciitis is a life-threatening condition that requires aggressive medical and surgical management. Broad-spectrum antibiotics with activity against all potential aerobic and anaerobic pathogens should be administered. Intravascular volume should be maintained with infusions of crystalloid, and electrolyte abnormalities should be corrected. Finally, and most importantly, the wound must be debrided and all necrotic tissue must be removed.

Severe Sepsis

- Septic shock in obstetric patients usually is associated with four specific infections: (1) septic abortion, (2) acute pyelonephritis, (3) chorioamnionitis, or (4) endometritis.[13]
- The most common organisms responsible for septic shock were the aerobic gram-negative bacilli, such as *E. coli, K. pneumoniae,* and *Proteus* spp.
- In the early stages of septic shock, patients are usually restless, disoriented, tachycardic, and hypotensive. Although hypothermia is occasionally present, most patients have a relatively high fever (39°C to 40°C).
- The differential diagnosis of septic shock in obstetric patients includes hypovolemic and cardiogenic shock, diabetic ketoacidosis, anaphylactic reaction, anesthetic reaction, and amniotic fluid or venous embolism.
- The first goal of treatment of septic shock is to correct the hemodynamic derangements precipitated by endotoxin.
- If fluid resuscitation is not successful, a vasopressor should be administered. The initial drug of choice is norepinephrine
- The second objective of treatment is to administer broad-spectrum antibiotics targeted against the most likely pathogens.[3]
- Indicated surgery never should be delayed because a patient is unstable; operative intervention may be precisely the step necessary to reverse the hemodynamic derangements of septic shock.
- Patients with septic shock require meticulous and aggressive supportive care.

TOXOPLASMOSIS
Epidemiology

- Universal screening of pregnant women for toxoplasmosis is not recommended in the United States at this time.[14] Testing is indicated, however, if clinical infection is suspected or if the patient is immunocompromised (e.g., HIV infection).

Diagnosis

- The diagnosis of toxoplasmosis in the mother can be confirmed by serologic and histologic methods. Serologic tests that suggest an acute infection include detection of immunoglobulin M (IgM)-specific antibody, demonstration of an extremely high IgG antibody titer (and low IgG avidity), and documentation of IgG seroconversion from negative to positive.

Congenital Toxoplasmosis

- About 40% of neonates born to mothers with acute toxoplasmosis show evidence of infection. Congenital infection is most likely to occur when maternal infection develops in the third trimester. However, fetal injury is most likely to be severe when maternal infection occurs in the first half of pregnancy.
- The most valuable tests for antenatal diagnosis of congenital toxoplasmosis are ultrasound and amniocentesis.[15-17]

Management

- Treatment is indicated when acute toxoplasmosis occurs during pregnancy. Treatment of the mother reduces the risk for congenital infection and decreases the late sequelae of infection.[15,17,18] Pyrimethamine is not recommended for use during the first trimester of pregnancy because of possible teratogenicity, although specific adverse fetal effects have not been documented. Sulfonamides can be used alone, but single-agent therapy appears to be less effective than combination therapy. In Europe, spiramycin has been used extensively in pregnancy with excellent success. It is available for treatment in the United States through the CDC but only after confirmation of maternal infection in a reference laboratory.
- Aggressive early treatment of infants with congenital toxoplasmosis is indicated and consists of combination therapy with pyrimethamine, sulfadiazine, and leucovorin for 1 year. Early treatment reduces but does not eliminate the late sequelae of toxoplasmosis, such as chorioretinitis.[19]
- In the management of the pregnant patient, prevention of acute toxoplasmosis is of paramount importance.

LISTERIOSIS

- *Listeria monocytogenes* can cause meningitis, encephalitis, bacteremia, and gastroenteritis
- Because *L. monocytogenes* can grow and multiply at temperatures as low as 0.5°C (or 32.9°F), refrigerating contaminated foods does not always prevent infection, but cooking contaminated foods at high temperatures consistently destroys the bacteria.
- Maternal symptoms can vary from flulike or "like food poisoning" to septicemia, meningitis, or pneumonia.
- An exposed pregnant woman with a fever higher than 38.1°C (100.6°F) and signs and symptoms consistent with listeriosis for which no other cause of illness is known should be simultaneously tested and treated for presumptive listeriosis.[20] Diagnosis is made primarily by blood culture, and placental cultures should be obtained in the event of delivery.
- An overall perinatal mortality rate of 50% due to late miscarriage, premature delivery, and stillbirth was recorded before the use of modern therapies.[21]
- The standard therapy for listeriosis is a combination of ampicillin and gentamicin or, for patients who are intolerant of β-lactam agents, trimethoprim-sulfamethoxazole.

🔊 *References for this chapter are available at* ExpertConsult.com.

CHAPTER 55

Mental Health and Behavioral Disorders in Pregnancy*

Katherine L. Wisner ■ Dorothy K.Y. Sit ■ Debra L. Bogen ■ Margaret Altemus
■ Teri B. Pearlstein ■ Dace S. Svikis ■ Dawn Misra ■ Emily S. Miller

KEY POINTS

- Mental health is fundamental to health. To the extent that maternal biopsychosocial exposures with negative impact on pregnancy outcomes can be diminished, eliminated, or replaced with positive factors, the risk of poor pregnancy outcome can be reduced.

- Major depression is a treatable illness that is the leading cause of disease burden among girls and women worldwide. The period prevalence of depression is 12.7% during pregnancy, and 7.5% of women have a new (incident) episode.

- A brief and efficient 10-item self-report screening instrument, the Edinburgh Postnatal Depression Scale, is available to screen for perinatal depression. For clinical practice screening, the cutoff score for probable major depression in postpartum women is 13 or more; for pregnant women, it is 15 or more.

- Women with postpartum depression should be evaluated for bipolar disorder—which is characterized not only by depression but also by episodes of hypomania, mania, or mixed states—before prescribing antidepressant treatment, because antidepressants without a mood stabilizer can result in symptomatic worsening.

- The first-line antidepressant choice for a pregnant or breastfeeding woman is the drug with established efficacy and tolerability. Specific congenital malformations in offspring exposed to antidepressant drugs (if any) are rare and the absolute risks are small.

- Abrupt discontinuation of any psychotropic medication creates a higher risk for recurrence than does gradual tapering and discontinuation (over at least 2 weeks).

- Postpartum psychosis is characterized by (1) rapid onset of hectic mood fluctuation, (2) marked cognitive impairment suggestive of delirium, (3) bizarre behavior, (4) insomnia, and (5) visual and auditory, and often unusual (tactile and olfactory), hallucinations. Women with acute-onset postpartum psychosis usually have BD.

- The first-line treatment for anorexia nervosa is normalization of eating and weight restoration. Cognitive behavioral therapy is the first-line treatment for bulimia nervosa. Antidepressant medications are the second-line treatment for bulimia nervosa, and they can also be useful adjuncts to therapy.

- Antipsychotic drug maintenance treatment and psychosocial support interventions aimed at maximizing function are the mainstays of treatment for schizophrenia.

- Concurrent maternal smoking, substance use, poor nutrition, and socioeconomic problems increase the risk for less optimal pregnancy outcomes.

- The perception of substance use disorders as afflictions solely of poor, minority, and young women is erroneous. Screening measures are available and easy to use, and multidisciplinary treatment intervention results in improved reproductive outcomes.

*Text for this chapter is available at ExpertConsult.com.

PART VII

Legal and Ethical Issues in Perinatology

Patient Safety and Quality Measurement in Obstetric Care*

William A. Grobman ■ Jennifer L. Bailit

KEY POINTS

- A proportion of adverse obstetric events have been shown to be preventable; this proportion varies with the clinical circumstances.
- Although multiple factors have been associated with the occurrence of adverse obstetric events, issues with communication have been implicated as a frequent contributor.
- Specific approaches that have been considered to enhance obstetric patient safety include checklists and protocols, simulation, and teamwork training.
- Further investigation is required to understand what approaches and combinations of approaches most improve clinical care and outcomes.
- Quality measures assess the degree to which maternal and neonatal care is optimized.
- Major categories of quality measures include structural, process, and outcome measures.

---

*Text for this chapter is available at ExpertConsult.com.

CHAPTER 57

Ethical and Legal Issues in Perinatology*

George J. Annas ▪ Sherman Elias†

KEY POINTS

- In *Roe v. Wade* (1973), the U.S. Supreme Court determined that a fundamental "right to privacy existed in the Fourteenth Amendment's concept of personal liberty" that is "broad enough to encompass a woman's decision whether or not to terminate a pregnancy" before fetal viability without state interference.
- In *Planned Parenthood of Southeastern Pennsylvania v. Casey* (1992), the U.S. Supreme Court reaffirmed the "core" of *Roe v. Wade* and ruled that before fetal viability, states cannot "unduly burden" a woman's decision to terminate a pregnancy (i.e., although consent and waiting periods may be constitutionally acceptable, states cannot regulate abortion in ways that will actually prevent women from obtaining them).
- *Roe* and *Casey* are critical to understanding the rights of obstetricians, which are derived from the rights of their patients, because they are the major sources of law regarding how far states can go to regulate decisions made in the obstetrician-patient relationship.
- *Roe* has been the source of political controversy since it was decided in 1973. Congress has enacted the Hyde Amendment every year since the mid-1970s, prohibiting the use of federal funds for almost all abortions, and its constitutionality has been upheld by the U.S. Supreme Court.
- The Hyde Amendment was the basis for another similar amendment, the Dickey-Wicker Amendment, which prohibited the use of federal funds for human embryonic stem cell research and was the basis for a temporary injunction that prohibited the NIH from funding such research in 2010 (overturned in 2011) under the Obama administration's human embryonic stem cell research rules.
- To protect patient privacy and autonomy, no information obtained in genetic counseling or screening should be disclosed to any third party without the patient's authorization.
- Self-determination and rational decision making are the central purposes of informed consent, and information on recommended procedures, risks, benefits, and alternatives should be presented in a way that furthers these purposes.
- The fetal-maternal relationship is a unique one that requires physicians to promote a balance of maternal health and fetal welfare while respecting maternal autonomy. Obstetricians should not perform procedures that are refused by pregnant women, although reasonable steps to persuade a woman to change her mind are appropriate.

---

*Text for this chapter is available at ExpertConsult.com.
† Deceased.

CHAPTER 58

Improving Global Maternal Health: Challenges and Opportunities*

Gwyneth Lewis ■ Lesley Regan ■ Chelsea Morroni ■ Eric R.M. Jauniaux

KEY POINTS

- Every day, 800 women die as a result of pregnancy or childbirth, and an additional 16,000 develop severe and long-lasting complications.
- Every day, 8000 newborn infants die and 7000 are stillborn, and more than half of these deaths are from maternal complications.
- Adolescent pregnancies account for 11% of all births worldwide, and these young girls and their infants are at far higher risk of death and complications than other mothers.
- Of all the maternal and neonatal deaths worldwide, 99% take place in developing countries.
- The leading obstetric causes of maternal death in developing countries are hemorrhage, puerperal sepsis, preeclampsia, unsafe abortion, obstructed labor, and embolism. HIV causes a growing number of deaths in countries where it is endemic.
- If all pregnant women and their babies could access the maternity care recommended by the WHO, the annual number of maternal deaths would fall by two- thirds—from 290,000 to 96,000—and newborn deaths would fall by more than three- quarters to 660,000 each year.
- If all women had control over their fertility and could access effective contraception, unintended pregnancies would drop by 70%, and unsafe abortions would drop by 74%.
- Apart from a lack of skilled health care and other resources, the quality of the care provided also varies widely. The clinical guidelines and protocols set forth by the WHO and professional organizations need to be urgently implemented, and their uptake audited, in developed as well as in developing countries.
- Safe motherhood for all women is enshrined as a basic human right by the UN, yet many societies have yet to recognize and address this, and they fail to provide the necessary resources to provide adequate reproductive health, maternity, and newborn care or to enact and enforce laws to support equality for women in all aspects of their life, which includes abolition of child marriage and other harmful traditional practices.
- A woman's life is always worth saving.

---

*Text for this chapter is available at ExpertConsult.com.

Normal Values in Pregnancy and Ultrasound Measurements

Henry L. Galan ■ Laura Goetzl

Pulmonary Function Tests, Mean Values

	First Trimester	Second Trimester	Third Trimester
Mean vital capacity (L)	3.8	3.9	4.1
Mean inspiratory capacity (L)	2.6	2.7	2.9
Mean expiratory reserve volume (L)	1.2	1.2	1.2
Mean residual volume (L)	1.2	1.1	1.0

Data from Gazioglu K, Kaltreider NL, Rosen M, Yu PN. Pulmonary function during pregnancy in normal women and in patients with cardiopulmonary disease. *Thorax.* 1920;25:445; and Puranik BM, Kaore SB, Kurhade GA, etal. A longitudinal study of pulmonary function tests during pregnancy. *Indian J Physiol Pharmacol.* 1994;38:129.

Liver/Pancreatic Function Tests

	First Trimester	Second Trimester	Third Trimester	Term
Total alkaline phosphatase (IU/L)	17-88	39-105	46-228	48-249
Gamma glutamyl transferase (IU/L)	2-37	2-43	4-41	5-79
Aspartate transaminase (AST, IU/L)	4-40	10-33	4-32	5-103
Alanine transaminase (ALT, IU/L)	1-32	2-34	2-32	5-115
Total bilirubin (mg/dL)	0.05-1.3	0.1-1.0	0.1-1.2	0.1-1.1
Unconjugated bilirubin (mg/dL)	0.1-0.5	0.1-0.4	0.1-0.5	0.2-0.6
Conjugated bilirubin (mg/dL)	0-0.1	0-0.1	0-0.1	—
Total bile acids (μM/L)	1.7-9.1	1.3-6.7	1.3-8.7	1.8-8.2
Elevated total bile acids (μM/L)	>10	>10	>10	>10
Lactate dehydrogenase (U/L)	78-433	80-447	82-524	—
Amylase (IU/L)	11-97	14-92	14-97	10-82
Lipase (IU/L)	5-109	8-157	21-169	—

Data from Bacq Y, Zarka O, Brechot JF, et al. Liver function tests in normal pregnancy: a prospective study of 103 pregnant women and 103 matched controls. *J Hepatol.* 1996;23:1030; Karensenti D, Bacq Y, Brechot JF, Mariotte N, Vol S, Tichet J. Serum amylase and lipase activities in normal pregnancy: a prospective case-control study. *Am J Gastroenterol.* 2001;96:697; Larsson A, Palm M, Hansson L-O, Axelsson O. Reference values for clinical chemistry tests during normal pregnancy. *BJOG.* 2008;115:874; Lockitch G. *Handbook of Diagnostic Biochemistry and Hematology in Normal Pregnancy.* Boca Raton, FL: CRC Press; 1993; van Buul EJA, Steegers EAP, Jongsma HW, et al. Haematological and biochemical profile of uncomplicated pregnancy in nulliparous women: a longitudinal study. *Neth J Med.* 1995;46:73; Girling JC, Dow E, Smith JH. Liver function tests in pre-eclampsia: importance of comparison with a reference range derived from normal pregnancy. *BJOG.* 1997;104;246; and Egan N. Reference standard for serum bile acids in pregnancy. *BJOG.* 2012;119;493.

Electrolytes, Osmolality, and Renal Function

	First Trimester	Second Trimester	Third Trimester	Term
Total osmolality (mOsm/kg)	267-280	269-289	273-283	271-289
Sodium (mEq/L)	131-139	129-142	127-143	124-141
Potassium (mEq/L)	3.2-4.9	3.3-4.9	3.3-5.2	3.4-5.5
Chloride (mEq/L)	99-108	97-111	97-112	95-111
Bicarbonate (meq/L)	18-26	18-26	17-27	17-25
Urea nitrogen (BUN, mg/dL)	5-14	4-13	3-13	4-15
Creatinine (mg/dL)	0.33-0.80	0.33-0.97	0.3-0.9	0.85-1.1
Serum albumin (g/dL)	3.2-4.7	2.7-4.2	2.3-4.2	2.4-3.9
Uric acid (mg/dL)	1.3-4.2	1.6-5.4	2.0-6.3	2.4-7.2
Urine volume (mL/24 hr)	750-2500	850-2,400	750-2700	550-3900
Creatinine clearance (mL/min)	69-188	55-168	40-192	52-208
Urine protein (mg/24 hr)	19-141	47-186	46-185	—
Urine protein/creatinine ratio (mg/mg); diagnosis of proteinuria	<0.3 Consider 24-hr collection when 0.15 to 0.29	<0.3 Consider 24-hr collection when 0.15 to 0.29	<0.3 Consider 24-hr collection when 0.15 to 0.29	<0.3 Consider 24-hr collection when 0.15 to 0.29

Data from Ezimokhai M, Davison JM, Philips PR, Dunlop W. Non-postural serial changes in renal function during the third trimester of normal human pregnancy. *Br J Obstet Gynaecol.* 1981;88:465; Higby K, Suiter J, Phelps JY, et al. Normal values of urinary albumin and total protein excretion during pregnancy. *Am J Obstet Gynecol.* 1994;171:984; Larsson A, Palm M, Hansson L-O, Axelsson O. Reference values for clinical chemistry tests during normal pregnancy. *BJOG.* 2008;15:874; Lockitch G. *Handbook of Diagnostic Biochemistry and Hematology in Normal Pregnancy.* Boca Raton, FL: CRC Press; 1993; Milman N, Bergholt T, Byg KE, Eriksen L, Hvas AM. Reference intervals for haematologic variables during normal pregnancy and postpartum in 434 healthy Danish women. *Eur J Haematol.* 2007;79:39; van Buul EJ, Steegers EA, Jongsma HW, et al. Haematological and biochemical profile of uncomplicated pregnancy in nulliparous women: a longitudinal study. *Neth J Med.* 1995;46:73; and American College of Obstetricians and Gynecologists. Task Force on Hypertension in Pregnancy. *Obstet Gynecol.* 2013;122:1122–1131.

Cholesterol and Lipids

	First Trimester	Second Trimester	Third Trimester	Term
Total cholesterol (mg/dL)	117-229	136-299	161-349	198-341
HDL (mg/dL)	40-86	48-95	43-92	44-98
LDL (mg/dL)	39-153	41-184	42-224	86-227
VLDL (mg/dL)	10-18	13-23	15-36	25-51
Triglycerides (mg/dL)	11-209	20-293	65-464	103-440

Data from Belo L, Caslake M, Gaffney D, et al. Changes in LDL size and HDL concentration in normal and preeclamptic pregnancies. *Atherosclerosis.* 2002;162:425; Desoye G, Schweditsch MO, Pfeiffer KP, Zechner R, Kostner GM. Correlation of hormones with lipid and lipoprotein levels during normal pregnancy and postpartum. *J Clin Endocrinol Metab.* 1987;64:704; Jimenez DM, Pocovi M, Ramon-Cajal J, Romero MA, Martinez H, Grande H. Longitudinal study of plasma lipids and lipoprotein cholesterol in normal pregnancy and puerperium. *Gynecol Obstet Invest.* 1988;25:158; Lain KY, Markovic N, Ness RB, Roberts JM. Effect of smoking on uric acid and other metabolic markers throughout normal pregnancy. *J Clin Endocrinol Metab.* 2005;90:5743; Lockitch G. *Handbook of Diagnostic Biochemistry and Hematology in Normal Pregnancy.* Boca Raton, FL: CRC Press; 1993.
HDL, high-density lipoprotein; LDL, low-density lipoprotein; TRI, trimester; VLDL, very-low-density lipoprotein.

Hematologic Indices, Iron, and B_{12}

	First Trimester	Second Trimester	Third Trimester	Term
White blood cells ($10^3/mm^3$)	3.9-13.8	4.5-14.8	5.3-16.9	4.2-22.2
Neutrophils ($10^3/mm^3$)	2.2-8.8	2.9-10.1	3.8-13.1	4.8-12.9
Lymphocytes ($10^3/mm^3$)	0.4-3.5	0.7-3.9	0.7-3.6	0.9-2.5
Monocytes ($10^3/mm^3$)	0-1.1	0-1.1	0-1.4	0-0.8
Eosinophils ($10^3/mm^3$)	0-0.6	0-0.6	0-0.6	—
Basophils ($10^3/mm^3$)	0-0.1	0-0.1	0-0.1	—
Platelet count ($10^9/L$)	149-433	135-391	121-429	121-397
Hemoglobin (g/dL)	11.0-14.3	10.5-13.7	11.0-13.8	11.0-14.6
Hematocrit (%)	33-41	32-38	33-40	33-42
Mean cell volume (fL)	81-96	82-97	81-99	82-100
Mean corpuscular hemoglobin (pg)	27-33	—	28-33	28-34
Free erythrocyte protoporphyrin (µg/g)	<3	<3	<3	<3
Ferritin (serum, ng/mL)	10-123	10-101	10-48	10-64
Total iron binding capacity (µg/dL)	246-400	216-400	354-400	317-400
Iron (µg/dL)	40-215	40-220	40-193	40-193
Folate (serum, ng/mL)	2.3-39.3	2.6-15	1.6-40.2	1.7-19.3
Transferrin saturation (%)	>16	>16	>16	>16
B_{12} (pg/mL)	118-438	130-656	99-526	—

Data from American College of Obstetricians and Gynecologists. Anemia in Pregnancy. ACOG Practice Bulletin No. 95. *Obstet Gynecol.* 112:201, 2008; Balloch AJ, Cauchi MN. Reference ranges in haematology parameters in pregnancy derived from patient populations. *Clin Lab Haemetol.* 1993;15:7; Lockitch G. *Handbook of Diagnostic Biochemistry and Hematology in Normal Pregnancy.* Boca Raton, FL: CRC Press; 1993; Malkasian GD, Tauxe WN, Hagedom AB. Total iron binding capacity in normal pregnancy. *J Nuclear Med.* 1964;5:243; Milman N, Agger OA, Nielsen OJ. Iron supplementation during pregnancy. Effect on iron status markers, serum erythropoietin and human placental lactogen. A placebo controlled study in 207 Danish women. *Dan Med Bull.* 1991;38:471; Milman N, Bergholt T, Byg KE, Eriksen L, Hvas AM. Reference intervals for haematologic variables during normal pregnancy and postpartum in 434 healthy Danish women. *Eur J Haematol.* 2007;79:39; Romslo I, Haram K, Sagen N, Augensen K. Iron requirements in normal pregnancy as assessed by serum ferritin, serum transferring saturation and erythrocyte protoporphryin determinations. *Br J Obstet Gynaecol.* 1983;90:101; Tamura T, Goldenberg RL, Freeberg LE, Cliver SP, Cutter GR, Hoffman HJ. Maternal serum folate and zinc concentrations and their relationship to pregnancy outcome. *Am J Clin Nutr.* 1992;56:365; van Buul EJ, Steegers EA, Jongsma HW, et al. Haematological and biochemical profile of uncomplicated pregnancy in nulliparous women; a longitudinal study. *Neth J Med.* 1995;46:73; Walker MC, Smith GN, Perkins SL, Keely EJ, Garner PR. Changes in homocysteine levels during normal pregnancy. *Am J Obstet Gynecol.* 1999;180:660.

Homocysteine, Vitamin, and Mineral Levels

	First Trimester	Second Trimester	Third Trimester	Term
Homocysteine (µmol/L)	4.1-7.7	3.3-11.0	3.9-11.1	4.7-12.8
Homocysteine (µmol/L), on folate	5.0-7.6	2.9-5.5	3.1-5.8	—
Vitamin D 25(OH)D (ng/mL)	>30	>30	>30	>30
Copper (µg/dL)	69-241	117-253	127-274	163-283
Selenium (µg/L)	98-160	85-164	84-162	84-144
Zinc (µg/dL)	51-101	43-93	41-88	39-71

Data from Izquierdo Alvarez S, Castañón SG, Ruata ML, et al. Updating of normal levels of copper, zinc and selenium in serum of pregnant women. *J Trace Elem Med Biol.* 2007;21:49; Ardawi MS, Nasrat HA, BA'Aqueel HS: Calcium-regulating hormones and parathyroid hormone-related peptide in normal human pregnancy and postpartum: a longitudinal study. *Eur J Endocrinol.* 1997;137:402; Dawson-Hughes B, Heany RP, Holick MF, et al. Estimates of optimal vitamin D status. *Osteopor Int.* 2005;16:713; Lockitch G. *Handbook of Diagnostic Biochemistry and Hematology in Normal Pregnancy.* Boca Raton, FL: CRC Press; 1993; Milman N, Bergholt T, Byg KE, Eriksen L, Hvas AM. Reference intervals for haematologic variables during normal pregnancy and postpartum in 434 healthy Danish women. *Eur J Haematol.* 2007; 79:39; Mimouni F, Tsang RC, Hertzberg VS, Neumann V, Ellis K. Parathyroid hormone and calcitor: changes in normal and insulin dependent diabetic pregnancies. *Obstet Gynecol.* 1989;74:49; Murphy MM, Scott JM, McPartlin JM, Fernandez-Ballart JD: The pregnancy-related decrease in fasting plasma homocysteine is not explained by folic acid supplementation, hemodilution, or a decrease in albumin in a longitudinal study. *Am J Clin Nutr.* 2002;76:614; Qvist I, Abdulla M, Jagerstad M, Svensson S. Iron, zinc and folate status during pregnancy and two months after delivery. *Acta Obstet Gynecol Scand.* 1986;65:15; Walker MC, Smith GN, Perkins SL, Keely EJ, Garner PR. Changes in homocysteine levels during normal pregnancy. *Am J Obstet Gynecol.* 1999;180:660.

Calcium Metabolism

	First Trimester	Second Trimester	Third Trimester	Term
Total calcium (mg/dL)	8.5-10.6	7.8-9.4	7.8-9.7	8.1-9.8
Ionized calcium (mg/dL)	4.4-5.3	4.2-5.2	4.4-5.5	4.2-5.4
Parathyroid hormone (pg/mL)	7-15	5-25	5-26	10-17

Data from Ardawi MSM, Nasrat HAN, BA'Aqueel HS. Calcium-regulating hormones and parathyroid hormone-related peptide in normal human pregnancy and postpartum: a longitudinal study. *Eur J Endocrinol.* 1997;137:402; Lockitch G. *Handbook of Diagnostic Biochemistry and Hematology in Normal Pregnancy.* Boca Raton, FL: CRC Press; 1993; Mimouni F, Tsang RC, Hertzberg VS, Neumann V, Ellis K. Parathyroid hormone and calcitrol changes in normal and insulin dependent diabetic pregnancies. *Obstet Gynecol.* 1989;74:49; Pitkin RM, Reynolds WA, Williams GA, Hargis GK. Calcium metabolism in normal pregnancy: a longitudinal study. *Am J Obstet Gynecol.* 1979; 133:781; Seki K, Makimura N, Mitsui C, et al. Calcium-regulating hormones and osteocalin levels during pregnancy: a longitudinal study. *Am J Obstet Gynecol.* 1991;164:1248.

Coagulation

	First Trimester	Second Trimester	Third Trimester	Term
Prothrombin time (sec)	8.9-12.2	8.6-13.4	8.3-12.9	7.9-12.7
International normalized ratio	0.89-1.05	0.85-0.97	0.81-0.95	0.80-0.94
Partial thromboplastin time (sec)	24.3-38.9	24.2-38.1	23.9-35.0	23.0-34.9
Fibrinogen (mg/dL)	278-676	258-612	276-857	444-670
D-dimer (µg/mL)	0.04-0.50	0.05-2.21	0.16-2.8	—
Antithrombin III (%)	89-112	88-112	81-135	82-138
Antithrombin III deficiency diagnostic criteria	<60%	<60%	<60%	<60%
Protein C, FA (%)	78-121	83-132	73-125	67-120
Protein-C deficiency diagnostic criteria	<60% FA	<60% FA	<60% FA	<60% FA
Protein S, total (%)	39-105	27-101	33-101	—
Protein S, free (%)	34-133	19-113	20-69	37-70
Protein S, FA (%)	57-95	42-68	16-42	—
Protein-S deficiency diagnostic criteria, FA%	NA	<30%	<24%	<24%
Factor II (%)	70-224	73-214	74-179	68-194
Factor V (%)	46-188	66-185	34-195	39-184
Factor VII (%)	60-206	80-280	84-312	87-336
Factor X (%)	62-169	74-177	78-194	72-208
von Willebrand factor (%)	—	—	121-258	132-260

Data from Cerneca F, Ricci G, Simeone R, et al. Coagulation and fibrinolysis changes in normal pregnancy. Increased levels of procoagulants and reduced levels of inhibitors during pregnancy induce a hypercoagulable state, combined with a reactive fibrinolysis. *Eur J Obstet Gynecol Reprod Biol.* 1997;73:31; Choi JW, Pai SH. Tissue plasminogen activator levels change with plasma fibrinogen concentrations during pregnancy. *Ann Hematol.* 1997;81:611; Faught W, Garner P, Jones G, Ivey B. Changes in protein C and protein S levels in normal pregnancy. *Am J Obstet Gynecol.* 1995;172:147; Francalanci I, Comeglio P, Liotta AA, Cellai AP, Fedi S, Parretti E. D-dimer concentrations during normal pregnancy, as measured by ELISA. *Thromb Res.* 1995;78:399; Lefkowitz JB, Clarke SH, Barbour LA. Comparison of protein S functional and antigenic assays in normal pregnancy. *Am J Obstet Gynecol.* 1996;175:657; Lockitch G. *Handbook of Diagnostic Biochemistry and Hematology in Normal Pregnancy.* Boca Raton, FL: CRC Press; 1993; Morse M. Establishing a normal range for d-dimer levels through pregnancy to aid in the diagnosis of pulmonary embolism and deep vein thrombosis. *J Thromb Haemost.* 2004;2:1202; Stirling Y, Woolf L, North WR, Sebhatchian MJ, Meade TW. Haemostasis in normal pregnancy. *Thromb Haemost.* 1984;52:176; Wickstrom K, Edelstam G, Lowbeer CH, Hansson LO, Siegbahn A. Reference intervals for plasma levels of fibroenectin, von Willebrand factor, free protein S and antithrombin during third trimester pregnancy. *Scand J Clin Lab Invest.* 2004;64:31; Inherited thrombophilias in pregnancy. Practice Bulletin No. 138. American College of Obstetricians and Gynecologists. *Obstet Gynecol.* 2013;122:706-717.

FA, functional activity.

Inflammation and Immune Function

	First Trimester	Second Trimester	Third Trimester	Term
C-reactive protein (mg/L)	0.52-15.5	0.78-16.9	0.44-19.7	—
C3 complement (mg/dL)	44-116	51-119	60-126	64-131
C4 complement (mg/dL)	9-45	10-42	11-43	16-44
Erythrocyte sedimentation rate (mm/h)	4-57	7-83	12-90.5	—
Immunoglobulin A (mg/dL)	21-317	23-343	12-364	14-338
Immunoglobulin G (mg/dL)	838-1410	654-1330	481-1273	554-1162
Immunoglobulin M (mg/dL)	10-309	20-306	0-361	0-320

Data from Saarelainen H, Valtonen P, Punnonen K, et al. Flow mediated vasodilation and circulating concentrations of high sensitive C-reactive protein, interleukin-6 and tumor necrosis factor-alpha in normal pregnancy—The Cardiovascular Risk in Young Finns Study. *Clin Physiol Funct Imaging.* 2009;29:347; Van den Brock NR, Letsky EA. Pregnancy and the erythrocyte sedimentation rate. *BJOG.* 2001;108:1164; Lockitch G. *Handbook of Diagnostic Biochemistry and Hematology in Normal Pregnancy.* Boca Raton, FL: CRC Press; 1993.

Endocrine Tests

	First Trimester	Second Trimester	Third Trimester	Term
Cortisol (μg/dL)	7-23	6-51	12-60	21-64
Aldosterone (ng/dL)	6-104	9-104	15-101	—
Thyroid-stimulating hormone (μIU/mL)	0.1-4.4	0.4-5.0	0.23-4.4	0.0-5.3
Thyroxine, free (ng/dL)	0.7-1.58	0.4-1.4	0.3-1.3	0.3-1.3
Thyroxine, total (μg/dL)	3.6-9.0	4.0-8.9	3.5-8.6	3.9-8.3
Triiodothyronine, free (pg/mL)	2.3-4.4	2.2-4.2	2.1-3.7	2.1-3.5
Triiodothyronine, total (ng/dL)	71-175	84-195	97-182	84-214

Data from Goland R, Jozak S, Conwell I. Placental corticotropin-releasing hormone and the hypercortisolism of pregnancy. *Am J Obstet Gynecol.* 1994;171:1287; Larsson A, Palm M, Hansson L-O, Axelsson O. Reference values for clinical chemistry tests during normal pregnancy. *BJOG.* 2008;15:874; Lockitch G. *Handbook of Diagnostic Biochemistry and Hematology in Normal Pregnancy.* Boca Raton, FL: CRC Press; 1993; Mandel SJ, Spencer CA, Hollowell JG. Are detection and treatment of thyroid insufficiency in pregnancy feasible? *Thyroid.* 2005;15:44; Price A, Obel O, Cresswell J, et al. Comparison of thyroid function in pregnant and non-pregnant Asian and western Caucasian women. *Clin Chim Acta.* 2001;308:91; Bliddal S, Feldt-Rasmussen U, Boas M, et al. Gestational-age-specific references ranges from different laboratories misclassifies pregnant women's thyroid status; comparison of two longitudinal prospective cohort studies. *Eur J Endocrinol.* 2013;170;329.

Umbilical Cord Blood Gas Values and Hematologic Parameters*

	Artery	Vein
pH	7.06-7.36	7.14-7.45
P_{CO_2} (mm Hg)	27.8-68.3	24.0-56.3
P_{O_2} (mm Hg)	9.8-41.2	12.3-45.0
Base deficit (mmol/L)	0.5-15.3	0.7-12.6
White blood cell count (109/L)		11.1-16.2
Red blood cell count (1012/L)		4.13-4.62
Hemoglobin (g/dL)		15.3-17.2
Hematocrit (%)		45.2-50.9
Mean corpuscular volume (fL)		107.4-113.3
Platelet count (109/L)		237-321
Reticulocyte count (109/L)		145.8-192.6

Data from Eskes TK, Jongsma HW, Houx PC. Percentiles for gas values in human umbilical cord blood. *Eur J Obstet Gynecol Reprod Biol.* 1983;14:341; Mercelina-Roumans P, Breukers R, Ubachs, J, Van Wersch J. Hematological variables in cord blood of neonates of smoking and non-smoking mothers. *J Clin Epidemiol.* 1996;49:449.
*Ranges represent 25th to 75th percentiles.

Crown-Rump Length (6-18 Weeks)

Crown-Rump Length (mm)	Menstrual Age (Weeks)	Crown-Rump Length (mm)	Menstrual Age (Weeks)	Crown-Rump Length (mm)	Menstrual Age (Weeks)
1	1	30	10.0	61	12.6
2	2	32	10.1	62	12.6
3	5.9	33	10.2	63	12.7
4	6.1	34	10.3	64	12.8
5	6.2	35	10.4	65	12.8
6	6.4	36	10.5	66	12.9
7	6.6	37	10.6	67	13.0
8	6.7	38	10.7	68	13.1
9	6.9	39	10.8	69	13.1
10	7.1	40	10.9	70	13.2
11	7.2	41	11.0	71	13.3
12	7.4	42	11.1	72	13.4
13	7.5	43	11.2	73	13.4
14	7.7	44	11.2	74	13.5
15	7.9	45	11.3	75	13.6
16	8.0	46	11.4	76	13.7
17	8.1	47	11.5	77	13.7
18	8.3	48	11.6	78	13.8
19	8.4	49	11.7	79	13.9
20	8.6	50	11.7	80	14.0
21	8.7	51	11.8	81	14.1
22	8.9	52	11.9	82	14.2
23	9.0	53	12.0	83	14.2
24	9.1	54	12.0	84	14.3
25	9.2	55	12.1	85	14.4
26	9.4	56	12.2	86	14.5
27	9.5	57	12.3	87	14.6
28	9.6	58	12.3	88	14.7
29	9.7	59	12.4	89	14.8
30	9.9	60	12.5	90	14.9

From Hadlock FP, Shah YP, Kanon DJ, Lindsey JV. Fetal crown-rump length: reevaluation of relation to menstrual age (5-18 weeks) with high-resolution real-time US. *Radiology.* 1992;182:501.

Head Circumference

Menstrual Age (Weeks)	Head Circumference (cm)				
	3rd	10th	50th	90th	97th
14.0	8.8	9.1	9.7	10.3	10.6
15.0	10.0	10.4	11.0	11.6	12.0
16.0	11.3	11.7	12.4	13.1	13.5
17.0	12.6	13.0	13.8	14.6	15.0
18.0	13.7	14.2	15.1	16.0	16.5
19.0	14.9	15.5	16.4	17.4	17.9
20.0	16.1	16.7	17.7	18.7	19.3
21.0	17.2	17.8	18.9	20.0	20.6
22.0	18.3	18.9	20.12	21.3	21.9
23.0	19.4	20.1	21.3	22.5	23.2
24.0	20.4	21.1	22.4	23.7	24.3
25.0	21.4	22.2	23.5	24.9	25.6
26.0	22.4	23.2	24.6	26.0	26.8
27.0	23.3	24.1	25.6	27.0	27.9
28.0	24.2	25.1	26.6	28.1	29.0
29.0	25.0	25.9	27.5	29.1	30.0
30.0	25.8	26.8	28.4	30.0	31.0
31.0	26.7	27.6	29.3	31.0	31.9
32.0	27.4	28.4	30.1	31.8	32.8
33.0	28.0	29.0	30.8	32.6	33.6
34.0	28.7	29.7	31.5	33.3	34.3
35.0	29.3	30.4	32.2	34.1	35.1
36.0	29.9	30.9	32.8	34.7	35.8
37.0	30.3	31.4	33.3	35.2	36.3
38.0	30.8	31.9	33.8	35.8	36.8
39.0	31.1	32.2	34.2	36.2	37.3
40.0	31.5	32.6	34.6	36.6	37.7

From Hadlock FP, Deter RL, Harrist RB, Park SK. Estimating fetal age: computer-assisted analysis of multiple fetal growth parameters. *Radiology*. 1984;152:497.

Abdominal Circumference

Menstrual Age (Weeks)	Abdominal Circumference (cm)				
	3rd	10th	50th	90th	97th
14.0	6.4	6.7	7.3	7.9	8.3
15.0	7.5	7.9	8.6	9.3	9.7
16.0	8.6	9.1	9.9	10.7	11.2
17.0	9.7	10.3	11.2	12.1	12.7
18.0	10.9	11.5	12.5	13.5	14.1
19.0	11.9	12.6	13.7	14.8	15.5
20.0	13.1	13.8	15.0	16.3	17.0
21.0	14.1	14.9	16.2	17.6	18.3
22.0	15.1	16.0	17.4	18.8	19.7
23.0	16.1	17.0	18.5	20.0	20.9
24.0	17.1	18.1	19.7	21.3	22.3
25.0	18.1	19.1	20.8	22.5	23.5
26.0	19.1	20.1	21.9	23.87	24.8
27.0	20.0	21.1	23.0	24.9	26.0
28.0	20.9	22.0	24.0	26.0	27.1
29.0	21.8	23.0	25.1	27.2	28.4
30.0	22.7	23.9	26.1	28.3	29.5
31.0	23.6	24.9	27.1	29.4	30.6
32.0	24.5	25.8	28.1	30.4	31.8
33.0	25.3	26.7	29.1	31.5	32.9
34.0	26.1	27.5	30.0	32.5	33.9
35.0	26.9	28.3	30.9	33.5	34.9
36.0	27.7	29.2	31.8	34.4	35.9
37.0	28.5	30.0	32.7	35.4	37.0
38.0	29.2	30.8	33.6	36.4	38.0
39.0	29.9	31.6	34.4	37.3	38.9
40.0	30.7	32.4	35.3	38.2	39.9

From Hadlock FP, Deter RL, Harrist RB, Park SK. Estimating fetal age: computer-assisted analysis of multiple fetal growth parameters. *Radiology.* 1984;152:497.

Femur Length

Gestational Age (Weeks)	Femur (mm)		
	5th	50th	95th
12	3.9	8.1	12.3
13	6.8	11.0	15.2
14	9.7	13.9	18.1
15	12.6	16.8	21.0
16	15.4	19.7	23.9
17	18.3	22.5	26.8
18	21.1	25.4	29.7
19	23.9	28.2	32.6
20	26.7	31.0	35.4
21	29.4	33.8	38.2
22	32.1	36.5	40.9
23	34.7	39.2	43.6
24	37.4	41.8	46.3
25	39.9	44.4	48.9
26	42.4	46.9	51.4
27	44.9	49.4	53.9
28	47.3	51.8	56.4
29	49.6	54.2	58.7
30	51.8	56.4	61.0
31	54.0	58.6	63.2
32	56.1	60.7	65.4
33	58.1	62.7	67.4
34	60.0	64.7	69.4
35	61.8	66.5	71.2
36	63.5	68.3	73.0
37	65.1	69.9	74.7
38	66.6	71.4	76.2
39	68.0	72.8	77.7
40	69.3	74.2	79.0

From Jeanty P, Cousaert E, Cantaine F, et al. A longitudinal study of fetal limb growth. *Am J Perinatol.* 1984;1:136.

Amniotic Fluid Index

Gestational Age (Weeks)	2.5th	5th	50th	95th	97.5th
16	73	79	121	185	201
17	77	83	128	194	211
18	80	87	133	202	220
19	83	90	138	207	225
20	86	93	141	212	230
21	88	95	144	214	233
22	89	97	146	216	235
23	90	98	147	218	237
24	90	98	148	219	238
25	89	97	148	221	240
26	89	97	148	223	242
27	85	95	148	226	245
28	86	94	148	228	249
29	84	92	147	231	254
30	82	90	147	234	258
31	79	88	146	238	263
32	77	86	146	242	269
33	64	83	145	245	274
34	72	81	144	248	278
35	70	79	142	249	279
36	68	77	140	249	279
37	66	75	138	244	275
38	65	73	134	239	269
39	64	72	130	226	255
40	63	71	125	214	240
41	63	70	119	194	216
42	63	69	112	175	192

From Moore TR, Gayle JE. The amniotic fluid index in normal human pregnancy. *Am J Obstet Gynecol.* 1990;162:1168.

Small Head Circumference Measurements

Age (Weeks)	−2 SD	−3 SD	−4 SD	−5 SD
20	145	131	116	101
21	157	143	128	113
22	169	154	140	125
23	180	166	151	136
24	191	177	162	147
25	202	188	173	158
26	213	198	183	169
27	223	208	194	179
28	233	218	203	189
29	242	227	213	198
30	251	236	222	207
31	260	245	230	216
32	268	253	239	224
33	276	261	246	232
34	283	268	253	239
35	289	275	260	245
36	295	281	266	251
37	301	286	272	257
38	306	291	276	262
39	310	295	281	266
40	314	299	284	270

From Chervenak FA, Jeanty P, Cantraine F, et al. The diagnosis of fetal microcephaly. *Am J Obstet Gynecol.* 1984;149:512.

SD, standard deviation.

Umbilical Artery Resistance Index and Systolic/Diastolic Ratio

GA (Weeks)	5th Percentile			50th Percentile			95th Percentile		
	S/D	PI	RI	S/D	PI	RI	S/D	PI	RI
19	2.93	1.02	0.66	4.28	1.3	0.77	6.73	1.66	0.88
20	2.83	0.99	0.65	4.11	1.27	0.75	6.43	1.62	0.87
21	2.7	0.95	0.64	3.91	1.22	0.74	6.09	1.58	0.85
22	2.6	0.92	0.62	3.77	1.19	0.73	5.85	1.54	0.84
23	2.51	0.89	0.61	3.62	1.15	0.72	5.61	1.5	0.83
24	2.41	0.86	0.6	3.48	1.12	0.71	5.38	1.47	0.82
25	2.33	0.83	0.58	3.35	1.09	0.69	5.18	1.44	0.81
26	2.24	0.8	0.57	3.23	1.06	0.68	5	1.41	0.8
27	2.17	0.77	0.56	3.12	1.03	0.67	4.83	1.38	0.79
28	2.09	0.75	0.55	3.02	1	0.66	4.67	1.35	0.78
29	2.03	0.72	0.53	2.92	0.98	0.65	4.53	1.32	0.77
30	1.96	0.7	0.52	2.83	0.95	0.64	4.4	1.29	0.76
31	1.9	0.68	0.51	2.75	0.93	0.63	4.27	1.27	0.76
32	1.84	0.66	0.5	2.67	0.9	0.61	4.16	1.25	0.75
33	1.79	0.64	0.48	2.6	0.88	0.6	4.06	1.22	0.74
34	1.73	0.62	0.47	2.53	0.86	0.59	3.96	1.2	0.73
35	1.68	0.6	0.46	2.46	0.84	0.58	3.86	1.18	0.72
36	1.64	0.58	0.45	2.4	0.82	0.57	3.78	1.16	0.71
37	1.59	0.56	0.43	2.34	0.8	0.56	3.69	1.14	0.7
38	1.55	0.55	0.42	2.28	0.78	0.55	3.62	1.12	0.7
39	1.51	0.53	0.41	2.23	0.76	0.54	3.54	1.1	0.69
40	1.47	0.51	0.4	2.18	0.75	0.53	3.48	1.09	0.68
41	1.43	0.5	0.39	2.13	0.73	0.52	3.41	1.07	0.67

From Acharya G, Wilsgaard T, Berntsen GK, Maltau JM, Kiserud T. Reference ranges for serial measurements of the umbilical artery Doppler indices in the second half of pregnancy. *Am J Ob Gyn.* 2005;192:937-944.
GA, gestational age; PI, pulsatility index; RI, resistance index; S/D, systolic/diastolic.

Middle Cerebral Artery Pulsatility Index

Age (Weeks)	5th	10th	50th	90th	95th
21	1.18	1.26	1.6	2.04	2.19
22	1.25	1.33	1.69	0.15	2.30
23	1.32	1.41	1.78	2.25	2.41
24	1.38	1.47	1.86	2.36	2.52
25	1.44	1.54	1.94	2.45	2.62
26	1.50	1.6	2.01	2.53	2.71
27	1.55	1.65	2.06	2.60	2.78
28	1.58	1.69	2.11	2.66	2.84
29	1.61	1.71	2.15	2.70	2.88
30	1.62	1.73	2.16	2.72	2.90
31	1.62	1.73	2.16	2.71	2.90
32	1.61	1.71	2.14	2.69	2.87
33	1.58	1.68	2.10	2.64	2.82
34	1.53	1.63	2.04	2.57	2.74
35	1.47	1.56	1.96	2.47	2.64
36	1.39	1.48	1.86	2.36	2.52
37	1.30	1.39	1.75	2.22	2.38
38	1.20	1.29	1.63	2.07	2.22
39	1.1	1.18	1.49	1.91	2.05

From Ebbing C, Rasmussen S, Kiserud T. Middle cerebral artery blood flow velocities and pulsatility index and the cerebroplacental pulsatility ratio: longitudinal reference ranges and terms for serial measurements. *Ultrasound Obstet Gynecol.* 2007;30:287.

Anatomy of the Pelvis*

Steven G. Gabbe

E-Fig. A2.1   Major components of the bony pelvis, frontal superior view

E-Fig. A2.2   Major ligaments and notches of the female pelvis, posterior view of the female pelvis

E-Fig. A2.3   Muscles of the pelvic diaphragm, oblique view

E-Fig. A2.4   Muscles of the pelvic diaphragm, superior view

E-Fig. A2.5   Muscles of the pelvic diaphragm, inferior view

E-Fig. A2.6   Fascial and peritoneal relationships of the pelvic diaphragm

E-Fig. A2.7   Muscles of the deep perineal space, inferior view

E-Fig. A2.8   Muscles of the superficial perineal space, from below

E-Fig. A2.9   Ischiorectal fossa, frontal section

E-Fig. A2.10 Ischiorectal fossa and urogenital diaphragm, sagittal section

E-Fig. A2.11 External anal sphincter as viewed in dorsal lithotomy position

E-Fig. A2.12 Cutaneous nerve supply to the perineum

E-Fig. A2.13 Superficial perineal blood supply and nerves as viewed in dorsal lithotomy position

E-Fig. A2.14 Vessels and nerves of the deep perineal space

E-Fig. A2.15 Major organs of the pelvis, sagittal section

E-Fig. A2.16 Anatomy of the fallopian tube and ovary, posterior view

E-Fig. A2.17 Anatomic regions of the uterus, lateral view

E-Fig. A2.18 Anatomic relationships of the uterus, lateral view

E-Fig. A2.19 Broad ligament and contained organs, frontal view

E-Fig. A2.20 Organs of the pelvis, posterior view

E-Fig. A2.21 Major vessels of the pelvis, frontal view

E-Fig. A2.22 Major vessels of the pelvis, lateral view

E-Fig. A2.23 Blood supply to the uterus, fallopian tube, and ovary

E-Fig. A2.24 Blood supply to the vagina

E-Fig. A2.25 Major lymphatics of the pelvis

E-Fig. A2.26 Major nerves of the pelvis, lateral view

E-Fig. A2.27 Afferent innervation of the female genital tract

E-Fig. A2.28 Changes in the uterus with age and parity

E-Fig. A2.29 Changes in the uterus caused by pregnancy and parturition

*Figures for Appendix B are available at ExpertConsult.com.

Glossary of Key Abbreviations*

*Appendix C is available at ExpertConsult.com.

A

Abdominal closure, 142
Abnormal axial lie, 112–113
Abnormal labor, 90, 91t
Abruptio placentae, 125, 184
Accelerations
  baseline heart rate, 75
  direct fetal scalp stimulation, 101
  fetal heart rate, 75
  transabdominal halogen light stimulation, 101
  vibroacoustic stimulation, 101
Acetaminophen, 44
Acidemia, 104–105
Acidosis, 296
Acid-suppressing drugs, 43
Acne vulgaris, 376
Acromegaly, 319
Active management, of labor, 87
Active phase, of labor, 91
Active/reactive periods, 3–6
Active smoking, 26
Acute fatty liver of pregnancy (AFLP), 346
Acute glomerulonephritis, 296
Acute leukemia, 367
Acute pancreatitis, 344
Acute pyelonephritis, 295
Acute renal disease, 295–297
  acute renal failure, 296
  glomerular disease, 296
  hemolytic-uremic syndrome (HUS), 296
  nephrotic syndrome, 297
  polycystic kidney disease, 296
  renal artery stenosis, 297
  urolithiasis, 295
  vesicoureteral reflux, 297
Acute respiratory distress syndrome, 295
Acute treatment care, 209
Acute vaginal bleeding, 128
Acyclovir, 43
Adaptive immunity
  maternal-fetal immunology, 8–10
    antibody isotypes, 9, 9f
    helper T-cell subsets, 9–10
    humoral immune responses, 8
    major histocompatibility complex
      (MHC), 8
    T cells, 9

Adiposity, 15
Adnexa, 53
Adolescents
  calcium, 35
  maternal weight gain recommendations, 32
  parenthood, 25
Adrenal glands, fetal development, 3–6
Adrenals disorders, 4–8, 320–321
  adrenal insufficiency, 320
  Cushing syndrome, 320
  pheochromocytoma, 321
  primary hyperaldosteronism, 321
β-Adrenergic receptor activation
  fetal glucagon secretion, 3.e2
  fetal insulin secretion, 3.e2
Adrenocorticotropic hormone (ACTH), 3–6
Advanced maternal age, 23
AEDs. *See* Antiepileptic drugs (AEDs)
Agent, 40
Alcohol, 26, 45–46
Alimentary tract, 4–7
  appetite, 4–6
  gallbladder, 4–7
  intestines, 4–7
  liver, 4–7
  mouth, 4–6
  nausea and vomiting of pregnancy, 4–7
  stomach, 4–6
Alkaline phosphatase activity, 4–7
Alveolar cells, 172
American College of Cardiology (ACC), 277
American College of Medical Genetics (ACMG),
  63
American College of Obstetricians and
  Gynecologists (ACOG), 10, 45, 63, 82, 93, 96,
  120, 180, 295, 311
Amino acids, 2–7
Aminoglycosides, 43
Amniocentesis, 60, 67
Amnion, 2.e2
Amnionicity, 235, 235t, 236f
Amniotic fluid abnormalities, 73
Amniotic fluid assessment, 248
Amniotic fluid index (AFI), 52, 77, 78f
Amniotic fluid volume (AFV), 3.e1, 52–53, 53f, 253
  amniotic fluid formation, 266, 265
  amniotic fluid index (AFI), 264, 265f

Note: 'Page numbers followed by "f" indicate figures, "t" indicate tables and "b" indicate boxes.'

Amniotic fluid volume (AFV) *(Continued)*
  amniotic fluid removal, 265
  definition, 263–265, 264f
  fetal fluid production, 3.e1
  fetal fluid resorption, 3.e1
  fetal swallowing, 3.e1
  fetal urine, 3.e1
  lung fluid, 3.e1
  maximum vertical pocket (MVP), 264, 264f
  normal range, human gestation, 3.e1, 3.e1f
  oligohydramnios, 265–267
    evaluation, 266
    fetal causes, 266b
    labor, 267
    maternal causes, 266b
    treatment, 266
  overview, 263
  polyhydramnios, 267
    evaluation, 267
    fetal causes, 267b
    maternal causes, 267b
    treatment, 267
  ultrasound assessment, 263–265, 264f
  water circulation, 3.e1
Analgesia, labor, 107–109
  inhaled nitrous oxide, 107
  neuraxial analgesic and anesthetic techniques,
    108–109
  paracervical block, 109
  placental transfer, 107
  sedatives, 107
  systemic opioid analgesia, 107
Androgenic steroids, 40
Anemia, 34, 35t, 162
Anesthesia, 180, 365
Aneuploidy screening
  chromosome abnormalities, 62–63
    cell-free DNA analysis, 63
    first- and second-trimester, 63
    first-trimester, 62
    multiple gestation, 63
    second-trimester serum, 62
    ultrasound, 63
  first trimester, 57, 58f
  second trimester, 57
Angiogenesis, 2–5
Angiotensin-converting enzyme inhibitors, 42, 302
Angiotensin receptor blockers, 42
Antenatal betamethasone, 162
Antenatal corticosteroids, 159, 206–207
  duration of benefit, 206
  fetal effects, 206
  glucocorticoids, 206
  maternal effects, 206
  risks, 207

Antenatal surveillance, 273
Antepartum fetal evaluation, 69–78.e1
  biophysical techniques, 74–76
    contraction stress test (CST), 74–75
    Doppler ultrasound, 76
    fetal profile, 76, 77t
    maternal assessment of evaluation activity, 74,
      75f
    nonstress test (NST), 75–76, 76f, 78f
  fetal well-being, 74–75
    clinical application of tests, 77, 78f
  perinatal mortality, 70–74, 70f
    causes, 70
    characteristics, 70
    identifying risk, 71, 71t–72t
    maternal characteristics, 72, 73f
    maternal comorbidities, 72–74
    timing, 71
  testing, 74
    clinical application, 77, 78f
    fetal state, 74
Antepartum fetal surveillance, 74
Antepartum fetal testing, 74
  fetal state, 74
Antepartum hemorrhage
  coagulopathy, 134–136
  genital tract lacerations, 131–133
  placenta accreta, 129
  placental abruption, 125–127, 126f
  placenta previa, 127–129, 128t
  retained products of conception, 133
  uterine atony, 130–131
  uterine inversion, 134
  uterine rupture, 133–134
  vasa previa, 129–130
Anterior pituitary, 318–319
  acromegaly, 319
  clinically nonfunctioning adenomas, 319
  hormone changes, 318
  hypopituitarism, 319
  lymphocytic hypophysitis, 319
  pituitary tumors, 318–319
  prolactinoma, 318–319
  Sheehan syndrome, 319
Antiasthmatics, 42
Antibiotics, 43, 206, 216
Antibodies
  infection control, 8
  isotypes, 9, 9f
Anticoagulants, 41, 46
Antidepressants, 41
Antiemetics, 42–43
Antiepileptic drugs (AEDs), 40
Antifungal agents, 44
Antihistamines, 43

Antihypertensive drugs, 42
Antihypertensives, 46
Antiinfective agents, 43
Antimicrobial peptides, 7
Antineoplastic drugs, 42
Antioxidants, 33
Antiphospholipid syndrome (APS), 337
  catastrophic antiphospholipid syndrome, 337
  clinical criteria, 338b
  diagnosis, 337
  treatment, 337
Antiretroviral agents, 44
Antithyroid drugs, 41–42
Antituberculosis, 43
Antiviral agents, 43–44
Anxiety disorders, 17, 410.e4
Aortic regurgitation, 277
Aortic stenosis, 277
Aortocaval compression, 110
Appetite, 4–6, 15
Arginine vasopressin (AVP), 3–5, 320
Arrhythmia, 76
Arterial blood pressure, 4.e1
ASB. *See* Asymptomatic bacteriuria (ASB)
Ashkenazi Jewish genetic diseases, 65, 66t
Aspartame, 45
Asphyxia, 75
Aspiration/aspiration prophylaxis, 110
Aspirin, 44
Asthma, 288–290
  allergic rhinitis, 290
  antenatal management, 290
  assessment and monitoring, 288
  avoidance/control, 288
  breastfeeding, 290
  diagnosis, 288
  gastroesophageal reflux, 290
  hospital and emergency department management, 290
  inhaled β_2-agonists, 289
  inhaled corticosteroids, 289
  labor and delivery management, 290
  leukotriene moderators, 290
  management, 288
  objective measures, 288
  omalizumab, 290
  oral corticosteroids, 290
  patient education, 288
  pharmacologic therapy, 289–290
  step therapy, 289, 289t
  theophylline, 290
Asymptomatic bacteriuria (ASB), 295
Asymptomatic placenta previa, 128
Atopic eczema, 376

Atopic eruption of pregnancy, 378–381
Atrial natriuretic factor, 3–5
Atrial natriuretic peptide (ANP), 4–6
Audible swallowing of milk, 172
Autoimmune progesterone dermatitis, 376
Autosomal deletions, 61, 61t
Autosomal trisomy, 60
Axilla, 172

B
Back pain, 28, 109
Back-to-work issues, 176
Balanced general anesthesia, 110
Bariatric surgery, 181
Barrier methods, 169
Basal plate, mature placenta, 2.e1, 2.e1f
B cells, 8
BDSMSs
Betamethasone, 16
Bilateral looped uterine vessel sutures, 131
Bilirubin encephalopathy, 162
Bimanual uterine massage, 130
Bipolar disorder, 410.e3
  atypical antipsychotics, 410.e3
  history across childbearing, 410.e3
  lamotrigine, 410.e3
  lithium, 410.e3
  prevention, 410.e3
  treatment, 410.e3
  valproic acid, 410.e3
Birth asphyxia, 160
  sequelae of, 160, 161b
Birth injuries, 160–161
  brachial plexus injuries, 161
  primary subarachnoid hemorrhage, 161
  upper arm palsy (Erb-Duchenne paralysis), 161
Birth spacing, 28
Bisphenol A (BPA), 15
  gender-specific effects, 15
  low-dose maternal exposure, 15
Bladder flap, 141
Bladder trauma, 184
Blastocyst, 2.e1, 2.e2f
Bleeding placenta previa, 128
Blood urea nitrogen (BUN), 296
Blood volume, 274
Blunt trauma, 183
  abruption, 183
  domestic violence, 183
  falls, 183
  intimate partner violence, 183
  motor vehicle crashes (MVCs), 183
Body mass index (BMI), 310

Body water metabolism, 4–6
  atrial natriuretic peptide, 4–6
  brain natriuretic peptide, 4–6
  osmoregulation, 4–6
  pregnancy-related renal and urologic changes, 4–6
  renin-angiotensin-aldosterone system, 4–6
  salt metabolism, 4–6
Bone mass, 17
Brachial plexus injuries, 161
Bradycardia, 75
Brain natriuretic peptide (BNP), 4–6
Brain programming, 17
Breast
  anatomic abnormalities, 175
  anatomy, 172
  development, 172
  nipple pain, 175
  previous breast surgeries, 175
Breast abscess, 175–176
Breast cancer, 365–366
Breastfeeding, 15, 166
  acute infections, 176
  choline, 35
  cognitive development, 173
  drugs, 46
    drugs usually compatible, 46
  glandular tissue, 172
  mother-infant bonding and reduces poor social
    adaptation, 174
  successful breastfeeding, 174b
  successful management, 174
  uterine involution, 172
Breast masses, 176
Breast milk, 173–174
  antibody, 9
  expression, 175
  human-specific oligosaccharides, 173
  immunochemical and cellular components, 162
  protective properties, 173
  somatic growth and cardiovascular
    pathophysiology, 173, 173t
Breast reconstruction, 366
Breech presentation, 116–117
  contemporary management, 117
  delivery for, frank/complete breech, 117
  labor mechanism and conduct, 116–117
  vaginal delivery, 116–117
Breech second twin, 118
Broad-spectrum first-generation cephalosporin, 295
Bronchopulmonary dysplasia (BPD), 204
Brow presentation, 115
  frontum anterior position, 115f
Budd-Chiari syndrome, 345
Bullous disorders, 376
Bupivacaine, 108

C
Caffeine, 37, 45
Calcium, 2–7
  hypertension, 35
  metabolism, skeleton, 4–9
Cannabis, 26, 45
Capillary sprouts/loops, 2–5
Carbamazepine, 40
Carbon dioxide, 2–7
Cardiac arrest implications, 186–187
Cardiac output (CO), 4.e1
Cardiac rhythm, 4.e3
Cardinal movements, 83, 84f
  descent, 83
  engagement, 83, 85f
  expulsion, 83
  extension, 83
  external rotation, 83
  flexion, 83
  internal rotation, 83
Cardiomegaly, 4.e1
Cardiomyopathy, 279
Cardiopulmonary transition, 158–160
  abnormalities, 160
    birth asphyxia, 160
    delivery room management of newborn, 160
    sequelae of birth asphyxia, 160
  circulatory transition, 159–160
  fetal breathing, 159
  first breath, 159
  pulmonary development, 158–159, 159f
Cardiovascular function, regulation of, 3–5
  autonomic regulation, 3–4
  fetal hemoglobin, 3–5
  hormonal regulation, 3–5
Cardiovascular system
  arterial blood pressure, 4.e1
  cardiac output (CO), 4.e1
  cardiac rhythm, 4.e3
  central hemodynamic assessment, 4.e2, 4.e2t
  heart, 4.e1
  labor and immediate puerperium, 4.e2
  maternal physiology, 4.e1
  normal changes, heart disease, 4.e2
  systemic vascular resistance, 4.e1
  venous pressure, 4.e2
Category II fetal heart rate tracings, algorithm, 103,
  104f
Cats, food contamination, 37
Cavitation, 57
Cell-free DNA (cfDNA), 63
  analysis, 63
Centers for Disease Control and Prevention
  (CDC), 185, 270, 382
Central hemodynamic assessment, 4.e2, 4.e2t

Central medullary respiratory chemoreceptors, 3–6
Central nervous system
  maternal physiology, 4–9
  tumors, 371
Cephalic prominence, 113, 113f
Cephalopelvic disproportion, 160
Cephalosporins, 43
Cerebral palsy (CP), 160, 161b
Cervical cancer, 369–370
Cervical cerclage
  effectiveness based on evidence, 201
  history, 200
  multiple gestations, 242
  physical examination, 200–201
  premature rupture, 201
  premature rupture of membranes (PPROM), 216
  ultrasound, 201
Cervical dilation
  active phase disorders, 91
  characteristics, 86f
Cervical effacement, 85
Cervical insufficiency
  activity restriction, 201
  acute cervical insufficiency, 200
  cerclage technique, 200–201
  cervical length (CL), 198
  Cervical Length Education and Review program, 199
  clinical diagnosis, 199
  criteria, 200b
  definition, 199
  diagnosis, 200
  history-indicated cerclage, 200–201
  membranes premature rupture, 201
  overview, 198–199
  patient history, 199
  pessary, 202
  physical examination, 200
  physical examination-indicated cerclage, 200–201
  preterm labor, 201
  progesterone, 202
  risks, 199, 201b
  short cervix, 199
  sonographic diagnosis, 199–200
  tests, 199
  transvaginal ultrasound (TVU), 198
  treatment, 200–202
  ultrasound-indicated cerclage, 201
Cervical ripening, 92
Cervix, 4–9, 53
Cesarean delivery (CD), 137–144.e1
  abnormal lie, 113
  anesthesia
    thoracic spinal nerve 4 (T-4), 107
  asymptomatic placenta previa, 129

Cesarean delivery (CD) (Continued)
  breech, 118
  compound presentation, 115
  forceps, 93
  incidence, 138
  indications for, 138–140
    fetal indications, 138
    maternal-fetal indications, 138, 139b–140b
    maternal indications, 138, 140b
    maternal request, 138–140
  intraoperative complications
    bladder injury, 143
    maternal mortality, 143
    ureteral injury, 143
    uterine lacerations, 143
  maternal postoperative morbidity
    endomyometritis, 143
    septic pelvic thrombophlebitis, 144
    thromboembolic disease, 143
    wound infection, 143
  multiparous women, 87
  nulliparous women, 87
  obstetric anesthesia, 109–111
    aspiration and aspiration prophylaxis, 110
    general anesthesia, 110
    left uterine displacement, 110
    neuraxial anesthesia, 110, 111b
    postoperative care, 111
  perinatal mortality rates (PMRs), 117
  placenta accreta (PA), 152
  placenta previa, 128
  prelabor, 118
  primary, 117
  prior indication, 146
  puerperium management, 167
  safe prevention, 139b–140b
  technique, 141–142
    abdominal closure, 142
    abdominal entry, 141
    abdominal skin incision, 141
    bladder flap, 141
    delivery of fetus, 142
    placental extraction, 142
    postpartum hemorrhage, 142
    precesarean antibiotics, 141
    precesarean thromboprophylaxis, 141
    site preparation, 141
    uterine incision, 141–142
    uterine repair, 142
  tubal sterilization, 144
    modified Pomeroy, 144
Chemoattractants, 8
Chemokines, 8. See also Cytokines.
  maternal-fetal tolerance, 12

Chemotherapy, 366
  alkylating agents, 364
  antimetabolites, 364
  antitumor antibiotics, 365
  general g effects, 364
  platinum agents, 365
  targeted therapies, 365
  vinca alkaloids, 365
Chlamydia
  diagnosis, 383
  epidemiology, 382–383
  pathogenesis, 383
  treatment, 383
Chlamydia trachomatis, 382, 384b
Cholecystitis, 344–345
Cholelithiasis, 344–345
Choline, 35
Chorioamnionitis, 75, 405–406
  diagnosis, 406
  epidemiology, 405
  management, 406
Choriocarcinoma, 373
Chorionicity, 233–234
Chorionic plate, mature placenta, 2.e1, 2.e1f
Chorionic villous surface area, 100
Chorionic villus sampling (CVS), 67
Chrionic hypertension
  antihypertensive therapy
    goals, 231
    safety, 231
  classification, 230–232
  definition, 230
  diagnosis, 230
  etiology, 230
  evaluation, 231–232
  high-risk hypertension, 232
  low-risk hypertension, 231–232
  maternal risks, 230
  perinatal risks, 230
  recommended management, 231–232
Chromatin packaging, 14
Chromosomal rearrangements
  inversions, 193
  translocations, 191–193
Chromosome abnormalities, 60–64
  aneuploidy screening, 62–63
    cell-free DNA analysis, 63
    first- and second-trimester, 63
    first-trimester, 62
    multiple gestation, 63
    second-trimester serum, 62
    ultrasound, 63
  autosomal deletions, 61, 61t
  Down syndrome, 61
  duplications, 61

Chromosome abnormalities *(Continued)*
  fetal death, 70
  prenatal diagnostic testing, 63–64
    accuracy of, 64
    cytogenetic testing, 63–64, 64f
  sex chromosome abnormalities, 62
    Klinefelter syndrome, 62
    monosomy X (45,X), 62
    polysomy X, girls, 62
    polysomy Y, boys, 62
  trisomy 21, 61
Chronic abruption, 125
Chronic disease, 27
Chronic hepatitis B, 345
Chronic hepatitis C, 345
Chronic leukemia, 367
Chronic mild hyperventilation, 4–5
Chronic renal disease, 297–299
  hemodialysis, 298
  management, 298
  pregnancy, 298
  renal function, 297–298
  renal transplant, 298–299
Chronic respiratory alkalosis, 4–5
Circulatory transition, 159–160
Cirrhosis, 16
Clarithromycin, 43
Classic forceps, 94
Clavulanate, 43
Clinical pelvimetry, 83
Coagulation system, 4.e4
Coagulopathy, 134–136
  clinical manifestations, 134
  definition, 134
  diagnosis, 134
  fluid resuscitation and transfusion,
    135–136
    fresh frozen plasma, 135–136
    packed red blood cells, 135
    platelet concentrates, 135
    volume resuscitation, 135
  incidence, 134
  management, 135
  pathogenesis, 134
  pathophysiology and clinical manifestations,
    135f
  risk factors, 134
Coarctation of the aorta, 279
Cocaine
  abruptio placentae, 45
  brain abnormality, 45
  brain systems, 17
  miscarriage, 45
Cochrane meta-analysis, 85
Codeine, 44

Collagen vascular diseases
    antiphospholipid syndrome (APS), 337
        catastrophic antiphospholipid syndrome, 337
        clinical criteria, 338b
        diagnosis, 337
        treatment, 337
    rheumatoid arthritis (RA), 338–340
        antirheumatic drugs, 339–340
        biologic agents, 339
        leflunomide, 340
        management, 339
        methotrexate (MTX), 340
        pregnancy considerations, 339
        sulfasalazine, 339
        tumor necrosis factor-α inhibitors, 339
    Sjögren syndrome (SS), 341
    systemic lupus erythematosus (SLE), 333–336
        azathioprine, 336
        clinical manifestations, 334
        cyclophosphamide, 336
        cyclosporine A, 336
        diagnosis, 334
        drug, 336
        epidemiology, 333–334
        etiology, 334
        glucocorticoids, 336
        hydroxychloroquine, 336
        lupus flare, 334
        lupus nephritis (LN), 334–335
        management, 335–336
        mycophenolate mofetil (MMF), 336
        neonatal lupus erythematosus, 335
        nonsteroidal antiinflammatory (NSAID), 336
        pregnancy complications, 335
    systemic sclerosis (SSc), 340
        diagnosis, 340
        management, 340
        pregnancy considerations, 340
Colloid osmotic pressure, 2–7
Colon cancer, 371
Colostrum, 172
Common liver diseases, 345–346
    acute fatty liver of pregnancy (AFLP), 346
    Budd-Chiari syndrome, 345
    chronic hepatitis B, 345
    chronic hepatitis C, 345
    intrahepatic cholestasis, 346
    liver transplantation, 345
Common patient-centered issues, 28
Complement system, 7
    maternal-fetal tolerance, 12
Complex maternal bowel injury, 184
Compound presentation, 115–116
    cesarean delivery, 115
    cord prolapse, 115

Compound presentation *(Continued)*
    persistent compound presentation, 116
    prolapsed extremity, 115
    upper extremity and vertex, 115, 116f
Confined placental mosaicism (CPM), 64, 193
Congenital heart disease, 278–279
    atrial septal defects (ASDs), 278
    coarctation of the aorta, 279
    Eisenmenger syndrome, 279
    Fontan procedure, 279
    isolated septal defects, 278
    patent ductus arteriosus, 278
    Tetralogy of Fallot, 278
    transposition of the great arteries (TGA), 278
    ventricular septal defects (VSDs), 278
Congenital malformations, 70, 75, 301
Congenital syphilis, 386–387
Conjoined twins, 240
Constipation, 36, 36b
Consumptive coagulopathy, 134
Contraception, 176, 309
Contraction stress test (CST), 74–75
    predictive value of, 75
Cord blood transplantation, 10
Cord clamping, 88
Cord prolapse, 113
Coronary artery disease, 303
Corticosteroids, 3.e2, 216
Cortisol, 3–6
Creatinine clearance (CCl), 4–5
CST. *See* Contraction stress test (CST)
Cushing syndrome, 320
    diagnosis of, 4–8
Cyclooxygenase (COX), 207
Cyclosporine A, 299
Cystic fibrosis (CF), 66
    counseling patients, 292
    effect of pregnancy, 291–292
    forced vital capacity, 291–292
    management, 292–293
    pulmonary involvement, 291
Cytochrome P450 enzymes, 2–6
Cytogenetic testing, 63–64, 64f
    fluorescence in situ hybridization (FISH), 63–64,
        64f
Cytokines
    fetal inflammatory response syndrome, 7
    IL-6, 7
    IL-1β and TNF-α, 7
    immune and inflammatory response, 7
    maternal-fetal tolerance, 12
    proinflammatory, 7
Cytomegalovirus infection, 396–397
    risks, 396
Cytotrophoblastic shell, 2.e1

D

Decongestants, 43
Defensins, 7
Delayed cord clamping, 209
Delayed pushing, 88
DeLee suction, 88
Deletion syndromes, 61, 61t
Delivery, 79–89.e2
  breech, 117
  episiotomy, 88–89
  vs. expectant management, 103–104, 104f
  fetal membranes, 88
  labor and method of, 109
  perineal injury, 88–89
  placenta, 88
  placenta previa, 128–129
  repair, 88–89
  spontaneous vaginal delivery, 88
  ultrasound, 89
Delivery room management of newborn, 160
Dendritic cells (DCs), maternal-fetal tolerance, 12
Dermatitis, 376
Descent, 83
Developmental origins, of adult health and disease,
    13–20.e1
  chromatin packaging, 14
  DNA methylation, 14
  endocrine programming, 18
  energy-balance programming, 15–17
    brain, 17
    environmental agents, 15
    hepatic, 16
    osteoporosis, 17
    pancreatic, 16–17
  epigenetic markers, changes, 14
  epigenetic phenomena, 14
  fetal nutrition and growth, 14–15
    folate deficiency, 14
    iodine deficiency, 14
    nutritional insufficiency, 15
    obesity, 14–15
  gestational programming, 13
    impact of, 14f
  glucocorticoids and prematurity, 18
  immune function, 18
  maternal stress and anxiety, 17
  noncoding RNAs, 14
  renal programming, 19
  sexuality programming, 18–19
Dexamethasone, 18
Diabetes insipidus, 320
Diabetes mellitus, 72, 193
  angiotensin-converting enzyme (ACE), 302
  antepartum fetal evaluation, 305, 306t–307t
  congenital malformations, 301

Diabetes mellitus *(Continued)*
  contraception, 309
  coronary artery disease, 303
  dietary recommendations, 305b
  fetal macrosomia, 301
  gestational diabetes mellitus detection, 303, 303t
  glucoregulation, 307
  human insulin, 304t
  hypoglycemia, 301
  insulin analogues, 304t
  ketoacidosis, 305, 306b
  labor and delivery, 307
  management, 307–308
  maternal classification, 301–303, 302t
  mode of delivery, 305–307
  mortality, 301
  neonatal hypoglycemia, 301
  overt diabetes, 303
  perinatal morbidity, 301
  postpartum follow-up, 308
  prepregnancy counseling, 308, 309b
  respiratory distress syndrome, 301
  retinopathy, 302–303
  risks, 301–303
  target plasma glucose levels, 304t
  timing of delivery, 305–307
  treatment, 307–308
  type 1 diabetes mellitus, 303–305, 304t
  type 2 diabetes mellitus, 303–305, 304t
Diagnosis
  asthma, 288
  cancer, 366
  cervical insufficiency, 200
  chlamydia, 383
  chorioamnionitis, 406
  chrionic hypertension, 230
  coagulopathy, 134
  eclampsia, 228
  gastrointestinal disorders, 347–349, 348b
  genital tract lacerations, 131
  gonorrhea, 384
  group B streptococcal infection, 403
  heart disease, 276
  herpesvirus, 397
  human immunodeficiency virus (HIV), 389–390,
    390f
  intrauterine growth restriction (IUGR), 247–249
  labor, 90–91
    abnormal, 90, 91t
    active phase, 91
    labor at term (Zhang), 91t
    latent phase, 90
    second stage, 91
    third stage, 91
  measles, 396t

Diagnosis *(Continued)*
  multiple gestations, 234–235
  placenta accreta, 129
  placental abruption, 125–127
    laboratory findings, 127
    radiology, 125, 126f
  placenta previa, 128, 128t
  postterm pregnancy, 271
  preeclampsia, 220
  preterm birth (PTB), 205, 205b
  puerperal endometritis, 406
  red cell alloimmunization, 259–260
  retained products of conception, 133
  rheumatoid arthritis (RA), 339
  syphilis, 385
  systemic lupus erythematosus
    (SLE), 334
  systemic sclerosis (SSc), 340
  toxoplasmosis, 408
  tuberculosis, 286–287
  uterine atony, 130
  uterine inversion, 134
  uterine rupture, 133–134
  vasa previa, 130
Diagnostic imaging
  surgery, 179–180
  trauma, 186, 187f
Dietary reference intakes (DRIs), 33
  calcium, 35
  folate, 34
  vitamin K, 34
  zinc, 35
Diffusion
  blood-blood barrier, 100
Diffusional exchange, 2–3
Digoxin, 42
Dimenhydrinate, 42
Diphenhydramine, 42
Direct fetal injuries, 184
Disorders of invasive placentation,
  151, 152f
Disseminated intravascular coagulation,
  296
DNA methylation, 14
dNK cells, 7
Documentation, 53
Domestic violence, 183
Domperidone, 176
Doppler heart rate monitoring, 115
Doppler ultrasound, 76, 253
Doppler velocimetry, 248–249, 252f, 255f
Dose effect, 40
Down syndrome, 61
  multiple serum markers, 63
Doxylamine, 4–7, 42

Drugs
  breast milk, 45–46
    compatible with breastfeeding, 46
    contraindicated, breastfeeding, 46
    significant effects (administer with caution), 46
    unknown effects on nursing infants, 46
  labeling, 39
  medical use, 40–44
    acid-suppressing drugs, 43
    androgenic steroids, 40
    antiasthmatics, 42
    antibiotics, 43
    anticoagulants, 41
    antiemetics, 42–43
    antiepileptic drugs (AEDs), 40
    antifungal agents, 44
    antihistamines, 43
    antihypertensive drugs, 42
    antiinfective agents, 43
    antineoplastic drugs, 42
    antiretroviral agents, 44
    antiviral agents, 43–44
    decongestants, 43
    digoxin, 42
    estrogens, 40
    immunosuppressants, 42
    induction of ovulation, 44
    isotretinoin, 40–41
    mild analgesics, 44
    progestins, 40
    psychoactive drugs, 41
    specific drugs, 40–44
    spermicides, 40
    sympathetic blocking agents, 42
    thyroid and antithyroid drugs, 41–42
    vitamin A, 41
  milk production, 176
Drugs of abuse
  alcohol, 45
  aspartame, 45
  caffeine, 45
  cannabis/marijuana, 45
  cocaine, 45
  narcotics and methadone, 45
  nicotine, 44
Ductal closure, 160
Ductus arteriosus, 3.e2, 159
Duplications, 61
Dystocia, 87

E

Early pregnancy loss (EPL)
  alcohol, 195
  autosomal trisomy, 191

Early pregnancy loss (EPL) *(Continued)*
  β-human chorionic gonadotropin (β-hCG), 190
  caffeine, 195
  cervical insufficiency, 194
  chemicals, 195
  chemotherapeutic agents, 195
  chromosomal rearrangements, 191–193
  cigarette smoking, 195
  contraceptive agents, 195
  diabetes mellitus, 193
  exogenous agents, 194–195
  formal evaluation, 196
  frequency, 190
  genetic counseling, 191
  infections, 194
  intrauterine adhesions, 193
  inversions, 193
  leiomyomas, 194
  luteal phase defects (LPD), 193
  management, 195–196
  maternal age, 190
  medications, 195
  mosaics, 193
  monosomy X, 191, 192t
  Müllerian fusion defects, 193–194
  numerical chromosomal abnormalities, 190–191
  obstetric outcome complications, 197
  placental anatomic characteristics, 190
  polyploidy, 191
  psychological factors, 195
  radiation agents, 195
  recommended evaluation, 196
  recurrent aneuploidy, 191
  recurrent early pregnancy loss (REPL), 190
  recurrent losses, 191
  second-trimester losses, 193
  sex chromosome polysomy, 191
  synechiae, 193
  thrombophilias, 194
  thyroid abnormalities, 193
  timing, 190
  translocations, 191–193
  trauma, 195
Early pregnancy markers, 73
Eating disorders, 410.e4
  MDE, 410.e4
Ebola, 401
Eclampsia
  cerebral pathology, 228–229
  definition, 217–218, 228
  diagnosis, 228
  intrapartum management, 230
  late postpartum eclampsia, 228
  maternal outcome, 229
  perinatal outcome, 229

Eclampsia *(Continued)*
  postpartum management, 230
  preventions, 229
    maternal injury, 229
    recurrent convulsions, 229
  time of onset, 228
  treatment, 229
Efavirenz, 44
Eisenmenger syndrome, 279
Elective induction of labor, 92
Electrolyte homeostasis, 3–5
Electronic fetal heart rate monitoring, 98–100
  benefits, 105
  external environment, 98
  fetal response to interrupted oxygen transfer,
      100–101
    injury threshold, 101
    mechanisms of injury, 101
  limitations, 105
  maternal blood, 99
  maternal heart, 99
  maternal lungs, 99
  maternal vasculature, 99
  oxygen transfer from environment to fetus, 98,
      99f
  placenta, 100
    chorionic villous surface area, 100
    diffusion across blood-blood barrier, 100
    interruption, placental blood vessels, 100
    intervillous space blood flow, 100
    intervillous space Pao₂, 100
  uterus, 100
Emergency department (ED), 185
Endocrine programming, 18
Endometrial cancer, 371
Endometrium
  cytotrophoblastic shell, 2–3
  first trimester, 2–3
  placenta accreta, 2–3
Endomyometritis, 143
Energy, 32
Energy-balance programming, 15–17
  brain, 17
  environmental agents, 15
    programmed obesity, 15
  hepatic, 16
  osteoporosis, 17
  pancreatic, 16–17
Engagement, 83
  breech presentation, 116
  fetal head, 83, 85f
Engorgement, 173
Enoxaparin, 41
Environmental exposures, 27
Environmental hazards, 47

Epidermal growth factor (EGF)
  embryonal implantation, 3.e2
Epidural analgesia, 109
Epidural anesthesia, 175
Epidural blood patch, 108
Epigenetic markers, changes in, 14
Epinephrine, uterine blood flow, 107
Episiotomy, 120
Erythromycin, 43
Escherichia coli, 295
Estrogens, 2–8, 40
Ethical/legal issues, perinatology, 413–413.e3
  abortion politics, 413.e1
  forced cesarean delivery, 413.e2
  genetic counseling, 413.e2
  human embryonic stem cell research funding,
      413.e1
  Obamacare, 413.e1
  prenatal diagnosis, 413.e2
  reproductive liberty, 413.e1
  screening, 413.e2
Exogenous agents, 194–195
  active maternal smoking, 195
  alcohol, 195
  caffeine, 195
  chemicals, 195
  chemotherapeutic agents, 195
  cigarette smoking, 195
  contraceptive agents, 195
  medications, 195
  passive maternal smoking, 195
  psychological factors, 195
  radiation, 195
  secondhand smoking, 195
  trauma, 195
Expulsion, 83
Extension, 83
External cephalic version (ECV), 113
  regional anesthesia, 119
  terbutaline, 119
External rotation, 83
Extravillous trophoblast (EVT), 2–3
Extubation, 110

F
Face presentation, 113–115, 113f
  labor mechanism, 114–115, 114f
Failed induction of labor, 92
Falls, trauma, 183
Fatty acids, 2–7
Fentanyl, 107
Fertility preservation, 372
Fetal activity periods, 3–6
Fetal adaptation, 74

Fetal alcohol spectrum disorders, 41
Fetal alcohol syndrome, 26
Fetal anemia, 75
Fetal baroreflex sensitivity, 3–4
Fetal biometry, 55b, 247–248
Fetal biophysical characteristics, 74
Fetal biophysical profile, 76, 77t
  management, 77t
  predictive value, 76
Fetal breathing, 3–6, 159
Fetal cardiovascular system, 3–5
  cardiovascular function, 3–5
    autonomic regulation, 3–4
    fetal hemoglobin, 3–5
    hormonal regulation, 3–5
  ductus arteriosus functions, 3.e2
  fetal heart. *See* Fetal heart
  left atrial filling, 3.e2
  single-lumen tube, 3.e2
  umbilical and hepatic circulation anatomy, 3.e2,
      3.e3f
  venous pathways, 3.e2
  well-oxygenated ductus venosus blood, 3.e2
Fetal central nervous system, 3–6
Fetal chin (mentum), 113
Fetal death, 73
  causes, 70
  characteristics, 70
  gestational cholestasis, 73
  vs. maternal age across gestation, 72, 73f
  risk factors for, 71t–72t
  timing, 71
Fetal development, 3–3.e7
  adrenal glands, 3–6
  amniotic fluid volume (AFV), 3.e1
    fetal fluid production, 3.e1
    fetal fluid resorption, 3.e1
    fetal swallowing, 3.e1
    fetal urine, 3.e1
    lung fluid, 3.e1
    normal range, human gestation, 3.e1, 3.e1f
    water circulation, 3.e1
  cardiovascular system, 3–5
    development, 3.e2, 3.e3f
    fetal heart, 3–4, 3.e3f
    regulation, cardiovascular function, 3–5
  central nervous system, 3–6
  gastrointestinal system. (*See* Fetal gastrointestinal)
      system
  growth and metabolism, 3.e1
    hormones, 3.e2
    substrates, 3.e1
  kidney, 3–5
  thyroid gland, 3–6
  umbilical blood flow, 3.e1

Fetal fibronectin (fFN), 213
Fetal fluid production, 3.e1
Fetal fluid resorption, 3.e1
Fetal gastrointestinal system, 3–6
  gastrointestinal tract, 3–5
  liver, 3–6
Fetal glucagon secretion, 3.e2
Fetal growth restriction, 73
Fetal head, 83, 85f
Fetal heart, 3–4
  and central shunts anatomy, 3.e2, 3.e3f
  coronary blood flow, 3–4
  ductus arteriosus oxygen tension, 3–4
  fetal heart rate (FHR), 3–4
  period variability, 3–6
  Starling mechanisms, 3–4
  vascular distribution, 3–4
  ventricular stroke volumes, 3–4
Fetal heart rate (FHR), 3–4
  standardized "ABCD" approach, 103
    clear obstacles to rapid delivery, 103
    corrective measures as indicated, 103, 104f
    determine decision-to-delivery time, 103
    oxygen pathway, 103
Fetal hydantoin syndrome, 40
Fetal hyperthyroidism, 316
Fetal injury, 184
Fetal kidney, 3–5
  atrial natriuretic factor, 3–5
  glomerular filtration rate (GFR), 3–5
  reduced concentrating ability, 3–5
Fetal laryngeal, 115
Fetal lie, 82, 112
Fetal liver free thyroxine metabolism, 3–6
Fetal macrosomia, 82, 301
Fetal malformations, 74
Fetal membranes, 88
Fetal monitoring, 185
Fetal mortality predictors, 184
Fetal movement, 74
Fetal/neonatal morbidity, 207
Fetal nutrition and growth, 14–15
  folate deficiency, 14
  iodine deficiency, 14
  nutritional insufficiency, 15
  obesity, 14–15
Fetal parasympathetic system, 3–4
Fetal-placental metastasis, 372
Fetal plasma renin, 3–5
Fetal reflex responses, 3–4
Fetal rejection, maternal-fetal tolerance, 12
Fetal swallowing, 3.e1
Fetal sympathetic system, 3–4
Fetal tachycardia, 74
Fetal thyroid, 3.e2

Fetal urine, 3.e1
Fetal water, 3–5
Fetal well-being assessment, 74–75,
    252–254
  clinical application of tests, 77, 78f
  condition-specific testing, 77, 78f
Fetoplacental circulation, 3.e1
Fetus (passenger), 82, 82f
Fick's law, 2–3
First breath, 159
First-degree tear, 88–89
First trimester, 2.e2
  antidepressants, 41
  arginine vasopressin (AVP), 3–5
  chromosome abnormalities, 60
  corticosteroids, 42
  doxycycline exposure, 43
  endometrium, 2–3
  folate and neural tube defects, 34
  iron, 34
  lithium, 41
  maternal circulation (MC), 2–3
  maternal-fetal relationship, 2–3
  medical management, 27
  microvilli, 2–5
  nutritional requirements, 33
  screening
    aneuploidy, 57, 58f, 62
  serum markers, 73
  smoking, 26
  thyroid-stimulating hormone, 4–7
  ultrasound, 50
    abnormal findings, 50
    dating, 54
    normal findings, 50
Fish oil supplementation, 33
Flexion, 83
Flow velocity waveforms, 49
Fluorescence in situ hybridization (FISH), 63–64,
    64f
Fluoroquinolones, 43
Focal syncytial necrosis, 2–5
Folate, 34
  adequate levels, 34
  embryonic neural tube closure, 34
  neural tube defects, 34
  supplementation, 34
Folic acid, 33
Fontan procedure, 279
Food contamination, 36–37
Footling breech, 118
Forceps
  classic forceps, 94
  classification, 94, 95f
  indications

Forceps *(Continued)*
  prolonged second stage, 93
  suspicion of immediate/potential fetal
    compromise, 93
  midforceps, 93
  outlet forceps, 93
  prerequisites for, 93, 94b
  rotational forceps, 94
  specialized forceps, 93
Fourth-degree tear, 88–89
Fraternal birth order effect, 19

G
Galactogogues, 176
Gallbladder, 4–7
Gas exchange, 4–5
Gastric emptying, pregnancy, 4–6
Gastrointestinal cancers, 371
Gastrointestinal disorders
  abdominal pain, 347, 348t–349t
  acute appendicitis, 351
  constipation, 349
  diagnosis, 347–349, 348b
  diagnostic testing, 349–354
  endoscopy, 349–354
  evaluation, 347–349
  gastroesophageal reflux, 350–351
  hematemesis, 349
  hemorrhoids, 352
  inflammatory bowel diseases (IBDs),
    352, 353t
  intestinal obstruction, 351–352
  intestinal pseudoobstruction, 352
  irritable bowel syndrome (IBS), 352–354
  nausea, 350
  peptic ulcer disease, 350–351
  radiologic imaging, 349
  red blood per rectum, 349
  risks, 350t
  vomiting, 350
General anesthesia, 110
  extubation, 110
  induction, 110
  intubation, 110
    failed intubation, 110
  nitrous oxide and oxygen, 110
  preoxygenation, 110
  volatile halogenated agent, 110
Genetic counseling, 191
Genetics
  counseling, 60
  history, 60
  red cell alloimmunization, 258
  thromboembolic disorders, 329

Genital tract lacerations, 131–133
  clinical manifestations, 131
  definition, 131
  diagnosis, 131
  incidence, 131
  management, 131–133
    retroperitoneal hematoma, 133
    vaginal hematoma, 131–133
    vulvar hematoma, 131
  pathogenesis, 131
  risk factors, 131
Genitourinary tract, 155
Gestational diabetes mellitus (GDM), 23, 303, 303t
Gestational hypertension
  definitions, 217
  features, 218
Gestational programming, 13
  impact of, 14f
Gestational trophoblastic disease, 372–373
Gestational weight gain (GWG), 4.e1, 4.e1t, 310–311
Ginger, 43
Global maternal health, 414–414.e7
  maternal health, 414.e1
    adolescent girls, 414.e1
    causes of the causes, 414.e2
    clinical causes, 414.e2
    death burden, 414.e1
    disability burden, 414.e1
    health system factors, 414.e2
    infants who die, 414.e1
    life and death, 414.e1
    lifetime risk, 414.e1
    morbidity, 414.e1
    mothers who survive, 414.e1
    United States, 414.e1
    vulnerability, 414.e2
    where mothers die, 414.e1
    why mothers die, 414.e2
    women's rights, 414.e2
  obstetric complications, 414.e3
    cesarean delivery, 414.e4
    eclampsia, 414.e4
    human immunodeficiency virus, 414.e4
    malaria, 414.e4
    obstetric fistula, 414.e4
    obstructed labor, 414.e4
    postpartum hemorrhage, 414.e3
    preeclampsia, 414.e4
    sepsis, 414.e4
  sexual and reproductive health, 414.e2
    contraception, 414.e3
    induced abortion, 414.e3
    mothers well-being, 414.e3
    unintended pregnancy, 414.e2
  volunteering to work overseas, 414.e5

Global maternal health *(Continued)*
    health care staff, 414.e5
    predeparture preparation, 414.e6
    realism, 414.e5
    research, 414.e5
    respect, 414.e5
Glomerular disease, 296
Glomerular filtration rate (GFR), 3–5
Glucocorticoids, 18, 206
Glucoregulation, 307
Glucose, 2–7
    fetal oxidative metabolism, 3.e1, 3–6
    milk production, 172
    pancreas and fuel metabolism, 4–8
Glucose transporter 1 (GLUT1), 2–7
Glycosuria, 295
Gonorrhea
    diagnosis, 384
    epidemiology, 383
    pathogenesis, 383
    treatment, 384–385
Graves disease, 314–316
Group B streptococcal infection, 403
    diagnosis, 403
    epidemiology, 403
    maternal complications, 403
    prevention, 403
Gynecologist, 174

H

Health maintenance, 167–168
    delayed postpartum hemorrhage, 167
    maternal-infant attachment, 168
    normal postpartum uterus, 167, 168f
    perineal and pelvic care, 167
    postpartum anemia, 167
    postpartum infection, 167
Heart disease
    aortic regurgitation, 277
    aortic stenosis, 277
    blood volume, 274
    cardiomyopathy, 279
    coarctation of the aorta, 279
    congenital heart disease, 275f, 278–279
    critical care, 280–281
    delivery, 276b
    diagnosis, 276, 279b
    Eisenmenger syndrome, 279
    Fontan procedure, 279
    general care, 276–278
    hemodynamic management, 281
    hemodynamic monitoring, 280
    hemodynamic parameters, 275f
    hypertrophic cardiomyopathy, 280

Heart disease *(Continued)*
    isolated septal defects, 278
    labor, 276b
    malignant ventricular arrhythmias, 280
    Marfan syndrome, 280
    maternal hemodynamics, 274
    mitral regurgitation, 277
    mitral stenosis, 277
    myocardial infarction (MI), 280
    patent ductus arteriosus, 278
    prosthetic valves, 277–278
    pulmonary hypertension, 280
    risks, 276
    Tetralogy Of Fallot, 278
    transposition of the great arteries, 278
    valvular disease, 277
Heat transfer, 161
Hematologic complications
    hemoglobinopathies, 326–327
    hemoglobin S, 326–327
    hemoglobin SC disease, 327
    thalassemia, 327, 328f
    thrombocytopenia, 323–324
        evaluation, 324
        fetal/neonatal alloimmune thrombocytopenia, 325
        gestational thrombocytopenia, 322–324
        glucocorticoids, 322–323
        hemolytic-uremic syndrome (HUS), 323–324
        idiopathic thrombocytopenic purpura (ITP), 322–323
        immune thrombocytopenic purpura (ITP), 323–324
        iron deficiency anemia, 325
        management, 324
        megaloblastic anemia, 325–326
        preeclampsia, 322–323
        therapy, 324
        thrombotic thrombocytopenic purpura (TTP), 322–324
    von Willebrand disease (vWD), 327–328
Hematologic malignancies, 367
Hemodialysis, 298
Hemoglobin electrophoresis, 65–66
Hemoglobinopathies, 65–66, 326–327
Hemolytic-uremic syndrome (HUS), 296
Hemorrhage
    antepartum, 125–136
        coagulopathy, 134–136
        genital tract lacerations, 131–133
        placenta accreta, 129
        placental abruption, 125–127, 126f
        placenta previa, 127–129, 128t
        retained products of conception, 133
        uterine atony, 130–131

Hemorrhage *(Continued)*
  uterine inversion, 134
  uterine rupture, 133–134
  vasa previa, 129–130
  classification, 124–125, 124t
    class 1, 124
    class 2, 124
    class 3, 125
    class 4, 125
  physiologic adaptation, 123, 124f
  physiologic response, 124t
  postpartum, 130
Hepatic disorders
  abdominal imaging, 343–344
    banding, 344
    endoscopic variceal sclerotherapy, 344
    informed consent, 344
    team approach, 344
    therapeutic endoscopic retrograde
      cholangiopancreatography, 344
  common liver diseases, 345–346
    acute fatty liver of pregnancy (AFLP), 346
    Budd-Chiari syndrome, 345
    chronic hepatitis B, 345
    chronic hepatitis C, 345
    intrahepatic cholestasis, 346
    liver transplantation, 345
  diagnosis, 343
  maternal jaundice, 343
  nausea, 343
  overview, 342
  pancreatobiliary disease, 344–345
    acute pancreatitis, 344
    cholecystitis, 344–345
    cholelithiasis, 344–345
  pruritus, 343
  right upper quadrant abdominal pain, 343
  vomiting, 343
Hepatic glucagon receptors, 3.e2
Hepatic programming, 16
Hepatitis, 398–401
  hepatitis A, 398
  hepatitis B, 398–399, 399f, 400t
  hepatitis C, 399, 400b
  hepatitis D, 400
  hepatitis E, 401
Herbal supplements, 37
Herpesvirus, 397
  diagnosis, 397
  treatment, 398t
High spinal anesthesia, 108
HIV, disable T-cell responses, 9
Hodgkin lymphoma (HL), 367
Hormones, fetal growth and metabolism, 3.e2
Human chorionic gonadotropin (hCG), 2–8

Human immunodeficiency virus (HIV), 389–393
  diagnosis, 389–390, 390f
  discordant couples, 393
  epidemiology, 389
  factors, 393
  intrapartum management, 393
  management, 390–393
  postpartum care, 393
  stages, 392t
  treatment, 390
Human insulin, 304t
Human leukocyte antigens (HLAs), 12
Human papillomavirus, 401
Humoral immune responses, 8
Hydatidiform mole, 372
Hyperemesis gravidarum, 28
Hyperextension, 118
Hyperparathyroidism, 313–314
Hyperstimulation, 81
Hypertension, 19
  calcium, 35
  reduced nephron number, 19
Hypertensive disorders
  chrionic hypertension. (*See* Chrionic hypertension)
  eclampsia. (*See* Eclampsia)
  gestational hypertension. (*See* Gestational
    hypertension)
  perinatal mortality, 72
  preeclampsia. (*See* Preeclampsia)
  severe hypertension. (*See* Severe hypertension)
Hyperthyroidism
  fetal hyperthyroidism, 316
  graves disease, 314–316
  left ventricular decompensation, 315
  methimazole (MMI), 315, 315f
  propylthiouracil (PTU), 315, 315f
  thyroid-stimulating hormone (TSH), 315
Hypertrophic cardiomyopathy, 17, 280
Hypervolemia, 4.e3
Hypofibrinogenemia, 127
Hypoglycemia, 301
Hypoparathyroidism, 314
Hypopituitarism, 319
Hypotension
  neuraxial analgesic/anesthetic techniques, 108
Hypothyroidism, 42, 316
  clinical hypothyroidism, 316
  subclinical hypothyroidism, 316
Hypoxemia, 3.e5, 3–4
  fetal adaptation, 74
  fetal movement, 74
Hypoxia
  fetal oxygen consumption, 3–6
  peripheral arterial chemoreceptors, 3–4
Hysterectomy, 131, 155

I

IL-6, 7
IL-8, 8
IL-1β, 7
Immediate puerperium, 4.e2
Immune system
adaptive immunity, 8–10
antibody isotypes, 9, 9f
helper T-cell subsets, 9–10
humoral immune responses, 8
major histocompatibility complex (MHC), 8
T cells, 9
fetal immune system, 10
cord blood transplantation, 10
innate immunity, 6–8
antimicrobial peptides, 7
chemokines, 8
complement system, 7
cytokines, 7
macrophages, 7
natural killer (NK) cells, 7
toll-like receptors (TLRs), 7, 8f
prenatal stress, 18
regulatory T cells, 10
Immunizations, advanced maternal age, 25
Immunoglobulin
IgA, 9
IgG, 9
IgM, 9
structure, 9, 9f
Immunoglobulin A (IgA), 9, 296
Immunoglobulins G (IgG), 9
Immunoglobulins M (IgM), 9
Immunosuppressants, 42
Impetigo herpetiformis, 376
Imprinted genes, 3.e2
Induction, 110
Infant feeding, 162
necrotizing enterocolitis, 162
neonatal hypoglycemia, 162
neonatal jaundice, 162
Infant growth, 176
Infant mortality, 204
Inflammatory skin diseases, 376
Influenza, 394
definition, 394
intranasal vaccine, 394
Initial prenatal visit, 27
Injectable contraception, 169
Innate immunity
maternal-fetal immunology, 7–8
antimicrobial peptides, 7
chemokines, 8
complement system, 7
cytokines, 7

Innate immunity *(Continued)*
macrophages, 7
natural killer (NK) cells, 7
toll-like receptors (TLRs), 7, 8f
Instrumented vaginal delivery/perineal repair, 109
local anesthesia, 109
monitored anesthesia care with sedation, 109
pudendal nerve block, 109
spinal (subarachnoid) block, 109
Insulin-like growth factor-1 (IGF-1), 2–5
fetal size increase, 3.e2
growth restriction, 3.e2
Insulin-like growth factor-2 (IGF)-2, 2–5
Insulin resistance
antenatal exposure, betamethasone, 16
extremes in weight, 16
type 2 diabetes, 16
Internal rotation, 83
Interrupted oxygenation
fetal response, 100–101
injury threshold, 101
mechanisms of injury, 101
placental causes, 100
fetal blood, 100
umbilical cord, 100
Intervillous space (IVS), 2.e1, 2.e2f, 2f–4f
blood flow, 100
first trimester, 2–3
oxygen concentration, 2–3
Pao_2, 100
Intestines, 4–7
Intraabdominal pressure, 180
Intrahepatic cholestasis, 73, 346
Intranasal oxytocin, 176
Intrapartum fetal evaluation, 97–105.e1
direct fetal heart rate, 98
electronic fetal heart rate monitoring, 98–100
external environment, 98
maternal blood, 99
maternal heart, 99
maternal lungs, 99
maternal vasculature, 99
oxygen transfer from environment to fetus, 98, 99f
placenta, 100
uterus, 100
electronic fetal monitoring
benefits, 105
limitations, 105
indirect fetal heart rate, 98
2008 National Institute of Child Health and Human Development consensus report, 101–105, 102t
expectant management *vs.* delivery, 103–104, 104f

Intrapartum fetal evaluation *(Continued)*
  physiology, 101–102
  standardized "ABCD" approach, fetal heart
    rate management, 103
  pattern recognition and interpretation, 101
  placental causes of interrupted oxygenation,
    100
    fetal blood, 100
    umbilical cord, 100
  uterine activity monitoring, 98
Intrauterine adhesions, 193
Intrauterine growth restriction (IUGR), 2–7, 52,
    64, 410.e6
  amniotic fluid assessment, 248
  amniotic fluid volume, 253
  arterial and venous doppler indices, 249
  asymmetric growth pattern, 246
  definition, 246
  delivery, 254–256
  diagnostic approach, 252, 249
  diagnostic tools, 247–249
  doppler ultrasound, 253
  doppler velocimetry, 248–249, 252f, 255f
  etiologies, 246
  fetal biometry, 247–248
  fetal compromise progression, 255, 254
  fetal manifestations, 246–247
  fetal well-being assessment, 252–254
  long-term outcomes, 254–256
  management, 251–252
  maternal manifestations, 246–247
  middle cerebral artery flow-velocity waveform,
    255f
  patterns, 246
  perinatal mortality, 245
  placental insufficiency, 249t
  prevention, 249
  reference ranges, 248
  regulation, 245–246
  screening, 249
  short-term outcomes, 254
  symmetric growth pattern, 246
  therapeutic options, 251–252
  timing of delivery, 254
  umbilical artery flow-velocity waveforms,
    252f
Intrauterine hyperglycemia, 16
Intraventricular hemorrhage (IVH), 164,
    204
Intubation, 110
  failed intubation, 110
Inversions, 193
Iodide, 42
Ionizing radiation, 47
  surgery, 179

Iron, 33
  anemia, diagnosis of, 34, 35t
  deficiency, 34
  oral supplements, 34, 35t
  prenatal care providers, 34
Iron absorption, duodenum, 4.e3
Iron metabolism, 4.e3
Iron requirements, of gestation, 4.e3
Isolated metabolic acidemia, 101, 104–105
Isolated respiratory acidemia, 101, 104–105
Isotretinoin, 39–41
IUGR. *See* Intrauterine growth restriction
    (IUGR)
IVS. *See* Intervillous space (IVS)

J
Jaundice, newborn, 176

K
Ketoacidosis, 305, 306b
Kleihauer-Betke (KB) test, 186
Klinefelter syndrome, 62

L
Labor, 79–89.e2
  augmentation, 149
  breech presentation, 116–117
  cardinal movements, 83, 84f
    descent, 83
    engagement, 83, 85f
    expulsion, 83
    extension, 83
    external rotation, 83
    flexion, 83
    internal rotation, 83
  definition, 80
  delivery management, 175
  diabetes mellitus, 307
  diagnosis, 90–91
    abnormal, 90, 91t
    active phase, 91
    labor at term (Zhang), 91t
    latent phase, 90
    second stage, 91
    third stage, 91
  effect of, 4.e2
  face presentation, 114–115, 114f
  induction, 92
    elective induction, 92
    failed induction, 92
    oxytocin, 92
    prostaglandins, 92

Labor *(Continued)*
  techniques for, 92
    transcervical balloon catheter, 92
  induction of, 148, 149t
  mechanics, 81–83
    fetus (passenger), 82, 82f
    maternal pelvis (passage), 82–83
    uterine activity (powers), 81
  neurologic disorders, 359
  normal progress, 85–88
    active management, 87
    active phase, 85
    cervical effacement, 85
    Cochrane meta-analysis, 85
    epidural use, 86
    first stage, 85
    interventions normal labor outcomes, 87
    latent phase, 85
    second stage, 85, 87–88
    third stage, 85
    Zhang partogram, 86f
  obstetric anesthesia, 107–109
    inhaled nitrous oxide, 107
    neuraxial analgesic and anesthetic techniques, 108–109
    paracervical block, 109
    placental transfer, 107
    sedatives, 107
    systemic opioid analgesia, 107
  physiology, 80
  ultrasound, 89
  uterine activity regulation, 80, 81f
Labor and delivery conduct, 209
  cesarean delivery, 209
  delayed cord clamping, 209
  intrapartum assessment, 209
Labor induction, 92
  elective induction, 92
  failed induction, 92
  postterm pregnancy, 273
  techniques for, 92
    oxytocin, 92
    prostaglandins, 92
    transcervical balloon catheter, 92
Lactation
  breast masses, 176
  endocrinology, 172
  hormonal changes, 173
  maternal nutrition, 175
  milk transfer, 172–173
  physiology, 175
  stages, 172
Lactic acid, accumulation, 100
Lacunae, 2.e1, 2.e2f
Large-for-gestational-age, 312

Last menstrual period (LMP), 39, 270
Latent labor, 90
Lead, 47
Left ventricular decompensation, 315
Leiomyomas, 194
Leopold maneuvers, sensitivity, 113
Leptin, 2–3, 2.e8
  downstream anorexigenic pathways, 15
  proopiomelanocortin neurons, 15
Leukocytes, 4.e3
Lindane, 44
IV lipid emulsion, 108
Lipids, 2–7
Lipid-soluble local anesthetics, 108
Lipolysis, 2–8
Lipopolysaccharide (LPS), TLR4 recognition, 8f
Listeriosis, 36, 408
Lithium
  discontinuation, 41
  polyhydramnios, 41
Lithotripsy, 295
Liver, 4–7
  transplantation, 345
Local anesthesia
  instrumented vaginal delivery/perineal repair, 109
Local anesthetics
  allergy, 108
  toxicity, 108
Long-acting reversible contraception, 169
Long-chain polyunsaturated fatty acids, 2–7
Lower reproductive tract
  cervix, 4–9
  vagina, 4–9
Low-molecular-weight heparins, 41
LPD. *See* Luteal phase defects (LPD)
Lumbar epidural analgesia/anesthesia, 108
Lung fluid, 3.e1
Lung volumes, nonpregnant and pregnant women, 4.e4, 4.e4f
Luteal phase defects, 193
Lymphocytic hypophysitis, 319

M
Macrophages, 7
Macrosomia, 57
  birth injuries, 160
Magnetic resonance imaging (MRI)
  placenta accreta (PA), 153
  surgery, 179
Major depressive episode (MDE), 410.e1
  DSM-V criteria, 410.e1b
  Edinburgh Postnatal Depression Scale, 410.e1
  low birthweight (LBW), 410.e1
  postpartum period, 410.e2, 410.e2t

Major depressive episode (MDE) *(Continued)*
preterm birth (PTB), 410.e1
selective serotonin reuptake inhibitors (SSRIs), 410.e1
side effects, 410.e1
treatment, 410.e1
Major histocompatibility complex (MHC), 8
Malignant diseases
acute leukemia, 367
anesthesia, 365
breast cancer, 365–366
breast reconstruction, 366
cancer therapy, 364–365
cancer treatment, 365
central nervous system tumors, 371
cervical cancer, 369–370
chemotherapy, 366
alkylating agents, 364
antimetabolites, 364
antitumor antibiotics, 365
general effects, 364
platinum agents, 365
targeted therapies, 365
vinca alkaloids, 365
choriocarcinoma, 373
chronic leukemia, 367
colon cancer, 371
diagnosis, 366
endometrial cancer, 371
fertility preservation, 372
fetal-placental metastasis, 372
gastrointestinal cancers, 371
gestational trophoblastic disease, 372–373
hematologic malignancies, 367
Hodgkin lymphoma (HL), 367
hydatidiform mole, 372
invasive
distant metastasis, 369
early-stage disease, 369
locally advanced disease, 369
invasive mole, 372
lactation, 366
local therapy, 366
melanoma, 368, 368f
method of delivery, 369
microinvasion, 369
neonatal outcomes, 371–372
non-Hodgkin lymphoma, 367
ovarian cancer, 370, 370f
partial hydatidiform mole, 372
placental site trophoblastic tumor, 373
postoperative adjuvant therapy, 370–371
pregnancy- related issues, 372–373
pregnancy termination, 366
prognosis, 366

Malignant diseases *(Continued)*
radiation therapy, 365
rectal cancer, 371
staging, 366
subsequent pregnancy, 366
surgery, 365
survival, 370
treatment, 366
upper gastrointestinal cancers, 371
urinary tract cancers, 371
vaginal cancer, 371
vulvar cancer, 371
Malignant melanoma, 376–378
Malignant ventricular arrhythmias, 280
Mallampati airway examination, 180
Malpresentations, 112–122.e1
abnormal axial lie, 112–113
breech presentation, 116–117
contemporary management, 117
delivery for, frank/complete breech, 117
labor mechanism and conduct, 116–117
vaginal delivery, 116–117
brow presentation, 115
frontum anterior position, 115f
clinical circumstances, 112
compound presentation, 115–116
cesarean delivery, 115
cord prolapse, 115
persistent compound presentation, 116
prolapsed extremity, 115
upper extremity and vertex, 115, 116f
face presentation, 113–115, 113f
labor mechanism, 114–115, 114f
shoulder dystocia, 119–120
ACOG Patient Safety Checklist, 120
anterior shoulder rotation, 120f
clinical diagnosis, 119
contemporaneous documentation, 120
delivery percentage, 119
episiotomy, 120
occurrence, 119
recurrence risks for, 119
unilateral brachial plexus palsies, 119
singleton gestation, 113
Term Breech Trial, 117–119
breech second twin, 118
external cephalic version, 118–119
footling breech, 118
hyperextension, 118
premature breech, 118
Managing medication exposure, 27
Manifestations, 40
Marfan syndrome, 280
Mastitis, 175–176
Maternal assessment of evaluation activity, 74, 75f

Maternal B cells, maternal-fetal tolerance, 11
Maternal characteristics, 72
  age, 72, 73f
  race, 72
Maternal circulation (MC), 2–3, 2.e1f, 2f–4f
  first trimester, 2–3
Maternal comorbidities, 72–74
  amniotic fluid abnormalities, 73
  diabetes mellitus, 72
  early pregnancy markers, 73
  fertility history and assisted reproductive
        technology, 73
  fetal growth restriction, 73
  fetal malformations, 74
  hypertensive disorders, 72
  intrahepatic cholestasis, 73
  obesity, 72
  postterm pregnancy, 74
  renal disease and systemic lupus erythematosus,
        73
  thrombophilia, 72
Maternal-fetal exchange
  units, 2.e1
Maternal-fetal immunology, 5–12.e1
  adaptive immunity, 8–10
    antibody isotypes, 9, 9f
    helper T-cell subsets, 9–10
    humoral immune responses, 8
    major histocompatibility complex
        (MHC), 8
    T cells, 9
  amelioration of rheumatoid arthritis, 12
  CD71+ cells, 10
  cord blood transplantation, 10
  innate immunity, 7–8
    antimicrobial peptides, 7
    chemokines, 8
    complement system, 7
    cytokines, 7
    macrophages, 7
    natural killer (NK) cells, 7
    toll-like receptors (TLRs), 7, 8f
  regulatory T cells, 10
  solid organ transplantation, 12
  tolerance of fetus, 10–12
    chemokines, 12
    complement, 12
    cytokines, 12
    dendritic cells and antigen presentation, 12
    fetal rejection, 12
    human leukocyte antigens, 12
    maternal B cells, 11
    maternal T cells, 10
    mechanisms, 10, 11f
Maternal Fetal Medicine Network trial, 33

Maternal-fetal tolerance, 10–12
  chemokines, 12
  complement, 12
  cytokines, 12
  dendritic cells and antigen presentation, 12
  fetal rejection, 12
  human leukocyte antigens, 12
  maternal B cells, 11
  maternal T cells, 10
  mechanisms, 10, 11f
Maternal gestational diabetes, 16
Maternal hemodynamics, 274
Maternal hypothyroidism, 4–7
Maternal-infant attachment, 168
Maternal oxygen consumption, 4–5
Maternal pelvis (passage), 82–83
Maternal physiology, 4–4.e10
  alimentary tract, 4–7
    appetite, 4–6
    gallbladder, 4–7
    intestines, 4–7
    liver, 4–7
    mouth, 4–6
    nausea and vomiting of pregnancy, 4–7
    stomach, 4–6
  body water metabolism, 4–6
    atrial natriuretic peptide, 4–6
    brain natriuretic peptide, 4–6
    osmoregulation, 4–6
    pregnancy-related renal and urologic changes,
        4–6
    renin-angiotensin-aldosterone system, 4–6
    salt metabolism, 4–6
  cardiovascular system, 4.e1
    arterial blood pressure, 4.e1
    cardiac output (CO), 4.e1
    cardiac rhythm, 4.e3
    central hemodynamic assessment, 4.e2, 4.e2t
    heart, 4.e1
    labor and immediate puerperium, 4.e2
    normal changes, heart disease, 4.e2
    systemic vascular resistance, 4.e1
    venous pressure, 4.e2
  central nervous system, 4–9
  endocrine changes, 4–8
    adrenals, 4–8
    pituitary, 4–8
    thyroid, 4–7, 4f–8f
  gestational weight gain (GWG), 4.e1
    recommendations, 4.e1t
  hematologic changes, 4.e3
    coagulation system, 4.e4
    iron metabolism, 4.e3
    leukocytes, 4.e3
    plasma volume, 4.e3

Maternal physiology *(Continued)*
  platelets, 4.e3
  red cell mass, 4.e3
  lower reproductive tract, 4–9
    cervix, 4–9
    vagina, 4–9
  microbiome, 4–10
    placental microbiome, 4–10
  pancreas and fuel metabolism, 4–9
    glucose, 4–8
    proteins and lipids, 4–9
  respiratory system, 4–5
    gas exchange, 4–5
    lung volume and pulmonary function, 4.e4, 4.e4f
    mechanical changes, 4.e4
    sleep, 4–5
    upper respiratory tract, 4.e4
  skeleton, 4–9
    calcium metabolism, 4–9
    and postural changes, 4–9
  skin, 4–9
  surgery, 179
  urinary system, 4–5
    anatomic changes, 4–5
    excretion of nutrients, 4–5
    renal hemodynamics, 4–5
    renal tubular function, 4–5
Maternal serum AFP (MSAFP), 67
Maternal smoking, 44
Maternal stress, 17
Maternal T cells, maternal-fetal tolerance, 10
Maternal weight gain recommendations, 31–32
  consuming healthy food, 31
  low/underweight preconception body mass index, 31
  overweight and obese prepregnancy body mass index, 31–32
  special populations, 32
    adolescents, 32
    multiple gestations, 32
McRoberts maneuver, 119
Mean corpuscular volume (MCV), 66
Measles, 394–396, 396t
Meclizine, 42
Meconium, 272
  aspiration syndrome, 88
Medical drug use, 40–44
  acid-suppressing drugs, 43
  androgenic steroids, 40
  antiasthmatics, 42
  antibiotics, 43
  anticoagulants, 41
  antiemetics, 42–43
  antiepileptic drugs (AEDs), 40

Medical drug use *(Continued)*
  antifungal agents, 44
  antihistamines, 43
  antihypertensive drugs, 42
  antiinfective agents, 43
  antineoplastic drugs, 42
  antiretroviral agents, 44
  antiviral agents, 43–44
  decongestants, 43
  digoxin, 42
  estrogens, 40
  immunosuppressants, 42
  induction of ovulation, 44
  isotretinoin, 40–41
  mild analgesics, 44
  progestins, 40
  psychoactive drugs, 41
  specific drugs, 40–44
  spermicides, 40
  sympathetic blocking agents, 42
  thyroid and antithyroid drugs, 41–42
  vitamin A, 41
Membrane rupture, failed induction, 92
Mendelian disorders, 64–66, 65t
  Ashkenazi Jewish genetic diseases, 65, 66t
  cystic fibrosis, 66
  hemoglobinopathies, 65–66
  newborn screening, 66
Meperidine, 107
Mercury exposure, 26
Mercury, hazards, 47
Metabolic acidosis, 100
Methadone, 45
Methamphetamine, 17
Methimazole (MMI), 41, 315, 315f
Methotrexate, 42
Methylprednisolone, 43
Metoclopramide, 43, 176
Metronidazole, 43
Microarray analysis (MA), 61
Microbiome, 4–10
  placental microbiome, 4–10
Microcephaly, 45
Microvilli, 2–5
Middle cerebral artery flow-velocity waveform, 255f
Midforceps, 93
Mild analgesics, 44
  acetaminophen, 44
  aspirin, 44
  nonsteroidal antiinflammatory agents, 44
Milk transfer, 172–173
  engorgement, 173
  errors, 173
  and infant growth, 176

Milk transfer *(Continued)*
  positions, 172
  sign of, 172
Mineralocorticoids, 3–6
Minerals, 34–35
  calcium, 35
  choline, 35
  iron, 34, 35t
  zinc, 35
Mitral regurgitation, 277
Mitral stenosis, 277
Mixed acidemia, 105
M-mode, 49
Monoamniotic twins, 240
Monosomy X, 62
Mood disorders
  bipolar disorder, 410.e3
    atypical antipsychotics, 410.e3
    history across childbearing, 410.e3
    lamotrigine, 410.e3
    lithium, 410.e3
    prevention, 410.e3
    treatment, 410.e3
    valproic acid, 410.e3
  major depressive episode (MDE), 410.e1
    DSM-V criteria, 410.e1b
    Edinburgh Postnatal Depression Scale, 410.e1
    low birthweight (LBW), 410.e1
    postpartum period, 410.e2, 410.e2t
    preterm birth (PTB), 410.e1
    selective serotonin reuptake inhibitors (SSRIs), 410.e1
    side effects, 410.e1
    treatment, 410.e1
Mortality
  diabetes mellitus, 301
  multiple gestations
    perinatal morbidity, 236, 237t
  postterm pregnancy, 271–272, 271f
Mosaicism, 193
Motor vehicle crashes (MVCs), 183
Mouth, 4–6
M-style mushroom vacuum extractor cup, 94, 96f
Multifactorial and polygenic disorders, 66–67
  neural tube defects, screening, 66–67
Multiple class-specific transporter proteins, 2–7
Multiple gestations
  antepartum management, 240–244, 243f
    antenatal testing, 243, 243
    bed rest, 242
    cerclage, 242
    discordant growth, 244
    fetal growth surveillance, 243–244
    hospitalization, 242
    maternal nutrition, 240

Multiple gestations *(Continued)*
    pessary, 242–243
    progesterone, 242
    spontaneous preterm birth, 241–243
    tocolysis, 242
    weight gain, 240
  birth outcomes, 237t
  chorionicity, 233–234
    amnionicity, 235, 235t, 236f
    determination, 235, 235t
    twin-twin transfusion syndrome (TTTS), 235
  complications, 236–239
  diagnosis, 234–235
  fetal risks, 235–236
  first-trimester multifetal pregnancy reduction, 237–238
  first-trimester pregnancies, 235t
  intrapartum management, 244
  intrauterine fetal demise (IUFD), 238
  issues, 236–239
  low birthweight (LBW), 236
  maternal complications, 236, 237t
  maternal risks, 235–236
  mode of delivery, 244
  perinatal morbidity, 236, 237t
  postterm pregnancy, 273
  second and third trimesters, 236f
  selective intrauterine growth restriction (sIUGR), 239
  timing of delivery, 244
  twin anemia-polycythemia sequence (TAPS), 239–240
    conjoined twins, 240
    monoamniotic twins, 240
    twin reversed arterial perfusion (TRAP) sequence, 240
  twin peak sign, 235, 235f
  twin-twin transfusion syndrome, 238–239
    diagnosis, 238
    laser therapy, 239
    management, 239
    quintero staging, 238t
    septostomy, 239
    serial amnioreduction, 239
    staging, 238
  vanishing twin, 236
  very low birthweight (VLBW), 236
  zygosity, 233–234
Multiple sclerosis (MS), 359–361
  breastfeeding, 360
  cerebral vein thrombosis, 361
  disease-modifying agents, 359–360
  headache, 360–361
  idiopathic intracranial hypertension, 360–361
  management, 360

Multiple sclerosis (MS) *(Continued)*
  migraine, 360
  postpartum period, 360
  prepregnancy counseling, 360
  reversible cerebral vasoconstriction, 361
  subarachnoid hemorrhage, 361
Mycophenolate mofetil, 42, 299
Myocardial infarction (MI), 280

N
Na$^+$/K$^+$ATPase, 2–7
Narcotic medications, 75
Narcotics, 45
Nasopharynx, 4.e4
National Center for Health Statistics, 70
2008 National Institute of Child Health and
    Human Development consensus report,
    101–105, 102t
  evaluating fetal status, 104
  expectant management *vs.* delivery, 103–104,
    104f
  physiology, 101–102
  standard fetal heart rate definitions, 102t
  standardized "ABCD" approach, fetal heart rate
    management, 103
    clear obstacles to rapid delivery, 103
    corrective measures as indicated, 103
    determine decision-to-delivery time, 103
    oxygen pathway, 103
Natural family planning methods, 169
Natural killer (NK) cells
  innate immunity, 7
  spiral artery remodeling, 2–3
Natural surfactant, 159
Nausea and vomiting, 4–7, 28
  antiemetics, 42
  ginger, 43
  managing strategies for, 36, 36b
  nutrition-related problems, 35–36, 36b
  vitamin B$_6$, 33
Necrotizing enterocolitis, 162
2014 Neonatal Encephalopathy Task Force
    consensus report, 101
Neonatal hematology, 162
  anemia, 162
  polycythemia, 162
  thrombocytopenia, 162
Neonatal hypoglycemia, 162, 301
Neonatal jaundice, 162
Neonatal morbidity, 272t
Neonatal thermal regulation, 161
Neonate, 157–164.e1
  birth injuries, 160–161
  cardiopulmonary transition, 158–160

Neonate *(Continued)*
  abnormalities, 160
  circulatory transition, 159–160
  fetal breathing, 159
  first breath, 159
  pulmonary development, 158–159, 159f
  clinical applications, 161
  delivery room, 161
  nursery, 161
  infant feeding, 162
  necrotizing enterocolitis, 162
  neonatal hypoglycemia, 162
  neonatal jaundice, 162
  innate host defense system, 173
  late preterm infant, 164
  neonatal hematology, 162
  anemia, 162
  polycythemia, 162
  thrombocytopenia, 162
  neonatal intensive care, 164
  neonatal thermal regulation, 161
  nursery care, 164
  care of parents, 164
  kangaroo care, 164
  perinatal infection, 163
  early-onset bacterial infection, 163
  respiratory distress, 163–164
  intraventricular hemorrhage, 164
  periventricular leukomalacia, 164
  threshold of viability, 164
Nephron number, 19
Nephrotic syndrome, 297
Nephrotoxic drugs, 19
Nerve injury, 108
Neural tube defects (NTDs), 34
  lead, 47
  screening for, 66–67
Neuraxial analgesic/anesthetic techniques, 108–109
  labor and method of delivery, 109
  labor and cesarean delivery rate, 109
  lumbar epidural analgesia/anesthesia, 108
  neuraxial blocks, complications, 108–109
  allergy to local anesthetics, 108
  back pain, 109
  high spinal /"total spinal" anesthesia, 108
  hypotension, 108
  local anesthetic toxicity, 108
  nerve injury, 108
  spinal headache, 108
Neuraxial anesthesia, 110, 111b
Neuraxial blocks, complications, 108–109
  allergy to local anesthetics, 108
  back pain, 109
  high spinal /"total spinal" anesthesia, 108
  hypotension, 108

Neuraxial blocks, complications (Continued)
  local anesthetic toxicity, 108
  nerve injury, 108
  spinal headache, 108
Neuraxial techniques, 109
Neurologic disorders, 355–362
  antepartum management, 358
  anticonvulsant medications, 356–358
  antiepileptic drugs, 356, 357t
  breastfeeding, 359
  carpal tunnel syndrome, 361–362
  delivery, 359
  epilepsy, 356–359
  labor, 359
  multiple sclerosis (MS), 359–361
    breastfeeding, 360
    cerebral vein thrombosis, 361
    disease-modifying agents, 359–360
    headache, 360–361
    idiopathic intracranial hypertension, 360–361
    management, 360
    migraine, 360
    postpartum period, 360
    prepregnancy counseling, 360
    reversible cerebral vasoconstriction, 361
    subarachnoid hemorrhage, 361
  obstetric and neonatal outcomes, 358
  postpartum period, 359
  preconception counseling, 358
  seizures, 356–359
  stroke, 361
    hemorrhagic stroke, 361
    ischemic stroke, 361
    vascular malformations, 361
  teratogenic effects, 356
  vitamin K, 358
Newborn screening, 66
Nicotine, 44
Nipple pain, 175
Nitrofurantoin, 43
Nitrous oxide, side effects, 107
Nonalcoholic fatty liver disease (NAFLD), 16
Noncoding RNAs, 14
Non-Hodgkin lymphoma, 367
Nonshivering thermogenesis, 161
Nonsteroidal antiinflammatory agents, 44
Nonsteroidal antiinflammatory drugs, 19
Nonstress test (NST), 75–76, 76f, 78f
  fetal heart rate patterns observable, 75
  patterns/findings
    arrhythmia, 76
    bradycardia, 75
    deceleration, 76
    sinusoidal pattern, 75
    tachycardia, 75

Norepinephrine, uterine blood flow, 107
Normeperidine, 107
Nuclei, 2–5
Nucleic acid amplification tests (NAATs), 383
Nulliparous labor, 86f
Numerical chromosomal abnormalities
  aneuploidy, 191
  autosomal trisomy, 191
  diandric triploidy, 191
  genetic counseling, 191
  monosomy X, 191
  nonmosaic triploidy, 191
  paternal meiosis, 191
  polyploidy, 191
  recurrent aneuploidy management, 191
  recurrent losses, 191
Nursery care, 164
  care of parents, 164
  kangaroo care, 164
Nutrients, 3.e1
  excretion of, 4–5
Nutrition, 30–37.e1
  dietary reference intakes (DRIs), 33
  energy, 32
  maternal weight gain recommendations, 31–32
    low/underweight preconception body mass
      index, 31
    overweight and obese prepregnancy body mass
      index, 31–32
    special populations, 32
  minerals, 34–35
    calcium, 35
    choline, 35
    iron, 34, 35t
    zinc, 35
  obstetric history, 30–31
  omega-3 fatty acids, 32–33
  problems, pregnancy, 35–37
    constipation, 36, 36b
    food contamination, 36–37
    heartburn and indigestion, 36, 36b
    nausea and vomiting, 35–36, 36b
  proteins, 32
  special nutritional considerations, 37
    caffeine, 37
    herbal supplements, 37
    vegetarian and vegan diets, 37
  tolerable upper intake level, 33
  vitamins, 33–34
    folate, 34
    vitamin A, 33
    vitamin B_6, 33
    vitamin C and E, 33
    vitamin D, 33
    vitamin K, 34

Nutrition-related problems, 35–37
   constipation, 36, 36b
   food contamination, 36–37
   heartburn and indigestion, 36, 36b
   nausea and vomiting, 35–36, 36b

O

Obesity, 14–15
   adult obesity, United States 2013, 31f
   breastfeeding, 15
   facilities, 312
   gestational weight gain, 310–311
   large-for-gestational-age, 312
   leptin resistance, 15
   neonate/child, 312
   perinatal mortality, 72
   postpartum considerations
      maternal, 311–312
   pregnancy complications
      early pregnancy, 311
      intrapartum complications, 311
      mid to late pregnancy, 311
   reproductive age women, 310–311
   surgery, 181
Oblique lie, 113
Obstetric anesthesia, 106–111.e1
   analgesia, for labor, 107–109
      inhaled nitrous oxide, 107
      neuraxial analgesic and anesthetic techniques,
         108–109
      paracervical block, 109
      placental transfer, 107
      sedatives, 107
      systemic opioid analgesia, 107
   cesarean delivery, 109–111
      aspiration and aspiration prophylaxis, 110
      general anesthesia, 110
      left uterine displacement, 110
      neuraxial anesthesia, 110, 111b
      postoperative care, 111
   instrumented vaginal delivery/perineal repair, 109
      local anesthesia, 109
      monitored anesthesia care with sedation, 109
      pudendal nerve block, 109
      spinal (subarachnoid) block, 109
   pain
      effects, 107
      pathways, 107
   personnel, 107
   stress, effects, 107
Obstetric care
   checklists, 412.e1
   communication enhancement, 412.e1
   measurement, 412.e1

Obstetric care (Continued)
   multifaceted approaches, 412.e1
   patient safety, 412.e1
   protocols, 412.e1
   quality measurement, 412.e1
   simulation, 412.e1
Obstetrician, 174
Obstetrician-gynecologist, 10
Obstetric ultrasound, 48–58.e1
   attenuation, 49
   biophysics, 48
   components of examination, 52–53
      amniotic fluid volume, 52–53, 53f
      anatomic survey, 51b, 53
      cervix, 53
      documentation, 53
      uterus and adnexa, 53
   depth and zoom, 49
   "entertainment" ultrasound examinations,
      57–58
   first-trimester ultrasound, 50
      abnormal findings, 50
      normal findings, 50
   focus, 49
   frequency, 49
   gain, 49
   gestational age, 54–57
      determination, 54, 54f
      standard measurements, 54, 54f
      ultrasound dating, 54–57
   malformations diagnosis, 57
      aneuploidy screening, 57, 58f
   modalities, 49–50
      color and pulse-wave Doppler, 49
      M-mode, 49
      three-dimensional ultrasound, 50
   power, 49
   safety, 57
      quantifying machine power output, 57
   scanning technique, 50
      orientation, 50
      using natural windows, 50
   second-trimester ultrasound, 51–52
      performing and interpreting diagnostic
         ultrasound examinations, 52
      types of examinations, 51–52, 51b
   third-trimester ultrasound, 51–52
      performing and interpreting diagnostic
         ultrasound examinations, 52
      types of examinations, 51–52, 51b
Occupational hazards, 47
OCT. See Oxytocin challenge test (OCT)
Oligohydramnios, 265–267
   evaluation, 266
   fetal causes, 266b

Oligohydramnios *(Continued)*
  labor, 267
  maternal causes, 266b
  treatment, 266
Omega-3 fatty acids, 32–33
Ondansetron, 43
Operative vaginal delivery, 93–96
  birth injuries, 160
  classification, 93
  indications, 93
  instruments, 93–94
    forceps, 93–94, 95f. *See also* Forceps.
    vacuum extraction devices, 94, 96f
  prerequisites, 93
  risks of, 94–96
    fetal risks, 96
    maternal risks, 94–95
Opioids, 410.e6, 410.e7b
  acute pain management, 410.e6
  analgesia
    disadvantage, 107
    fentanyl, 107
    meperidine, 107
    remifentanil, 107
    sedation and sense of euphoria,
      107
  neonatal abstinence syndrome,
    410.e6
Optimizing care, 27
Oral acyclovir, 397
Oral contraceptives
  teratogenic risk, 39
Oral hormonal contraception, 169
Orthostatic hypotension, 124
Osmoregulation, 4–6
Osteoporosis programming, 17
Outlet forceps, 93
Ovarian cancer, 370, 370f
Overt diabetes, 303
Ovine fetal plasma AVP, 3–4
Ovulation, 166
Oxidative stress, 2f–6f
Oxygen
  electronic fetal heart rate monitoring
    fetal umbilical venous blood, 98
    hemoglobin tendency, 99
    interruption, 99–100
    transfer from environment to fetus,
      98, 99f
Oxytocin
  epidural analgesia, 109
  labor, 92
    failed induction, 92
  nipple stimulation, 172
Oxytocin challenge test (OCT), 74

P
Pain
  effects, 107
  pathways, 107
Pancreatic programming, 16–17
Paracervical block, 109
Parathyroid disorders
  hyperparathyroidism, 313–314
  hypoparathyroidism, 314
  primary parahyperthyroidism (PHPT), 313
  therapy, 314
Partial hydatidiform mole, 372
Parvovirus, 394, 395f, 395t
Passage, 82–83
Passenger, 82, 82f
Passive smoking, 26
Patent ductus arteriosus, 278
Patient-controlled analgesia, 107
Patient Protection and Affordable Care Act, 23
Peak flowmeters, 4.e4
Pelvicalyceal dilation, 4–5
Pelvic fracturesPemphigoid gestationis (PG), 184,
  378, 380f
Penicillins, 43
Peptic ulcer disease, 4–6
Peptide hormones, 2–8
Perinatal events, infant mortality, 70
Perinatal morbidity, 204, 271–272
  diabetes mellitus, 301
  multiple gestations, 236, 237t
  postterm pregnancy, 271–272
  preterm birth (PTB), 204
Perinatal mortality, 70–74, 70f
  causes, 70
  characteristics, 70
  identifying risk, 71, 71t–72t
  intrauterine growth restriction (IUGR), 245
  maternal characteristics, 72
    age, 72, 73f
    race, 72
  maternal comorbidities, 72–74
    amniotic fluid abnormalities, 73
    diabetes mellitus, 72
    early pregnancy markers, 73
    fertility history and assisted reproductive
      technology, 73
    fetal growth restriction, 73
    fetal malformations, 74
    hypertensive disorders, 72
    intrahepatic cholestasis, 73
    obesity, 72
    postterm pregnancy, 74
    renal disease and systemic lupus erythematosus, 73
    thrombophilia, 72
  timing, 71

Perinatal mortality rates (PMRs), 117
Perinatology
  ethical/legal issues, 413–413.e3
    abortion politics, 413.e1
    forced cesarean delivery, 413.e2
    genetic counseling, 413.e2
    human embryonic stem cell research funding,
      413.e1
    Obamacare, 413.e1
    prenatal diagnosis, 413.e2
    reproductive liberty, 413.e1
    screening, 413.e2
Peripheral arterial chemoreceptors, 3–4
Periventricular leukomalacia, 164
Perturbations, 4–7
Pfannenstiel abdominal incision, 141
Phagocytes, 7
Phenothiazines, 42
Phenylephrine, 108
Pheochromocytoma, 321
Physiologic changes, 165–166
  cardiovascular system, 166
  coagulation, 166
  immunity, 166
  ovarian function, 166
  renal function, 166
  thyroid function, 166
  urinary tract, 166
  uterus, 165–166
  weight loss, 166
Pituitary disorders, 4–8
  anterior pituitary, 318–319
    acromegaly, 319
    clinically nonfunctioning adenomas, 319
    hormone changes, 318
    hypopituitarism, 319
    lymphocytic hypophysitis, 319
    pituitary tumors, 318–319
    prolactinoma, 318–319
    Sheehan syndrome, 319
  posterior pituitary, 320
    arginine vasopressin (AVP), 320
    diabetes insipidus, 320
Pituitary tumors, 318–319
Placenta
  anatomy, 2–3
    amnion, 2.e2
    development, 2.e1, 2.e2f
    endometrium, first trimester, 2–3
    extravillous trophoblast and physiologic
      conversion, 2–3, 2f–4f
    maternal-fetal relationship, first
      trimester, 2–3
    mature placenta, 2.e1, 2.e1f
    spiral arteries, 2–3, 2f–4f

Placenta (Continued)
    villous trees, 2–3
    yolk sac, 2.e2
  delivery, 88
  electronic fetal heart rate monitoring, 100
    chorionic villous surface area, 100
    diffusion across blood-blood barrier, 100
    interruption, placental blood vessels, 100
    intervillous space blood flow, 100
    intervillous space Pao$_2$, 100
  endocrinology
    estrogens, 2–8
    human chorionic gonadotropin (hCG), 2–8
    leptin, 2–8
    placental growth hormone, 2–8
    placental lactogen, 2–8
    pregnancy-associated plasma protein A, 2–9
    progesterone, 2–8
  extracoelomic cavity, 2–5, 2.e2f, 2f–6f
  fetal development
    bilirubin elimination, 3–5
    water and electrolyte homeostasis, 3–5
  histology
    placental vasculature, 2–5
    villous membrane, 2–5
  interrupted oxygenation
    fetal blood, 100
    umbilical cord, 100
  intrauterine growth restriction (IUGR), 2–7
  nutrient supply, 2–7
  opioids, 107
  radioactive iodine, 4–7
  secondary yolk sac, 2–5, 2.e2f
  selective barrier, 2–6
  sex differences, placental development and
    function, 2–9
  substance-specific transport
    amino acids, 2–7
    calcium, 2–7
    glucose, 2–7
    lipids, 2–7
    respiratory gases, 2–7
    water and ions, 2–7
  umbilicoplacental circulation, vasomotor control,
    2–8
Placenta accreta (PA), 2–3, 129, 151–156
  clinical manifestations, 129
  definition, 129
  diagnosis, 129
  epidemiology, 152–153
    magnetic resonance imaging, 153
    primary uterine pathology, 152, 152b
    secondary uterine pathology, 152, 152b
    ultrasound imaging, 152, 153f–154f
  incidence, 129

Placenta accreta (PA) *(Continued)*
  management, 129, 153–155
    conservative management, 155
    reproductive outcomes, 155
    surgical management, 155
  pathogenesis, 129, 151
  vs. placenta percreta, 151
  risk factors, 129
Placental abruption, 125–127
  classification system, 126f
  clinical manifestations, 125
  definition, 125
  diagnosis, 125–127
    laboratory findings, 127
    radiology, 125, 126f
  incidence, 125
  management, 127
  neonatal outcome, 127
  pathogenesis, 125
  risk factors, 125
Placental blood vessels, interruption, 100
Placental extraction, 142
Placental growth hormone, 2–8
Placental lactogen, 2–8
Placental migration, 127
Placental oxidative stress, 2–3
Placental site trophoblastic tumor, 373
Placental vasculature, 2–5
Placenta malfunction, 73
Placenta previa, 127–129
  clinical manifestations, 127
  definition, 127
  delivery, 128–129
  diagnosis, 128
    radiology, 128, 128t
  incidence, 127
  management, 128
    asymptomatic, 128
    bleeding, 128
  pathogenesis, 127
  risk factors, 127
Plasma exchange, 296
Plasma proteins, 7
Plasma volume, 4.e3
Platelets, 4.e3
Polycythemia, 162
Polyhydramnios, 41, 52, 267
  evaluation, 267
  fetal causes, 267b
  maternal causes, 267b
  treatment, 267
Polymorphic eruption of pregnancy, 378, 381f
Polypeptides, 2–5
Polysomy X, girls, 62
Polysomy Y, boys, 62

Pomeroy technique, 144
Poor weight gain, infancy, 16
Postcesarean endomyometritis, 143
Posterior arm delivery, 119
Posterior pituitary, 320
  arginine vasopressin (AVP), 320
  diabetes insipidus, 320
Postmaturity, 272
Postnatal surfactant, 159
Postoperative adjuvant therapy, 370–371
Postpartum care, 393
Postpartum follow-up, 308
Postpartum hematocrit, 4.e3
Postpartum hemorrhage, 130
  etiologies, 130
  normal blood loss, 130
  postpartum hemorrhage, 130
  prevention, 142
Postpartum psychological reactions, 169–170
  postpartum posttraumatic stress disorder, 170
Postpartum thyroid dysfunction, 317, 317f, 317b
Postpartum visit components
  birth spacing, 28
  counseling, medical conditions and obstetric
    complications, 29
Postterm pregnancy, 74
  antenatal surveillance, 273
  definition, 270
  diagnosis, 271
  etiology, 270
  expectant management, 273
  fetal growth, 272
  incidence, 270
  labor induction, 273
  last menstrual period (LMP), 270
  long-term neonatal outcomes, 273
  management, 273
  maternal complications, 272
  meconium, 272
  mortality, 271–272, 271f
  multiple gestation, 273
  neonatal morbidity, 272t
  perinatal morbidity, 271–272
  postmaturity, 272
Posttraumatic stress disorder, 17
Powers, 81
Precesarean antibiotics, 141
Precesarean thromboprophylaxis, 141
Preconception health counseling, 23–27
  advanced maternal age, 23
  genetic and family history, 26
  immunizations, 25
  substance abuse and hazards, 26–27
  teen pregnancies, 25
  weight gain, 25

Preeclampsia, 2f–4f, 4.e3, 299
  advanced maternal age, 23
  angiotensin II, 4.e1
  antiplatelet agents, 221
  ascites, 218–219
  capillary leak syndrome, 218–219
  cocaine use, 26
  definitions, 217–218
  diagnosis, 220
  endovascular trophoblast migration, 220
  expectant management, 225
  facial edema, 218–219
  features, 218
  fetal syndrome, 218, 219f
  gestational hypertension-preeclampsia (GH-PE),
      224–225
    antepartum management, 224–225
    bed rest, 224
    blood pressure medications, 224–225
    fetal and maternal surveillance, 225
    hospitalization, 224
  gestational proteinuria, 218–219
  hematologic changes, 221
  hemolysis, elevated liver enzymes, and low
      platelets (HELLP) syndrome
    clinical findings, 222
    differential diagnosis, 222
    expectant management, 222
    hepatic complications, 224
    intrapartum management, 223–224
    laboratory criteria, 221–222
    management, 222, 223f
    maternal and perinatal outcome, 222–223
    postpartum management, 224
    recommended management, 223
  hepatic function, 221
  incidence, 218
  inflammation, 220
  intrapartum management, 226
  laboratory abnormalities, 221–225
  low-dose aspirin (LDA), 221
  maternal outcomes, 227
  maternal syndrome, 218, 219f
  mode of delivery, 227
  oxidative stress, 33
  pathophysiology, 219–220
  perinatal outcomes, 227
  placental oxidative stress, 2–3
  postpartum management, 227
  prediction, 220
  prevention, 221, 226
  pulmonary edema, 218–219
  recommended management, 225–227
  renal function, 221
  risk factors, 219

Preeclampsia (Continued)
  severe hypertension, 226–227
  soluble fms-like tyrosine kinase 1 (sFlt-1), 220
  spiral arterioles, 219
  vascular endothelial activation, 220
Pregnancy-associated plasma protein A, 2–9
Pregnancy prevention, 169
  barrier methods, 169
  injectable contraception, 169
  long-acting reversible contraception, 169
  natural family planning methods, 169
  oral hormonal contraception, 169
  sterilization, 169
Pregnancy-related hemodynamic changes, 123
Preimplantation genetic diagnosis (PGD),
      68, 191
Prelabor cesarean delivery, 118
Prelabor hematocrit, 4.e3
Premature breech, 118
Premature rupture of membranes (PROM)
  anatomy, 213
  clinical courses, 214
    maternal risks, 214
  etiology, 213
  fetal and neonatal risks, 214
  fetal fibronectin (fFN), 213
  management, 214–216
    antibiotic administration, 216
    cervical cerclage, 216
    corticosteroid administration, 216
    general considerations, 214–215
    neuroprotection magnesium sulfate, 216
    previable, 216
    at term, 215
    tocolysis, 216
    23-31 weeks, 215
    32-36 weeks, 215
  maternal risks, 214
  overview, 212
  physiology, 213
  preterm birth (PTB), 213
  risks, 213t, 214
  Streptococcus bacteriuria, 213
  vitamin C, 213
Prenatal care
  common patient-centered issues, 28
  components, 23, 24t–25t, 27
  daily iron supplementation, 34
  definition, 23
  goals of, 23
  initial prenatal visit, 27
  prenatal record, 28
  prepared parenthood and support groups, 28
  repeat prenatal visits, 27–28
  risk assessment, 27

Prenatal diagnostic testing, 63–64
  accuracy of, 64
    de novo structural abnormalities, 64
  cytogenetic testing, 63–64
    fluorescence in situ hybridization, 63–64, 64f
Prenatal genetic diagnosis
  amniocentesis, 67
    twin pregnancies, 67
  chorionic villus sampling (CVS), 67
  fetal blood sampling, 67
Prenatal record, 28
Prenatal stress, 18
Preoxygenation, 110
Prepregnancy counseling, 308, 309b
Prerequisites, forceps, 93, 94b
Preterm birth (PTB), 203–211.e1
  acute treatment care, 209
  antenatal corticosteroids, 206–207
  antibiotics, 206
  benefit duration, 206
  bronchopulmonary dysplasia, 204
  causes, 203
  cervical length (CL), 205
  cesarean delivery, 209
  clinical uses, 211
  cochrane meta-analyses, 207
  complications, 203
  cyclooxygenase (COX), 207
  definitions, 203
  delayed cord clamping, 209
  delivery frequency, 204, 204f
  diagnosis, 205, 205b
  diagnostic tests, 205
  efficacy, 207
  fetal effects, 206
  fetal/neonatal morbidity, 207
  glucocorticoids, 206
  infant mortality, 204
  intrapartum assessment, 209
  intraventricular hemorrhage (IVH), 204
  labor and delivery, 209
    conduct, 209
  long-term outcomes, 204
  low birthweight (LBW) infants, 204
  maternal effects, 206
  maternal transfer, 206
  necrotizing enterocolitis (NEC), 204
  neurologic morbidity, 207
  patent ductus arteriosus, 204
  perinatal morbidity, 204
  preterm premature rupture of membranes
    (PPROM), 206
  prevention, 209–211
  primary prevention, 211
  public and professional policies, 211

Preterm birth (PTB) (Continued)
  public educational interventions, 211
  respiratory distress syndrome (RDS), 204, 207
  risks, 207
  secondary prevention, 209–210
    cervical cerclage, 210
    maternal activity modification, 210
    nutritional supplements, 210
    before pregnancy, 209
    progestogens, 210, 210t
  social determinants, 211
  tocolysis, 207–209
    atosiban, 208
    calcium channel blockers, 208
    contraindications, 208
    cyclooxygenase inhibitors, 208
    magnesium sulfate, 208
    maternal effects, 208
    β-mimetic tocolytics, 208
    pharmacology, 208
    treatment maintenance, 209
  treatment, 205–209
Primary cesarean delivery, 117
Primary hyperaldosteronism, 321
Primary parahyperthyroidism (PHPT), 313
Primary subarachnoid hemorrhage, 161
Progesterone, 2–8
  smooth muscle relaxation, 4–5
Progestins, 40
Programmed obesity, 15
Progress, of labor, 85–88
  active phase, 85
  cervical effacement, 85
  Cochrane meta-analysis, 85
  epidural use, 86
  first stage, 85
  interventions normal labor
    outcomes, 87
  latent phase, 85
  second stage, 85, 87–88
  third stage, 85
  Zhang partogram, 86f
Prolactin, function, 4–8
Prolactinoma, 318–319
Prolapsed extremity, 115
Prolonged labor, 115
Propylthiouracil (PTU), 42, 46, 315,
  315f
Prostaglandins, labor induction, 92
Prosthetic valves, 277–278
Proteins, 32
Protraction disorder, 91
Prurigo of pregnancy, 379t, 381
Pruritic folliculitis of pregnancy, 381
Pruritus, 343, 378

Psychoactive drugs
  antidepressants, 41
  lithium, 41
Puerperal endometritis
  clinical presentation, 406
  diagnosis, 406
  epidemiology, 406
  management, 406
  prevention, 407
  severe sepsis, 407
  wound infection, 407
Puerperium management, 166–167
  cesarean delivery, 167
  home nursing visits, 166
  physical activity, 167
  sexual activity, 167
  Tdap, 167
  vaccines, 166
Pulmonary edema, 4.e2
Pulmonary function, 4.e4, 4.e4f
Pulmonary hypertension, 280
Pulmonary vascular resistance (PVR), 160
  ductus arteriosus, 159
Pyelonephritis, 295

Q
Quiet/nonreactive periods, 3–6

R
Radioactive iodine, 4–7
Reciprocal translocations, 193
Recurrent early pregnancy loss (REPL), 190–191
Red blood cell (RBC), 296
Red cell alloimmunization
  amniocentesis, 259
  clinical management, 260, 261f
    first affected pregnancy, 260
    previously affected fetus/infant, 260
  diagnostic methods, 259–260
  fetal blood sampling, 260
  fetal blood typing, 259
  fetal/neonatal hemolytic disease, 258
  genetics, 258
  hemolytic disease, non-RhD Antibodies, 262
  historic perspectives, 257
  history, 258
  incidence, 258
  indications, 258–259
  intrauterine transfusion, 260–262
    complications, 260
    neonatal transfusions, 262
    neurologic outcome, 262
    outcome, 260

Red cell alloimmunization (Continued)
    technique, 260
    therapeutic options, 262
    treatment modalities, 262
  maternal antibody determination, 259
  nomenclature, 257
  pathophysiology, 258
  preparations, 258
  RhD hemolytic disease, 258–260
  ultrasound, 260
Red cell mass, 4.e3
Reflex stimulation, 3–4
Regional anesthesia, 119
Regulatory T cells, 10
Remifentanil, 107
Renal biopsy, 298
Renal disease, 73
  acute renal disease, 295–297
    acute renal failure, 296
    glomerular disease, 296
    hemolytic-uremic syndrome
      (HUS), 296
    nephrotic syndrome, 297
    polycystic kidney disease, 296
    renal artery stenosis, 297
    urolithiasis, 295
    vesicoureteral reflux, 297
  altered renal physiology, 294–295
  asymptomatic bacteriuria (ASB), 295
  chronic renal disease, 297–299
    hemodialysis, 298
    management, 298
    pregnancy, 298
    renal function, 297–298
    renal transplant, 298–299
  Escherichia coli, 295
  pyelonephritis, 295
Renal hemodynamics, 4–5
Renal hypoplasia, 19
Renal programming, 19
Renal transplant, 298–299
Renal tubular function, 4–5
Renin-angiotensin-aldosterone system, 4–6
Renin-angiotensin II, 3–5
Repeat prenatal visits, 27–28
Respiratory activity, 159
Respiratory disease
  asthma, 288–290
    allergic rhinitis, 290
    antenatal management, 290
    assessment and monitoring, 288
    avoidance/control, 288
    breastfeeding, 290
    diagnosis, 288
    gastroesophageal reflux, 290

Respiratory disease *(Continued)*
 hospital and emergency department
  management, 290
 inhaled β_2-agonists, 289
 inhaled corticosteroids, 289
 labor and delivery management, 290
 leukotriene moderators, 290
 management, 288
 objective measures, 288
 omalizumab, 290
 oral corticosteroids, 290
 patient education, 288
 pharmacologic therapy, 289–290
 pregnancy effects, 288
 step therapy, 289, 289t
 theophylline, 290
 bacterial pneumonia, 283–284
 bacteriology, 283
 Haemophilus influenzae, 283
 Klebsiella pneumoniae, 283
 pneumonia, 282–283
 restrictive lung disease, 291–293
  cystic fibrosis (CF), 291–293
  sarcoidosis, 291
 Staphylococcus aureus, 283
 streptococcal pneumonia, 283
 Streptococcus pneumoniae, 283
 tuberculosis, 285–287
  BCG vaccine, 287
  clinical risk factors, 286b
  diagnosis, 286–287
  high-risk factors, 286b
  Mycobacterium tuberculosis, 287
  prevention, 287
  treatment, 287
 viral pneumonia, 284–285
  influenza virus, 284–285
  varicella virus, 285
Respiratory distress
 neonate, 163–164
  intraventricular hemorrhage, 164
  periventricular leukomalacia, 164
Respiratory distress syndrome (RDS), 159, 301
Respiratory gases, 2–7
Respiratory muscle function, 4.e4
Respiratory system, 4–5
 gas exchange, 4–5
 lung volume and pulmonary function, 4.e4, 4.e4f
 mechanical changes, 4.e4
 sleep, 4–5
 upper respiratory tract, 4.e4
Restitution, 83
Restrictive lung disease, 291–293
 cystic fibrosis (CF), 291–293
 sarcoidosis, 291

Retained products of conception, 133
 clinical manifestations, 133
 definition, 133
 diagnosis, 133
 incidence, 133
 management, 133
 pathogenesis, 133
 risk factors, 133
Retinopathy, 302–303
Retrograde ureteral stents, 155
Retroperitoneal hematoma, 133
Retroperitoneal hemorrhage, 183
Retroplacental hematomas, 125
Rhesus factor (Rh) testing, 186
Rheumatoid arthritis (RA), 338–340
 amelioration of, 12
 antirheumatic drugs, 339–340
 biologic agents, 339
 leflunomide, 340
 management, 339
 methotrexate (MTX), 340
 pregnancy considerations, 339
 sulfasalazine, 339
 tumor necrosis factor-α inhibitors, 339
Risks
 chrionic hypertension, 230
 cytomegalovirus infection, 396
 diabetes mellitus, 301–303
 gastrointestinal disorders, 350t
 heart disease, 276
 multiple gestations
  fetal risks, 235–236
  maternal risks, 235–236
 obesity, 311–312
 operative vaginal delivery, 94–96
  fetal risks, 96
  maternal risks, 94–95
 postterm pregnancy, 272
 preeclampsia, 219
 premature rupture of membranes (PPROM), 214
 preterm birth (PTB), 207
 thromboembolic disorders, 330, 332
 tuberculosis, 286b
Rotational forceps, 94
Rotational maneuvers, 119
Rubella, 396
Rushed delivery, 116–117

S

Salt metabolism, 4–6
Scanning technique, 50
 orientation, 50
 using natural windows, 50
Schizophrenia, 410.e4

Screening
aneuploidy, 62–63
cell-free DNA analysis, 63
first- and second-trimester, 63
first-trimester, 62
multiple gestation, 63
second-trimester serum, 62
ultrasound, 63
neural tube defects, 66–67
Secondary yolk sac, 2–5, 2.e2f
Second-degree tear, 88–89
Second trimesters
amniocentesis, 67
baseline heart rate, 75
iron, 34
painless vaginal bleeding, 127
screening
aneuploidy, 57
serum markers, 73
serum screening
aneuploidy, 62
ultrasound, 51–52
performing and interpreting diagnostic
ultrasound examinations, 52
types of examinations, 51–52, 51b
ureters and renal pelvis dilation, 4–5
Sedatives, 107
Selective arterial embolization, 131
Septic pelvic thrombophlebitis, 144
Sertraline, 46
Serum creatinine, 4–5
Serum urate levels, 295
Severe hypertension, 297
definitions, 217
Sex chromosome abnormalities, 62
Klinefelter syndrome, 62
monosomy X (45,X), 62
polysomy X, girls, 62
polysomy Y, boys, 62
Sexuality programming, 18–19
Sheehan syndrome, 319
Shoulder dystocia, 119–120
ACOG Patient Safety Checklist, 120
anterior shoulder rotation, 120f
birth injuries, 160
clinical diagnosis, 119
contemporaneous documentation, 120
delivery percentage, 119
episiotomy, 120
occurrence, 119
recurrence risks for, 119
unilateral brachial plexus palsies, 119
Single-gene disorders, 64–66, 65t
Ashkenazi Jewish genetic diseases, 65, 66t
cystic fibrosis, 66

Single-gene disorders (Continued)
hemoglobinopathies, 65–66
newborn screening, 66
Singleton gestation, management of, 113
Sinusoidal pattern, 75
Sirolimus, 299
Sjögren syndrome (SS), 341
Skin disease, 374–381
acne vulgaris, 376
atopic eczema, 376
atopic eruption of pregnancy, 378–381
autoimmune progesterone dermatitis, 376
cutaneous manifestations, 376–378
bullous disorders, 376
malignant melanoma, 376–378
skin tumors, 376
dermatitis, 376
impetigo herpetiformis, 376
inflammatory skin diseases, 376
pemphigoid gestationis (PG), 378, 380f
physiologic skin changes, 374, 375b
polymorphic eruption of pregnancy, 378, 381f
prurigo of pregnancy, 379t, 381
pruritic folliculitis of pregnancy, 381
pruritus, 378
specific dermatoses, 378–381
Skin-to-skin contact, 168
Skin tumors, 376
Sleep, respiratory system, 4–5
Smoking
active smoking, 26
maternal smoking, 44
passive smoking, 26
Smooth muscle relaxation, 4–5
Specialized forceps, 93
Special nutritional considerations, 37
caffeine, 37
herbal supplements, 37
vegetarian and vegan diets, 37
Special ultrasound modalities, 49–50
color and pulse-wave Doppler, 49
M-mode, 49
three-dimensional ultrasound, 50
Spermicides, 40
Spinal headache, 108
Spiral arteries, 2.e3, 2–3, 2.e4f, 2f–3f
Spirometry, 4.e4
Spontaneous vaginal delivery, 88
Standard fetal heart rate definitions, 102t
Starling mechanisms, 3–4
Sterilization, 169
Steroid hormones, 2–8
Stillbirth, 196–197
definition, 196
genetic factors, 196

Stillbirth *(Continued)*
  maternal evaluation, 197, 197b
  multifactorial disorders, 196
  polygenic disorders, 196
  risks, 196
  subsequent pregnancies, 197
Stomach, 4–6
Streptococcus bacteriuria, 213
Stress, 107
Stroke, 361
  hemorrhagic stroke, 361
  ischemic stroke, 361
  vascular malformations, 361
Subgaleal hemorrhage, 96
Substance abuse and hazards, 26–27
  active and passive smoking, 26
  alcohol, 26
  cannabis, 26
  cocaine use, 26
  environmental exposures, 27
  mercury exposure, 26
  poor obstetric outcomes, 26
Substance-related disorders, 410.e5
  acute pain management, 410.e6
  alcohol, 410.e5
  alcohol withdrawal management, 410.e5
  cannabis, 410.e6
  cocaine, 410.e6
  drugs of abuse, 410.e5
  methamphetamine, 410.e6
  neonatal abstinence syndrome, 410.e6
  opioids, 410.e6
  smoking, 410.e5
  treatment, 410.e5
Substrates, fetal growth and metabolism, 3.e1
Sulfonamides, 43
Sulpiride, 176
Sumatriptan, 44
Surfactant deficiency, 158
Surgery
  adnexal masses, 180–181
  anesthesia, 180
    pregnancy physiology, 180
    teratogenicity, 180
  bariatric surgery, 181
  complications, 181
  contrast in pregnancy, 179
  diagnostic imaging, 179–180
  early second trimester, 180
  fetal monitoring, 180
  first trimester, 179
  gravid uterus, 179
  intrauterine growth restriction, 181
  ionizing radiation, 179
  laparoscopy, 180

Surgery *(Continued)*
  low osmolarity iodinated contrast media, 179
  magnetic resonance imaging, 179
  maternal physiology, 179
  nonobstetric surgery, 180
  obesity, 181
  pregnancy, 181
  reduced absorptive capacity, 181
  regional anesthesia, 181
  right lower quadrant pain, 179
  trauma, 186–188
    cardiac arrest, 186–187
    nonobstetric surgery, 186
    perimortem cesarean section, 186–187
    uterine rupture, 186
  ultrasound, 179
Sympathetic blocking agents, 42
  angiotensin-converting enzyme (ACE)
      inhibitors, 42
  angiotensin receptor blockers, 42
Symphysis pubis, 83
Syncytial knots, 2–5
Syncytiotrophoblast, 2.e1, 2.e2f
  calcium levels, 2–7
  epidermal growth factor (EGF), 3.e2
  epithelium transport, 2–6
  metabolic rate, 2–5
  microvilli, 2–5
  multiple class-specific transporter proteins, 2–7
  $Na^+/K^+ATPase$, 2–7
Syphilis
  diagnosis, 385
  epidemiology, 385
  pathogenesis, 385
  treatment, 386
  Treponema pallidum, 386b
Systemic lupus erythematosus (SLE), 333–336
  azathioprine, 336
  clinical manifestations, 334
  cyclophosphamide, 336
  cyclosporine A, 336
  diagnosis, 334
  drug, 336
  epidemiology, 333–334
  etiology, 334
  fetal loss, 73
  glucocorticoids, 336
  hydroxychloroquine, 336
  lupus flare, 334
  lupus nephritis (LN), 334–335
  management, 335–336
  mycophenolate mofetil (MMF), 336
  neonatal lupus erythematosus, 335
  nonsteroidal antiinflammatory (NSAID), 336
  pregnancy complications, 335

Systemic opioid analgesia, 107
  patient-controlled analgesia, 107
Systemic sclerosis (SSc), 340
  diagnosis, 340
  management, 340
  pregnancy considerations, 340
Systemic vascular resistance, 4.e1

T

Tachycardia, 124
  etiology, 75
Tachypnea, 124
Tachysystolem defined, 81
Tacrolimus, 299
TAPS. *See* Twin anemia-polycythemia sequence
  (TAPS)
T cells, 9
Teen pregnancies, 25
Tenney-Parker change, 2–5
Teratogenicity, 180
Teratology
  all-or-none effect, 39
  malformations, 39
  principles, 39–40
    agent, 40
    dose effect, 40
    genotype and interaction with environmental
      factors, 39
    manifestations, 40
    mechanisms of, 39
    timing of exposure, 39
Terbutaline, 119
Term Breech Trial, 117–119
  breech second twin, 118
  external cephalic version, 118–119
  footling breech, 118
  hyperextension, 118
  premature breech, 118
Terminal villi, 2–3
  capillary sprouts/loops, 2–5
Tetracyclines, 43
Tetralogy Of Fallot, 278
TGA. *See* Transposition of the great arteries (TGA)
Thalassemia, 327, 328f
T-helper 1 (Th1) subset, 9–10
  intracellular bacterial infections, 10
T-helper 2 (Th2) subset, 9–10
Third-degree tear, 88–89
Third trimester
  baseline heart rate, 75
  blood gas values of pregnancy, 4–5
  glomerular filtration rate (GFR), 3–5
  iron, 34
  painless vaginal bleeding, 127

Third trimester *(Continued)*
  placenta previa, 128
  ultrasound, 51–52
    performing and interpreting diagnostic
      ultrasound examinations, 52
    types of examinations, 51–52, 51b
  ultrasound dating, 54
Thoracic spinal nerve 4 (T-4), 107
Three-dimensional (3D) ultrasound, 50
Thrombocytopenia, 162, 323–324
  evaluation, 324
  fetal/neonatal alloimmune thrombocytopenia, 325
  gestational thrombocytopenia, 322–324
  glucocorticoids, 322–323
  hemolytic-uremic syndrome (HUS), 323–324
  idiopathic thrombocytopenic purpura (ITP),
    322–323
  immune thrombocytopenic purpura (ITP), 323–324
  iron deficiency anemia, 325
  management, 324
  megaloblastic anemia, 325–326
  preeclampsia, 322–323
  therapy, 324
  thrombotic thrombocytopenic purpura (TTP),
    322–324
Thromboembolic disorders, 143
  venous thromboembolism (VTE), 329
    acute deep venous thrombosis, 332
    antiphospholipid syndrome (APS), 330
    associations, 330–332
    computed tomographic pulmonary
      angiography, 331
    coumarin, 332
    D-dimer assays, 330–331
    diagnostic procedures radiation exposure, 332
    epidemiology, 329
    fetal exposure, 332
    genetics, 329
    imaging, 330
    incidence, 329
    inherited thrombophilias, 330
    lower extremity eval, 331
    low-molecular-weight heparin, 332
    maternal exposure, 332
    pathophysiology, 329
    perioperative prevention, 332
    prophylactic anticoagulation recommendations,
      332
    pulmonary embolus, 332
    risks, 330–332
    spiral computed tomographic pulmonary
      angiography, 331
    suspected pulmonary embolus, 331, 331f
    unfractionated heparin, 332
    ventilation-perfusion scanning, 330–331

Thrombophilia, 72
  ACOG bulletin, 194
  acquired, 194
  antiphospholipid syndrome, 194
  first-trimester losses, 194
  inherited, 194
  second-trimester pregnancy, 194
Thyroid, 4–7, 4f–8f, 41–42
  diseases, 314–317
    hyperthyroidism. *See* Hyperthyroidism
    hypothyroidism. *See* Hypothyroidism
    postpartum thyroid dysfunction, 317, 317f,
      317b
    thyroid cancer, 316
    thyroid gland single nodule, 316
Thyroid gland, fetal development, 3–6
Thyroid gland single nodule, 316
Thyroid-stimulating hormone, 4–7, 315
Thyrotropin-releasing hormone (TRH), 3–6
Thyroxine-binding globulin, 4–7
TNF-α, 7
Tocolysis, 207–209
  atosiban, 208
  calcium channel blockers, 208
  contraindications, 208
  cyclooxygenase inhibitors, 208
  magnesium sulfate, 208
  maternal effects, 208
  β-mimetic tocolytics, 208
  multiple gestations, 242
  pharmacology, 208
  premature rupture of membranes (PPROM), 216
  preterm birth (PTB), 207–209
  treatment maintenance, 209
  vaginal bleeding, 128
Tolerable upper intake level, 33
Toll-like receptors (TLRs), 7, 8f
Total spinal anesthesia, 108
Total thyroxine, 4–7
Total triiodothyronine, 4–7
Toxoplasmosis, 37, 407–408
  congenital toxoplasmosis, 408
  diagnosis, 408
  epidemiology, 407
  management, 408
  treatment, 408
Tracheal edema, 115
Transcervical balloon catheter, 92
Transient gestational thyrotoxicosis, 4–7
Transposition of the great arteries (TGA), 278
Transverse lie, 113
Trauma
  abruptio placentae, 184
  anatomic and physiologic changes, 182–183
  bladder and urethral trauma, 184

Trauma *(Continued)*
  blunt trauma, 183
  cardiac arrest implications, 186–187
  complex maternal bowel injury, 184
  considerations, 183
  diagnostic imaging, 186, 187f
  direct fetal injuries, 184
  domestic violence, 183
  falls, 183
  fetal injury, 184
  fetal mortality predictors, 184
  FHR tracing, 185
  fractures, 183–184
  gunshot and stab wounds, 184
  gunshot wounds, 184
  incidence, 182
  intimate partner violence, 183
  Kleihauer-Betke (KB) test, 186
  laboratory testing, 186
  management considerations, 185–186
    Centers for Disease Control and Prevention
      (CDC), 185
    emergency department (ED), 185
    fetal monitoring, 185
    initial approach, 185
  maternal anatomic and physiologic changes, 183
  motor vehicle crashes (MVCs), 183
  pelvic fractures, 184
  penetrating trauma, 184
  perimortem cesarean section, 186–187
  prevention, 187–188
  retroperitoneal hemorrhage, 183
  Rhesus factor (Rh) testing, 186
  surgery, 186–188
  thermal injuries, 184
  traumatic injuries, 186–188
  uterine contraction monitoring, 185
  uterine rupture, 186
Treatment
  bipolar disorder, 410.e3
  cancer, 366
  cervical insufficiency, 200–202
  chlamydia, 383
  diabetes mellitus, 307–308
  eclampsia, 229
  gonorrhea, 384–385
  herpesvirus, 398t
  human immunodeficiency virus (HIV), 390
  major depressive episode (MDE), 410.e1
  oligohydramnios, 266
  polyhydramnios, 267
  preterm birth (PTB), 205–209
  red cell alloimmunization, 262
  substance-related disorders, 410.e5
  syphilis, 386

Treatment *(Continued)*
  toxoplasmosis, 408
  tuberculosis, 287
Treponema pallidum, 386b
Trial of labor after cesarean (TOLAC), 145
  candidates for, 145
  counseling, 149–150
    cost-effectiveness, 150
  induction of labor, 148, 149t
  interpregnancy interval, 148
  labor augmentation, 149
  management, 149
  maternal demographics, 146
  other risks, 149
  prior cesarean deliveries, 148, 148t
  prior vaginal delivery, 148
  sonographic evaluation of uterine scar, 149
  success rates for, 146–147, 146f
  uterine closure technique, 148
  uterine rupture, 147–149
Trisomy 21, 61
True mosaicism, 64
TTTS. *See* Twin-twin transfusion syndrome (TTTS)
Tubal sterilization, 144
  modified Pomeroy, 144
Tuberculosis, 285–287
  BCG vaccine, 287
  clinical risk factors, 286b
  diagnosis, 286–287
  high-risk factors, 286b
  Mycobacterium tuberculosis, 287
  prevention, 287
  treatment, 287
Turner syndrome, 62
Twin anemia-polycythemia sequence (TAPS), 239–240
  conjoined twins, 240
  monoamniotic twins, 240
  twin reversed arterial perfusion (TRAP) sequence, 240
Twin Birth Study, 118
Twin pregnancies, 67
Twin reversed arterial perfusion (TRAP) sequence, 240
Twin-twin transfusion syndrome (TTTS), 235, 238–239
  diagnosis, 238
  laser therapy, 239
  management, 239
  quintero staging, 238t
  septostomy, 239
  serial amnioreduction, 239
  staging, 238
Type 1 diabetes mellitus, 303–305, 304t
Type 2 diabetes mellitus, 303–305, 304t
Typhoid vaccination, 18

U
Ultrasound
  amniotic fluid disorders, 263–265
  aneuploidy screening, 63
  bradycardia, 75
  dating, 54–57
    assessing fetal growth, 54
    diagnosing abnormal growth, 57
    fetal weight estimation, 55, 55f–56f, 55b
    macrosomia, 57
  delivery, 89
  "entertainment" ultrasound examinations, 57–58
  gestational age determination, 54–57
    determination, 54, 54f
    standard measurements, 54, 54f
    ultrasound dating, 54–57
  labor, 89
  malformations diagnosis, 57
    aneuploidy screening, 57, 58f
  placenta accreta
    lower uterine segment at 10 weeks gestation, 153f
    lower uterine segment at 20 weeks gestation, 154f
    lower uterine segment at 22 weeks gestation, 153f
    lower uterine segment at 38 weeks gestation, 154f
    "moth-eaten" appearance, 153f
    myometrial interface, 152
  red cell alloimmunization, 260
  safety, 57
    quantifying machine power output, 57
  surgery, 179
  twin gestations, 67
Umbilical artery flow-velocity waveforms, 252f
Umbilical blood flow, 3.e1
Umbilical cord, 2.e1, 2.e2
  blood gas determination, 104–105
  pulmonary vascular resistance (PVR), 160
Umbilicoplacental circulation, vasomotor control, 2–8
Unfractionated heparin, 41
Uniparental disomy, 64
Upper arm palsy (Erb-Duchenne paralysis), 161
Upper gastrointestinal cancers, 371
Upper genital tract infections
  chorioamnionitis
    diagnosis, 406
    epidemiology, 405
    management, 406
  listeriosis, 408
  puerperal endometritis
    clinical presentation, 406
    diagnosis, 406

Upper genital tract infections *(Continued)*
  epidemiology, 406
  management, 406
  prevention, 407
  severe sepsis, 407
  wound infection, 407
  toxoplasmosis, 407–408
    congenital toxoplasmosis, 408
    diagnosis, 408
    epidemiology, 407
    management, 408
    treatment, 408
Upper respiratory tract, 4.e4
Urethral trauma, 184
Urinary bladder catheterization, 141
Urinary incontinence, 95
Urinary system
  maternal physiology, 4–5
    anatomic changes, 4–5
    excretion of nutrients, 4–5
    renal hemodynamics, 4–5
    renal tubular function, 4–5
Urinary tract cancers, 371
Urinary tract infections, 403–405
  acute cystitis, 404–405
  acute pyelonephritis, 405
  acute urethritis, 403
  asymptomatic bacteriuria, 404–405
  Chlamydia trachomatis, 403
  Escherichia coli, 403
  Neisseria gonorrhoeae, 403
Urine production, fetal kidney, 3–5
Urolithiasis, 295
Uterine activity (powers), 81
Uterine atony, 130–131
  clinical manifestations, 130
  definition, 130
  diagnosis, 130
  incidence, 130
  pathogenesis, 130
  prevention and management, 130–131
    bilateral looped uterine vessel sutures, 131
    bimanual uterine massage, 130
    selective arterial embolization, 131
    surgical intervention, 131
    uterine tamponade, 131
    uterotonic therapy, 131, 132t
  risk factors, 130
Uterine compression sutures, 131
Uterine contraction monitoring, 185
Uterine incision, 141–142
Uterine inversion
  clinical manifestations, 134
  definition, 134
  diagnosis, 134
  incidence, 134

Uterine inversion *(Continued)*
  management, 134
  pathogenesis, 134
  risk factors, 134
Uterine involution, 172
Uterine macrophages, 7
Uterine relaxing agent, 118
Uterine repair, 142
Uterine rupture, 133–134, 186
  clinical manifestations, 133–134
  definition, 133
  diagnosis, 133–134
  incidence, 133
  management, 134
  pathogenesis, 133
  risk factors, 133
Uterine scar, 151
Uterine tamponade, 131
Uteroplacental bed, 3.e1
Uterotonic therapy, 131, 132t
Uterus, 53

V
Vacuum extraction devices, 94, 96f
Vacuum extractor application, 93, 94b
  indications
    prolonged second stage, 93
    suspicion of immediate/potential fetal
      compromise, 93
Vagina, 4–9
Vaginal birth after cesarean (VBAC) delivery,
    145–150.e1
  birthweight, 147
  cervical examinations, 147
  labor status, 147
  multiple prior cesarean deliveries, 147
    postterm pregnancy, 147
    twin gestation, 147
  previous/unknown incision type, 147
  prior vaginal delivery, 147
  trial of labor after cesarean (TOLAC)
    candidates for, 145
    induction of labor, 148, 149t
    interpregnancy interval, 148
    labor augmentation, 149
    management, 149
    maternal demographics, 146
    other risks, 149
    prior cesarean deliveries, 148, 148t
    prior vaginal delivery, 148
    sonographic evaluation of uterine scar, 149
    success rates, 146–147, 146f
    uterine closure technique, 148
    uterine rupture, 147–149
Vaginal bleeding, 125

Vaginal breech delivery (Piper forceps), 94
Vaginal cancer, 371
Vaginal delivery
  breech presentation, 116–117
  descent, 114, 114f
  engagement, 114, 114f
  internal rotation, 114, 114f
  operative vaginal delivery. *See* Operative vaginal
    delivery
Vaginal hematoma, 131–133
Valproate, 40
Valproic acid, 40
Valvular disease, 277
Vanishing twin, 236
Variants of uncertain significance (VOUS), 63
Varicella virus, 285, 397–398
Varicella zoster immune globulin (VZIG), 397
Vasa previa, 129–130
  clinical manifestations, 130
  definition, 129
  diagnosis, 130
  incidence, 129
  management, 130
  pathogenesis, 129
  risk factors, 129
Vasoconstrictive effects, 3.e1
Vasodilatory effects, 2–8
Vegan diets, 37
Vegetarian, 37
Velamentous cord insertion, 129
Venous pressure, 4.e2
Venous thromboembolism, 141
Very low birthweight (VLBW), 236
Vesicoureteral reflux, 297
Vibroacoustic stimulation, 75
Villous membrane, 2–5
Villous stromal core, 2–5
Villous trees, 2–3, 2.e1f
  intervillous space (IVS), 2.e1
  terminal villi, 2–3
Viral infections, 389
  cytomegalovirus infection, 396–397
    risks, 396
  Ebola, 401
  hepatitis, 398–401
    hepatitis A, 398
    hepatitis B, 398–399, 399f, 400t
    hepatitis C, 399, 400b
    hepatitis D, 400
    hepatitis E, 401
  herpesvirus, 397
    diagnosis, 397
    treatment, 398t
  human immunodeficiency virus (HIV),
    389–393
    diagnosis, 389–390, 390f

Viral infections *(Continued)*
    discordant couples, 393
    epidemiology, 389
    factors, 393
    intrapartum management, 393
    management, 390–393
    postpartum care, 393
    stages, 392t
    treatment, 390
  human papillomavirus, 401
  Influenza, 394
    definition, 394
    intranasal vaccine, 394
  measles, 394–396, 396t
  parvovirus, 394, 395f, 395t
  rubella, 396
  varicella, 397–398
Viral pneumonia
  influenza virus, 284–285
  varicella virus, 285
Vitamin A, 33
  birth defects, 41
Vitamin B$_6$, 33
  antiemetics, 42
Vitamin C, 33, 213
Vitamin D, 33
Vitamin E, 33
Vitamin K, 34, 358
Volatile halogenated agent, 110
Vomiting, 343
von Willebrand disease (vWD),
  327–328
Vulvar cancer, 371
Vulvar hematoma, 131

W
Warfarin embryopathy, 41
Water, 2–7
Weight gain, advanced maternal age, 23
Well-woman visits, 23
White blood cell (WBC), 4.e3
World Health Organization, 310, 382
Worsening proteinuria, 297
Wound infection, 143

Y
Yolk sac, 2.e2

Z
Zhang partogram, 86f
Zidovudine, 44, 393
Zinc, 35
Zygosity, 233–234